The Cat

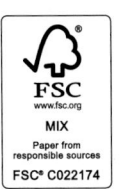

Dedication

To Bjarne's son Øyvind (1993–2010),

The cats' best friend

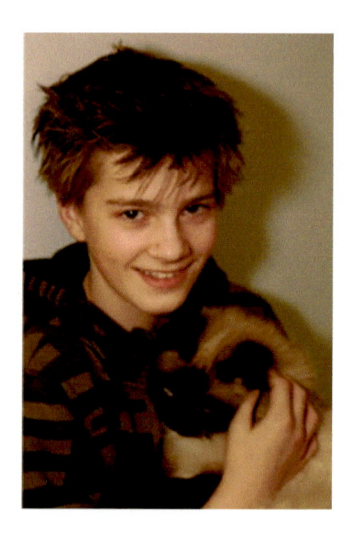

Øyvind Braastad

The Cat

Behaviour and Welfare

Bjarne O. Braastad

Faculty of Biosciences, Norwegian University of Life Sciences, Norway

Anne McBride

Department of Psychology, University of Southampton, UK

Ruth C. Newberry

Faculty of Biosciences, Norwegian University of Life Sciences, Norway

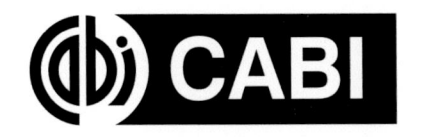

CABI is a trading name of CAB International

CABI
Nosworthy Way
Wallingford
Oxfordshire OX10 8DE
UK

CABI
200 Portland Street
Boston
MA 02114
USA

Tel: +44 (0)1491 832111
E-mail: info@cabi.org
Website: www.cabi.org

Tel: +1 (617)682-9015
E-mail: cabi-nao@cabi.org

© Bjarne O. Braastad, Anne McBride and Ruth C. Newberry 2022. All rights reserved. No part of this publication may be reproduced in any form or by any means, electronically, mechanically, by photocopying, recording or otherwise, without the prior permission of the copyright owners.

The views expressed in this publication are those of the author(s) and do not necessarily represent those of, and should not be attributed to, CAB International (CABI). Any images, figures and tables not otherwise attributed are the author(s)' own. References to internet websites (URLs) were accurate at the time of writing.

CAB International and, where different, the copyright owner shall not be liable for technical or other errors or omissions contained herein. The information is supplied without obligation and on the understanding that any person who acts upon it, or otherwise changes their position in reliance thereon, does so entirely at their own risk. Information supplied is neither intended nor implied to be a substitute for professional advice. The reader/user accepts all risks and responsibility for losses, damages, costs and other consequences resulting directly or indirectly from using this information.

CABI's Terms and Conditions, including its full disclaimer, may be found at https://www.cabi.org/terms-and-conditions/.

A catalogue record for this book is available from the British Library, London, UK.

ISBN-13: 9781789242317 (paperback)
    9781789242324 (ePDF)
    9781789242331 (ePub)

DOI: 10.1079/9781789242331.0000

Commissioning Editor: Caroline Makepeace
Editorial Assistant: Lauren Davies
Production Editor: Shankari Wilford

Typeset by: SPi, Pondicherry, India
Printed and bound in the UK by Severn, Gloucester, UK

Contents

About the Authors ... ix
Preface ... xi
Acknowledgements ... xiii

1. The Origin of Cats – How Did the Cat Become Tame and Domesticated? ... 1
   The Cat in Ancient Times ... 2
   The Cat Spreads Out ... 4
   The Cat Was Persecuted in the Middle Ages ... 6
   Emergence of Cat Breeds ... 6
   Further Reading ... 10

2. The Development of Kittens and Their Relationship with Their Mother and Siblings ... 11
   Heat, Mating and Gestation ... 11
   Maternal Behaviour ... 13
   Development of the Senses ... 15
   Behavioural Development ... 16
   New Home from 12 Weeks of Age – How to Achieve a Good Start ... 21
   Further Reading ... 24

3. The Cat's Personality – Individual Variation and Breed Characteristics ... 25
   What Is the Typical Behaviour of Cats? ... 25
   Differences in Personality ... 25
   Age Differences ... 26
   Sex Differences ... 27
   Genes and Behaviour ... 27
   Breed Differences in Behaviour ... 29
   Environment and Experience ... 30
   Further Reading ... 34

4. The Cat's Language – Communication ... 35
   How Animals Communicate ... 35
   Sound Signals – Acoustic Communication ... 36
   Body Language – Visual Communication ... 41
   Odour Language – Olfactory Communication ... 46
   Touch Language – Tactile Communication ... 49
   Communicating with Cats ... 49
   Further Reading ... 51

5. Social Behaviour of Cats ... 52
   Basics of Social Behaviour ... 52
   The Female Cat's Social Behaviour ... 56
   The Male Cat's Social Behaviour ... 57
   Multiple Cats in the Same Residence ... 60
   A Cat and Dog Together ... 61
   Further Reading ... 61

6. The Cat as a Predator	**63**
Predatory Behaviour	63
Effects on the Fauna	65
Further Reading	69
7. The Cat's Ability to Navigate	**70**
Tales of Cat Wanderings	70
Research on the Cat's Orientation Ability	71
The Cat's Behaviour in Unfamiliar Terrain	72
How Can the Cat Navigate in Unfamiliar Terrain?	73
How Can You Find a Lost Cat?	74
Taking Your Cat on Holiday	77
Further Reading	78
8. Motivation, Behavioural Needs and Emotions	**79**
Motivation and Behavioural Needs	79
How the Cat's Emotions Control Behaviour	81
Further Reading	87
9. Animal Welfare – How to Ensure the Cat's Welfare	**88**
Animal Welfare - What Is it Really?	88
Indicators of Animal Welfare	89
Ethical Obligation to Ensure Animal Welfare	90
Homeless Cats – What Can We Do about Them?	90
Health and Diseases	96
Health Problems in Pedigree Cats	96
Breeding Effects on Anatomy, Health and Behaviour	96
Requirements for the Cat's Environment and Care	98
What Are You Going to Do with the Cat during Holidays?	103
Requirements for Cat Boarding and Cat Shelters	104
Cat Assaults	106
Further Reading	106
10. Learning and Training	**107**
Habituation	107
Learning by Association	108
Operant Conditioning	115
Latent (Hidden) Learning	121
Social and Imitation Learning	121
Learning by Insight	122
Summary	122
Further Reading	122
Videos	122
11. Problem Behaviours in Cats	**123**
Introduction	123
What is Problem Behaviour in Cats?	123
Who is the Behaviour a Problem for – the Cat or the Human?	124
Preventing and Addressing Problem Behaviours – General Principles for All Cases, for All Cats and for All of Life	127
Emotional States	131
Scenting or Marking Behaviours	137
Inappropriate Toileting	138
Feline Cognitive Dysfunction	139

Attachment-related Problems	140
Pica and Over-grooming	140
Aggression	142
Inappropriate Play	146
Summary of Approaches to Prevent and Address Problem Behaviour	147
Conclusion	150
Further Reading	150

12. People and Cats — 151
What Characterizes Cat Owners?	151
Personality, Attachment and Cat Ownership	153
The Changing Landscape of Cat Keeping	155
Pets and Housing	157
Cats, COVID-19 and the Future	160
Further Reading	162

13. The Cat's Contribution to Human Health — 163
Research on the Health Effects of Pets	163
Cats and Our Physical Health	164
Cats and Our Mental Health	166
Pet Cats May Positively Affect Children's Development	168
Animal-assisted Therapy	169
Further Reading	173

14. Conclusions: How to Develop a Harmonious, Well-functioning Adult Cat — 174
Breeding	174
From Kittenhood to Adulthood	175

Literature — 179

Index — 185

Supplementary materials for this book can be accessed at: www.cabi.org/the-cat-behaviour-and-welfare/

About the Authors

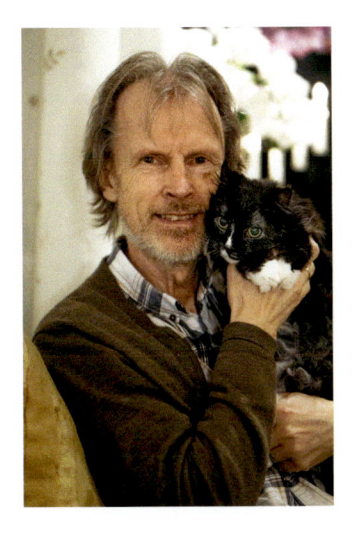

Bjarne O. Braastad is Professor Emeritus of Ethology (Behavioural Biology) in the Faculty of Biosciences at the Norwegian University of Life Sciences, where he worked for 37 years until 2020. He was born on a farm with several animal species, including five cats. For his MSc degree in ethology, he studied homing behaviour in cats, while his PhD in neurobiology was on development of visual brain cortex in cats. Since 1979, Bjarne has been researching and teaching in animal behaviour and animal welfare, and during 2001–2015 on animal-assisted interventions using farm animals for humans with mental health issues (termed 'green care'). Bjarne's research work has comprised most farmed species, including salmon, and a wide variety of ethological topics like prenatal stress, housing of farm animals, maternal behaviour, cognitive neurobiology and human–animal interactions. Bjarne has supervised a number of Master's projects on cat behaviour. He has a keen interest in dissemination of scientific knowledge to animal owners and the general public – in newspapers, magazines, radio, TV, on the internet, as well as through talks at meetings, particularly addressing cat owners. In 2013 he received his university's Research Dissemination Award for this work. He is an Honorary Member of the Society for Norwegian Ethologists. In 1982, he initiated the founding of the Norwegian Association of Cat Owners. Bjarne and his wife raised two sons. The younger one died at the age of 16 from acute leukaemia. This cat book is dedicated to him. Bjarne and his wife are enthusiastic folk dancers and Bjarne chairs the local folkdance group.

Anne McBride, also published as E.A. McBride, has a psychology degree and PhD in animal behaviour from University College London. She has had a few cat teachers, notably Corky (named for her corkscrew-shaped tail that had been broken in several places), a small, black non-pedigree, unwanted kitten brought to the vet's to be euthanized, where a young Anne was working as a Saturday helper. Instead, Corky found a home for the next 14 years. An Animal Behaviour and Training Council Registered Clinical Animal Behaviourist, she has been practising since 1987, and developed and ran for 20 years the first postgraduate course in this field at the University of Southampton. She continues to teach about human–animal interactions at Southampton and elsewhere, including teaching some of Bjarne's students about animal learning and training – with sessions to help them practise their skills by training new behaviours to cows! Her degree, experience as a clinician, and of life and people generally, and her strong interest in the 'hows and whys', are central to her main goal in life; namely, to help others become creative yet critical thinkers in respect of animal (and human) behaviour and welfare. Her second goal is to grow older whilst never truly growing up, by continuing to learn and laugh all the way to the end.

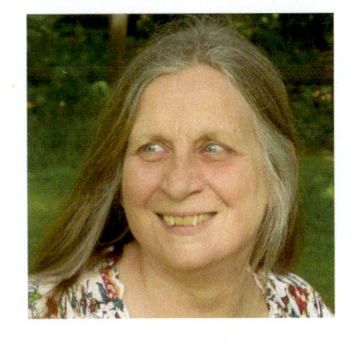

Ruth C. Newberry is a Professor of Ethology in the Faculty of Biosciences at the Norwegian University of Life Sciences. Her early years were spent on a farm near Ottawa, which had a resident cat colony. Before the cats were neutered, she saw first-hand the communal nursing of Tinkerbell and her adult daughter, and the comings and goings of the resident tomcat. As a zoology student at the University of Edinburgh, she was encouraged by Jane Goodall's writings to pursue the study of animal behaviour, leading to her PhD research in the Edinburgh Pig Park observing communal nursing in pig nests. After several years investigating chicken behaviour at the Agassiz Research Station in British Columbia, she journeyed south to join Washington State University's colleges of veterinary medicine and agriculture. There she conducted studies on a wide range of animals including cats. Having finally habituated to cowboy hats in her classroom, the northern lights beckoned once more, this time to Norway. Here, since 2013, her research has focused on methods of environmental enrichment that foster harmonious social development and positive welfare. Ruth is a Past President and Honorary Fellow of the International Society for Applied Ethology, and a member of several scientific advisory committees on animal welfare. A confirmed cat person meeting the personality traits described in Chapter 12, she has shared her home with a succession of beloved cats – Annapurra Katman, Cinnamon Daintree, Siena Kitkatla, to name a few – whose unique personalities have provided inspiration during the writing of this book.

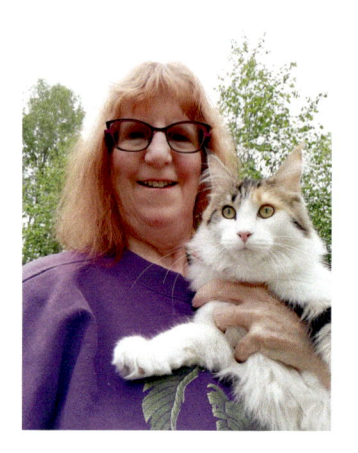

Jane Williams gained her Master's at the University of Southampton. Her first degree is in zoology from the University of Nottingham and she has an MA in Education from the Open University. Jane is Animal Behaviour and Training Council Registered as a clinical animal behaviourist, and an animal training instructor. Jane was the ABTC Chair (2018–20) and is currently a trustee and its Secretary (2020–22). She has been a full member of the Association of Pet Behaviour Counsellors since 2009, and she was its Chair (2017–20). She is currently an APBC committee member responsible for applications and assessments. Jane sees feline behaviour cases regularly, remotely and within her practice in the east of England. Jane has delivered talks for veterinary practices, rescue centres and owners on feline welfare and behaviour. She has presented at the Cats Protection Conference (September 2021) and provided consultancy services in feline behaviour for drug manufacturers and pet retailers, and written articles on stress reduction in companion animals during veterinary treatment and visits. Jane has several published articles in the field of reptile husbandry and welfare – tortoises being an area of special interest. Jane lives in Essex with 30 tortoises, six dogs, Harry the rabbit and another equally animal-mad human. She was a cat owner for many years, including phases of being a multi-cat household, and hopes to be one again in the not too distant future.

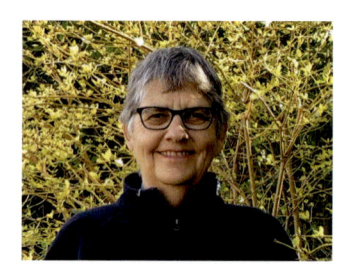

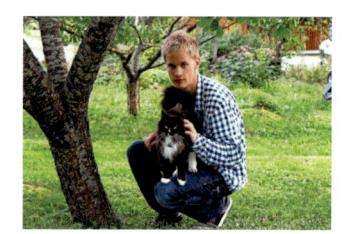

Audun Braastad, son of Bjarne, is a photographer educated at Bilder – Nordic School of Photography in 2012. He has been a photographer and video journalist for several newspapers and NTB Scanpix, the photo stock at the Norwegian News Agency. Audun photographs at weddings and does portrait photography. In 2020 he obtained a Bachelor's degree in digital marketing at Kristiania University College. Audun is a keen cat lover who does not miss an opportunity to catch good portraits of cats he encounters.

Preface

The cat is the most popular companion animal in large parts of the world, including western Europe and North America. This does not surprise the cat lover at all. On a scale from 1 to 10, regarding how closely attached a cat owner is to his or her cat, Norwegian research tells us that half of us give the top score of 10. The cat provides us with comfort and entertainment – and who can fail to be impressed by the beautiful appearance and graceful movements of the cat?

This book gives you the necessary knowledge to give your cat a rich life together with you. You will learn about behavioural development, cat language and social behaviour, navigation skills, the cat as a predator, cat keeping, and how the cat can help you to achieve better physical and mental health. The book will help you understand your cat better so that you can develop a closer social bond. Knowledge gives confidence and when you know the cat's natural behaviour and needs, you will understand why a cat may bite or urinate on the living room carpet. This knowledge will help you to solve the problem – but above all, you will know how to prevent such problems from occurring in the first place.

Ethology is the study of animal behaviour. It is the part of biology that deals with what animals do and why they do it. All behaviour can be explained by considering how behaviour in a particular situation can help the animal function in an optimal manner. The animal is acting out of its own interest, but we can do a lot to help the cat and the owner share common interests. Then one can develop a harmonious relationship where both parties thrive.

All people responsible for cats require sufficient competence to keep them. People who sell or give away a cat should also be able to provide information to the new owner about conditions needed to care for that cat in an appropriate way. An instruction manual should really come with the cat. This book provides knowledge that a cat owner needs to ensure the cat's welfare.

The subject material of the book is based on scientific research, so the reader can trust that the text gives as good an understanding of the cat as possible based on today's knowledge. The book is therefore applicable not just to cat owners but also to students, biologists, veterinarians, and animal nurses and technicians. At the end of each chapter, there is some further reading from scientific sources. We also contribute to the text from our own experience with cats which, when combined, adds up to nearly 200 years!

In Chapter 4, a QR code gives access to vocalizations of cats. With a smart phone, you can scan the links to access the clips. Throughout the book, there are links and QR codes to enable you to access relevant YouTube videos.

Supplementary material about the 'Good Manners' or 'Learn to Earn' programme as well as Bjarne's lecture slides can be accessed at: www.cabi.org/the-cat-behaviour-and-welfare/

Bjarne O. Braastad, Anne McBride and Ruth C. Newberry
May 2022

Acknowledgements

Thank you very much to everyone who has contributed to the book with photographs of cats, and a special thanks to photographer Audun Braastad for providing a large number of cat photos and editing most other Norwegian photos. Jane Williams kindly contributed to Chapter 11 on problem behaviours, including some cases and photos, for which we are very thankful. We are grateful to Caroline Makepeace, the Editorial Director at CABI, for her inspiring way of leading us through the process of making this book. Additional thanks are sent to Alison Smith, Lauren Davies and Shankari Wilford from the CABI team.

Last, but not least, thanks a lot to our respective spouses, Elin, Richard and Tony, and to our pets, for all their support and patience when we were busy writing this book.

1 The Origin of Cats – How Did the Cat Become Tame and Domesticated?

Our cherished pet cats have not always been domesticated. They resemble a lot of small wild cats from Africa and Eurasia, and still retain many similarities with them. Because domestic cats are now found all over the world, including places with resident populations of small wildcat species, we are not sure precisely where, when and how the domestic cat originated, but genetic, archaeological and historical studies provide good indications.

According to the International Union for Conservation of Nature, the domestic cat is classified as a species, in Latin called *Felis catus*, which can be distinguished from six wild species of *Felis* including the European wildcat (*Felis silvestris*; Fig. 1.1), the African wildcat (*Felis lybica*, Fig. 1.2) and the Chinese mountain cat (*Felis bieti*). There is uncertainty about this classification, and it may change based on future research. Some texts place the domestic cat as a subspecies of *Felis silvestris* known as *Felis silvestris catus*, with the European wildcat, African wildcat and Chinese mountain cat forming other subspecies of *Felis silvestris* with which the domestic cat is known to interbreed. Domestic cats can also potentially interbreed with other small cat species found in Africa and Asia. They can even be crossed with certain small wildcat species found in South and Central America but, with only 36 instead of the usual 38 chromosomes, fertile offspring are unlikely.

The European wildcat has been one candidate for ancestry of the domestic cat. Resembling a large brown tabby domestic cat, the European wildcat can be found in low numbers scattered across the temperate forests of Europe and western Asia. Once widespread in Great Britain, an isolated population still exists in Scotland, although on the verge of extinction in its pure form due to hybridization with feral domestic cats. Occasional reports of big black wildcats in Scotland, called Kellas cats, have turned out to be hybrids between the European wildcat and the domestic cat. The European wildcat is a really wild cat – timid, aggressive and solitary, and even the kittens are almost impossible to tame. These behavioural characteristics seem to be the opposite of those that would make a wildcat an obvious candidate for domestication; that is, easily tamed, sociable and functioning well in close contact with people.

The African wildcat is a more promising candidate for domestication. While there have been few studies of this species in the wild, African wildcats can be found living close to villages, and can be easily tamed if taken in as kittens. Although usually solitary, females are occasionally seen in groups with members of successive litters, as is also sometimes seen in domestic cats. The older offspring may then assist their mother in supplying food for their younger siblings. The African wildcat typically inhabits semi-arid areas and is found throughout much of Africa excluding the central Sahara and tropical rainforest. Not restricted to Africa, its range extends through the Middle East and across Asia to western China. The closely-related Chinese mountain cat is a large, blue-eyed wildcat adapted to life on the Tibetan Plateau, where it is not known for tractability. There are, however, other species of small wildcat in addition to the African wildcat that can be easily tamed.

The question arises whether domestic cats could have arisen from multiple domestication events in different parts of the world, involving more than one species of wildcat. The answer is yes and no. There is some evidence for early domestication of the mainland leopard cat, *Prionailurus bengalensis*, in China around 5000 years ago. However, those early domestic cats appear to have died out, as it has been discovered that the domestic cats found in China today can be traced back to African wildcats of Middle East origin. A DNA analysis of 979 wild and domestic cats from Europe, the Middle East, Africa and Asia showed that, in fact, all the tested domestic cats were derived from the African wildcat.

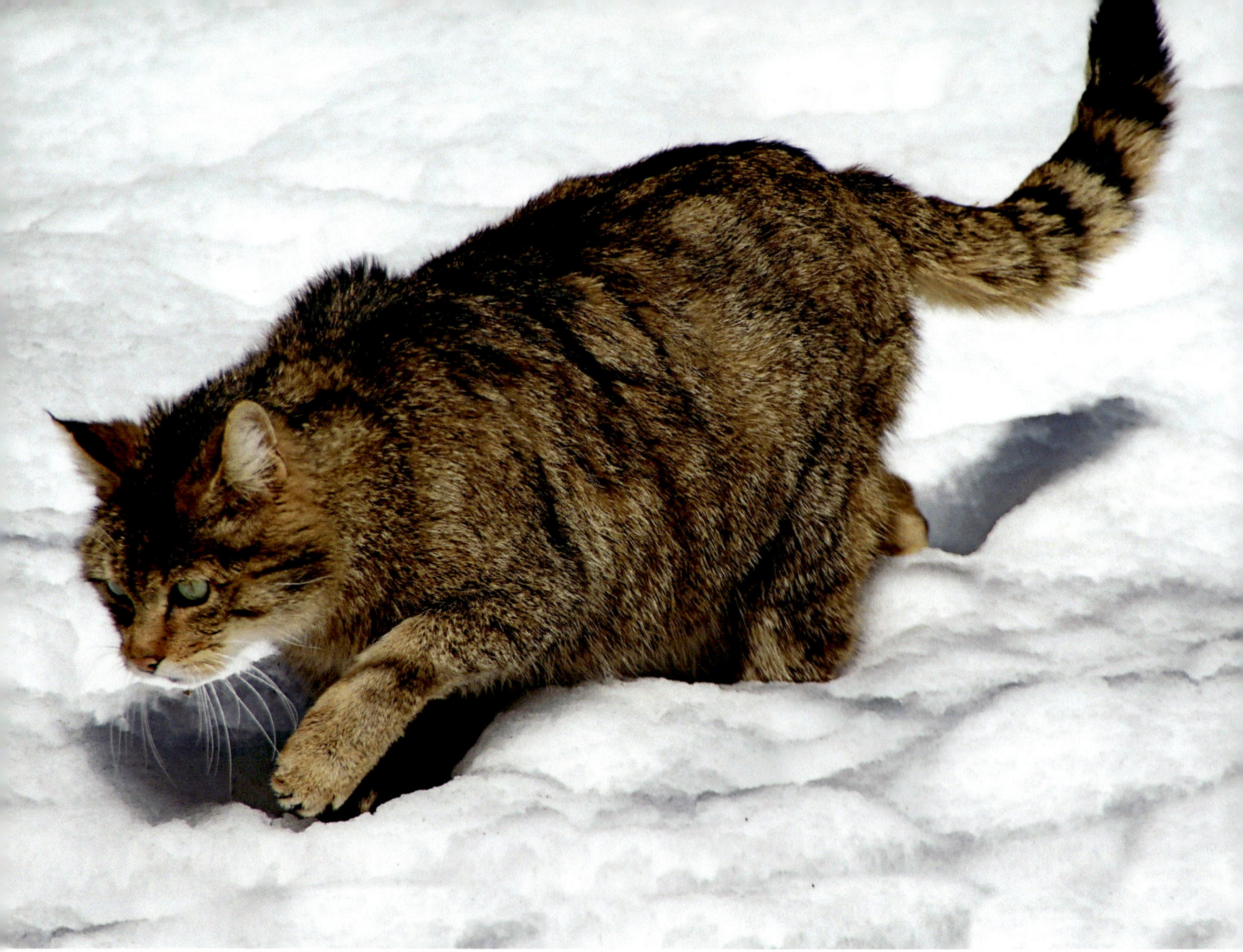

Fig. 1.1. European wildcat, *Felis silvestris*. (Photo: Aconcagua (Stefan Reicheneder), used by permission of Creative Commons Attribution-ShareAlike licence CC BY-SA 3.0, https://commons.wikimedia.org/wiki/File:European_Wildcat_Nationalpark_Bayerischer_Wald_03.jpg)

The analysis further indicated that they were descended from a subspecies of African wildcat found in the Fertile Crescent, the belt of land extending from the Egyptian Nile to Palestine and Mesopotamia where agriculture is believed to have originated roughly 12,000 years ago. Further research has shown that the Chinese mountain cat is not the original source of today's domestic cats in Asia, although it has subsequently interbred with domestic cats.

The relatively new cat breed, the Bengal cat, is derived from deliberate crossing of the domestic cat with the mainland leopard cat, a trend that started in the 1960s (Fig. 1.3). Joining the Bengal cat are several other new synthetic breeds created by crossing domestic cats with other wildcat species. See Chapter 9 for discussion of ethical issues arising from this practice.

The Cat in Ancient Times

The very earliest sign of cats living with humans comes from a 9500-year-old archaeological site in Cyprus. Excavations unearthed an approximately eight-month-old cat of the African wildcat type that had been buried in its own small pit just 40 cm from a person, aligned in the same direction. Cats have never lived wild in Cyprus, so it must be humans who brought the cat to this Mediterranean island. The fact that the cat was buried intact alongside a person suggests that the person had a strong relationship with this cat. Similarly, in Israel, dogs were being buried with people 12,000 years ago.

The area in the Middle East where the domestic cat originated is considered the cradle of civilization, where people gave up their hunter-gatherer lifestyle and began to cultivate the soil. Mice and other small rodents lived well on the stores of cereals that humans cultivated and harvested. These prey animals attracted wildcats that had spotted a rich food source. The humans no doubt welcomed this unexpected help. The cats and the people enjoyed a mutual benefit. It is likely that those cats that thrived and reproduced the most in human settlements were those that were the least fearful of people and the most willing to tolerate the proximity of livestock, dogs and other cats. Over generations, this natural selection for tameness and sociability would have led to the genetic divergence of domestic cats from their wild ancestors. These cats were friendly and funny, and interacting with them in kittenhood would have further accentuated their friendliness. It is no surprise that some cats became pets, enjoying the care and protection of their owners even when they grew old and were no longer efficient mousers.

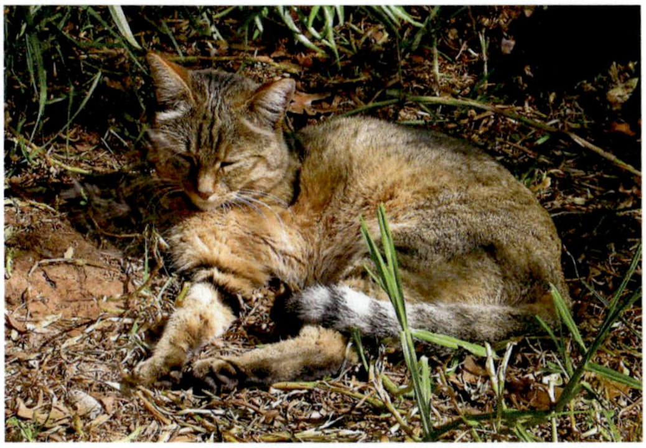

From the above, we can see that rather than humans 'domesticating' the cat, cats essentially domesticated themselves. While domestic cats are typically smaller than the African wildcat, and have a smaller brain, they are quite adept at training their owners to be their obedient servants. It suffices to scratch on the wall by the door to have the owner rushing to open the door. In Chapter 10, we shall see how we can easily train cats to avoid any unwanted behaviour. This allows us to live with them in harmony, continuing a close association that began at least 10,000 years ago.

Fig. 1.2. African wildcat, *Felis lybica*. (Photo: Sonelle, used by permission of Creative Commons Attribution-ShareAlike licence CC BY-SA 3.0, https://commons.wikimedia.org/wiki/File:AfricanWildCat.jpg)

The divine cat

The ancient Egyptians worshipped cats and kept many in captivity. A 4000-year-old wall painting in the tomb of Baqet III depicts a cat facing a rat, indicating that the cat was valued as a rat catcher. Where

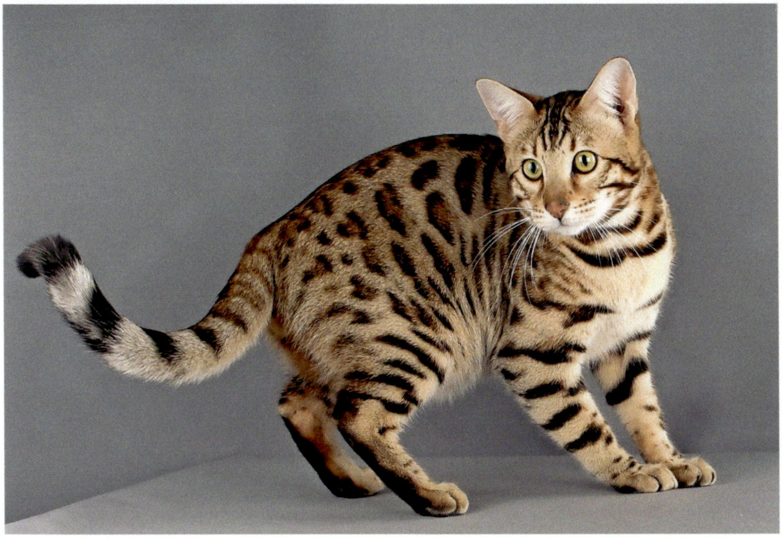

Fig. 1.3. The Bengal cat has become a popular breed in North America and Europe in recent decades. It is derived from crossing the mainland leopard cat with domestic shorthair cats. (Photo: Maria Myrland, 2019)

rats are found, it is not surprising that they attract snakes who eat them. The cat is also good at killing small snakes, as a source of prey or perhaps because snakes pose a threat to their kittens. This was probably known to the Egyptians 3500–4000 years ago when they carved 'magic knives' of ivory, decorated with cat figures to repel venomous snakes.

The Egyptians had many gods. In one myth, the sun god Ra, in the guise of a great tomcat, slays the serpent god Apophis. Around 3200–3500 years ago, cats were associated with the goddess Hathor, especially when she presented herself as Nebethetepet. This goddess represented sexual energy, and the association with the cat may relate to the fact that female cats can mate multiple times and bear offspring with different fathers in a single litter.

The most famous cat god was Bastet, who was associated with fertility, birth, protection and care of children. Initially, she was depicted with a lion head but about 2700–3000 years ago, this was replaced by a cat head signifying a more friendly deity (Fig. 1.4).

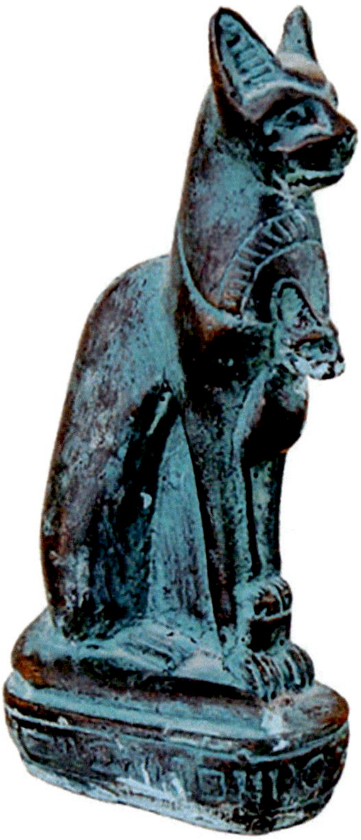

Many cats were kept in temples and sacrificed in the name of Bastet. Veneration of Bastet centred on the city of Bubastis in the south-eastern Nile delta but eventually spread throughout Egypt. The famous Greek historian Herodotus described the Bastet cult when he travelled in Egypt *c*.450 BCE. He recounted that festival worshippers at the temple of Bubastis arrived from miles around bearing cat mummies as offerings. When a family cat died, the people of the house shaved off their eyebrows to show their grief. Rich cat owners embalmed their dead cats and buried them in special cat cemeteries with bronze statuettes of cats as grave monuments. In some cases, a cat mummy was buried together with a human mummy. If someone happened to kill a cat, there was great concern. This was considered a serious crime and cat murderers risked lynching.

Herodotus also described incidences where male cats killed kittens. This would have caused their mother to come into heat, allowing her to be mated by the infanticidal male. Today, infanticide by males is a recognized phenomenon in the behavioural ecology of many species, and it is especially well known in lions. It is reported occasionally in feral domestic cats. Herodotus can thus be regarded as one of the first cat ethologists.

The Cat Spreads Out

As a result of the domestic cat being so useful, it was forbidden to export cats from ancient Egypt. Special agents were sent out to buy back and bring home cats that had been illegally exported. However, cats gradually spread out from the Fertile Crescent along trade routes. Various archaeological and historical sources show that domestic cats existed in the Indus Valley 4500–5000 years ago, in the Minoan culture of Crete 3100–3500 years ago and in Greece and southern Italy around 2500 years ago. The Greeks and Romans used ferrets and weasels to catch mice and rats, which initially limited the need for cats. However, the value of cats caught on and, with the expansion of the Roman Empire, cats spread through Europe, including England, where they are first described around 350 CE.

The cat arrives in Scandinavia

It is unclear when cats first arrived in Scandinavia, but cat bones have been found in Danish burial sites dating from about 1 to 375 CE. This suggests that

Fig. 1.4. The Egyptian god Bastet, a popular souvenir for tourists. (Photo: Bjarne O. Braastad, 2011)

cats spread north from areas of Roman occupation. However, cats remained uncommon until the Viking Age (*c.*850–1050 CE), when they were brought by Vikings returning home from travels to the south. In Iceland and elsewhere in Scandinavia, cat skins became a valuable commodity used to make gloves and other garments. According to a law established by the Norwegian King Magnus Lagabøte in 1274 CE, cat skins were a valid means of payment, with the skin of an adult male cat being worth three fox skins. Cats were important for controlling mice and rats both on land and on the Viking ships, but they also developed symbolic value. In Norse mythology, the goddess of fertility, Freya, was described as driving a wagon pulled by two cats (Fig. 1.5). Present-day cats in Scandinavia are often bigger than those kept by the Vikings, probably due to better nutrition and adaptation to colder climates.

Cats around the world

Based on historical records, domestic cats of Middle East origin were present in China during the Tang dynasty (618–907 CE) and in Japan in 889 CE, when Emperor Uda wrote of his joy in owning a black cat. Cats were valued for protecting silkworm cocoons from predation by rats. They are thought to have spread south and east with the early Arab maritime traders. In Madagascar, which had no indigenous wildcat species, domestic cats became the ancestors of today's wild forest cats. This occurred through the process known as feralization, which works in the opposite direction to domestication. Over generations of natural selection, populations of domesticated animals no longer supported by people become increasingly adapted to living in the local natural habitat and revert to wildtype behaviour and colouration. However, this only happens if conditions are favourable in terms of weather, food and ability to withstand native predators.

The Vikings took cats on their travels to Greenland and may have taken them as far as Vinland (now Newfoundland), though no sign remains. Columbus also carried cats aboard his ships. Cats became established in European settlements in the Americas in the 16th to 18th centuries. Cats were brought to Australia and New Zealand by European settlers in the late 18th century, although possibly earlier by Indonesian traders. In Australia, thousands of cats were released in the 19th century to control rabbits, native rats and infestations of mice at gold-mining settlements.

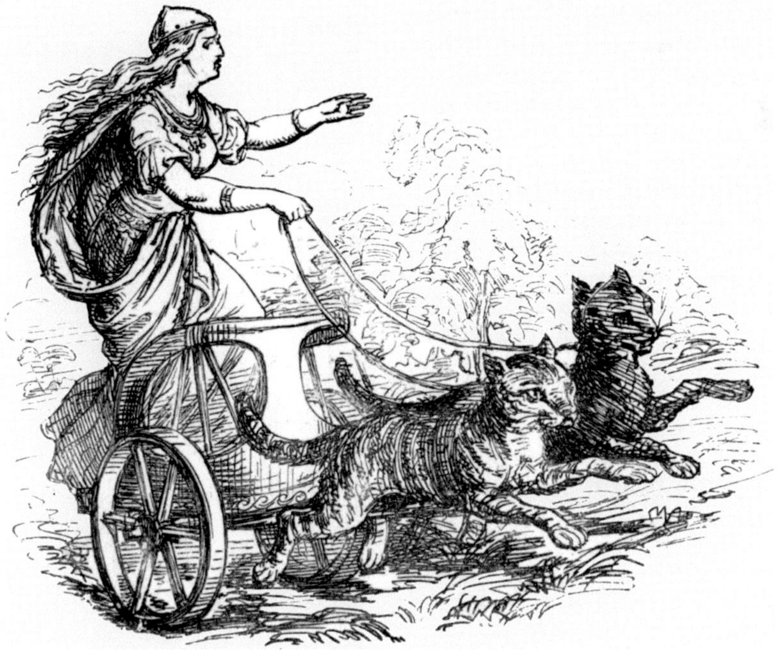

Fig. 1.5. The Norse goddess, Freya, on her cat-drawn wagon. (Illustration: Ludwig Pietsch, 1860. Public domain, https://commons.wikimedia.org/wiki/File:Freyja_riding_with_her_cats_(1874).jpg)

How many cats are there?

Today, the cat is the most popular pet in the world based on numbers owned, with an estimated 373 million owned cats and a further 480 million stray and feral cats (in 2018). The countries with the highest numbers of cats are the USA (74.1 million) and China (53.1 million). The European Pet Food Industry (FEDIAF, 2021) estimates that there are 113 million domestic cats living in Europe, Russia and Turkey, with 26% of households owning at least one cat. There were around 22.9 million cats in Russia, 12 million in the UK and 780,000 in Norway. In the UK, cats are found in about one in four homes, and in Norway, one in five households have a cat. These are only rough estimates, and the actual numbers may be much higher. The estimates vary greatly depending on the methods used to collect the data and do not account for all cats.

The Cat Was Persecuted in the Middle Ages

As we have seen, cats were worshipped in ancient Egypt. They were also admired in Muslim countries, unlike dogs, which were considered unclean. Alas, cats were persecuted by the Christian priesthood in Europe during the Middle Ages. Cats did not conform to the dogma that animals were created to serve man – they were independent and not overly attentive to the wishes and demands of people. This was seen as evidence of their allegiance to the devil.

Black cats, especially, were linked to witchcraft due to the belief that witches could transform themselves into cats at night and sneak about unseen doing the devil's work. Single women who kept cats and did not conform to social conventions were easily accused of being witches. In England, hundreds of female cat owners were executed between 1560 and 1700 CE because of friendship with cats. When they were burnt at the stake after sham trials, their cats were often burnt with them. In France, cats could themselves be placed on trial for witchcraft. Cats were burned alive during festivals or, in Ypres, Belgium, tossed from the bell tower. In Japanese mythology, it was thought that a cat's supernatural proclivities were signified by a long tail. To prevent kittens from becoming demons, their tails were cut off.

Perhaps an underlying biological explanation for the persecution of cats lies in their role in transmitting zoonotic diseases such as rabies and toxoplasmosis, and a periodic need to reduce cat over-population. On the other hand, any reduction in cat numbers might have facilitated the spread of Bubonic plague by flea-carrying rats. Clearly, medieval views about cats were steeped in superstition, with people burning cats for good luck while wearing their fur as a cure for rheumatism. Even today, people hold varied attitudes about the habits of cats and many cat owners struggle with their relationships with neighbours and landlords, as we address in Chapter 12.

Emergence of Cat Breeds

Even today, most domestic cats do not belong to any particular breed. They are the product of so-called random breeding by cats that have found their own mates without human intervention. These cats are termed non-pedigree cats, house cats or, in the UK, domestic short-haired cats. As with feral cats and strays (that are rarely pedigree cats), they express basic anatomical and behavioural characteristics that are not very different from those of wildcats.

During the early stages of domestication, most cats had wildtype mackerel (striped) tabby (Fig. 1.6) or black coats that camouflaged them from wild predators when hunting at night. However, association with people facilitated the survival of cats deviating from the wildtype, such as cats with patches of white fur, a typical signature of domestication. The blotched (swirl) coat pattern referred to as classic tabby (Fig. 1.7) was first noted in domestic cats in Turkey during the early Ottoman Empire (13th century). It subsequently spread to other regions of the world although it did not become common until the 19th century. The other two tabby coat patterns, spotted (Fig. 1.8) and ticked (producing faint tabby markings), probably spread in a similar manner.

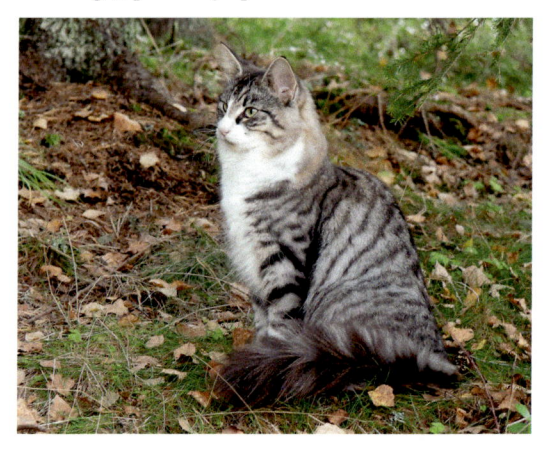

Fig. 1.6. A mackerel tabby Norwegian forest cat. (Photo: Maria Myrland, 2019)

The orange coat colour is determined by a sex-linked gene on the X chromosome. So males having the orange allele on their single X chromosome are always orange, while females can be orange if both their Xs carry the orange allele or tortoiseshell (orange mixed with black or tabby) if one X chromosome carries the orange allele. It appears that the Vikings favoured orange cats and were responsible for their dispersal along trade routes from Miklagard (today's Istanbul) to northern Europe.

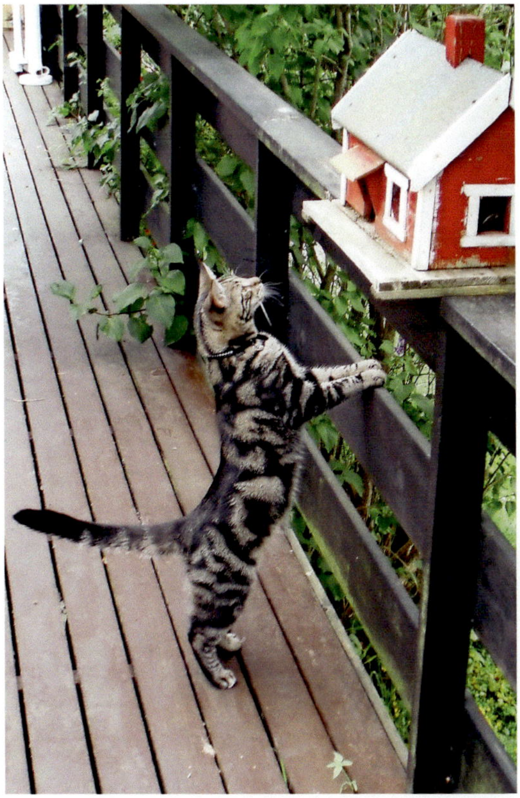

The Siamese and Persian are among the earliest known breeds, already distinct several hundred years ago. However, deliberate selective breeding of fancy breeds for specific traits only began in the 19th century when the rules of inheritance became better understood. Five breeds were exhibited at the first cat show at London's Crystal Palace in 1871 while over 40 breeds are recognized today, with the number of breeds varying between breed registries. This number continues to rise. The defining characteristics of breeds can also differ between breed registries and be amended over time. The popularity of cat breeds varies between regions and is influenced by changing fashions and attraction of buyers to novel and unusual traits (Table 1.1). Many of the recently developed breeds have emerged as a result of selection for particular mutations, such as the hairless Sphynx, or the Ragdoll that hangs passively while being picked up.

Genetic defects can easily be propagated when selecting for specific mutations within a narrow gene pool. Therefore, it is important to ensure broad genetic diversity within the breeding population of each breed so that one can breed in a favourable direction in terms of health and behaviour. In Chapter 9 we look more closely at welfare problems that can arise as an unintended consequence of pedigree breeding.

Relationships between cat breeds

Comprehensive DNA studies show that cat breeds can be divided into four main groups based on genetic relatedness: Europe, Asia, the Mediterranean basin, and East Africa, with differences between these populations arising due to geographical separation. The American breeds cluster with the European breeds, in keeping with their European descent. Thus, the Norwegian forest cat is closely related to the American Maine coon, but also to the Siberian cat, a type of forest cat found in Russia. Among the Asian breeds, the Siamese, Balinese and Oriental shorthair are closely related to each other and are also crossbred today, so they are considered to belong to the same gene pool.

Around 20 breeds are referred to as 'natural breeds' as they are thought to pre-date the cat fancy of the 19th century, having originally been derived from the local landrace cats in different regions of the world. Nowadays, some of these breeds bear relatively little genetic evidence of their historical roots,

Fig. 1.7. A classic tabby cat. (Photo: Grete Nakling, 2019)

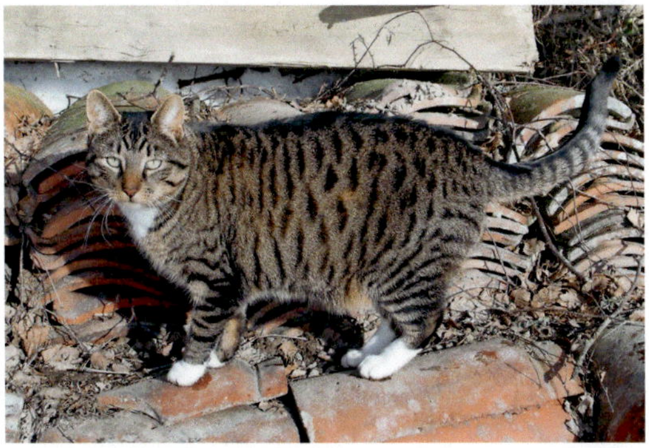

Fig. 1.8. A spotted tabby cat. (Photo: Maria Myrland, 2019)

Table 1.1. The most popular cat breeds in 2021.

Rank	The Cat Fanciers' Association registrations (international)	The Governing Council of the Cat Fancy registrations (UK)	Association of Pedigree Cat Clubs (NRR) registrations (Norway)	Cat insurance contracts (Anicom – Japan)
1	Ragdoll	British shorthair	Maine coon	Scottish fold
2	Maine coon	Ragdoll	Siberian	Mixed-breed cat
3	Exotic shorthair	Maine coon	Ragdoll	Munchkin
4	Persian	Siamese	British shorthair	American shorthair
5	Devon rex	Burmese	Sacred Birman	Norwegian forest cat
6	British shorthair	Persian	Norwegian forest cat	Ragdoll
7	Abyssinian	Oriental shorthair	Neva masquerade	British shorthair
8	American shorthair	British longhair	Bengal	Minuet (Persian hybrid)
9	Scottish fold	Birman	Persian	Siberian
10	Sphynx	Russian	Devon rex	Bengal

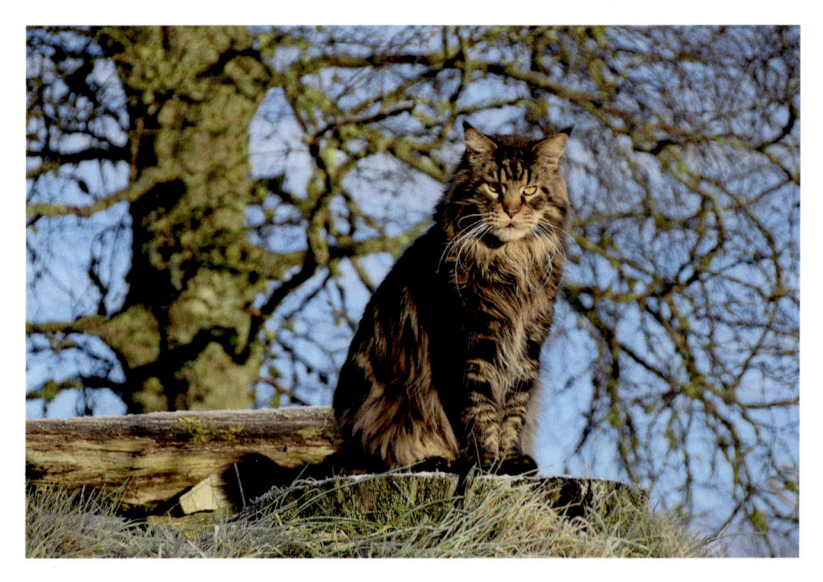

Fig. 1.9. The Maine coon is currently the most popular cat breed in Norway. This is an American forest cat derived from European forest cats. The picture shows a brown tabby Maine coon. (Photo: Jim Bertelsen, 2019).

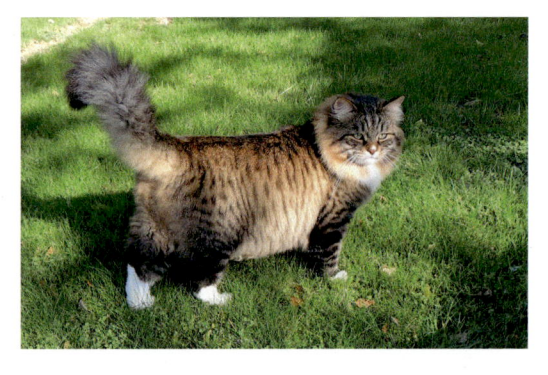

Fig. 1.10. The Siberian is a Russian forest cat that is increasing in popularity in Scandinavia. (Photo: Kari Granaas Hansen, 2019)

having been heavily crossed with other breeds to achieve a certain appearance. For example, based on their DNA, the Persian is placed among the European breeds along with the Exotic shorthair and Himalayan, with other relatives being the British shorthair and Scottish fold. Also found in the European group are the Abyssinian and Somali cats. These breeds are related to the hairless Sphynx cat, which is, in turn, closely related to the Devon rex. Although reputed to originate from the temples of Burma, the Sacred Birman was reconstructed in post-World War II France by crossing two remaining cats with Persian and Siamese cats.

In the Mediterranean basin group, the Egyptian mau is related to the Turkish angora while the Turkish

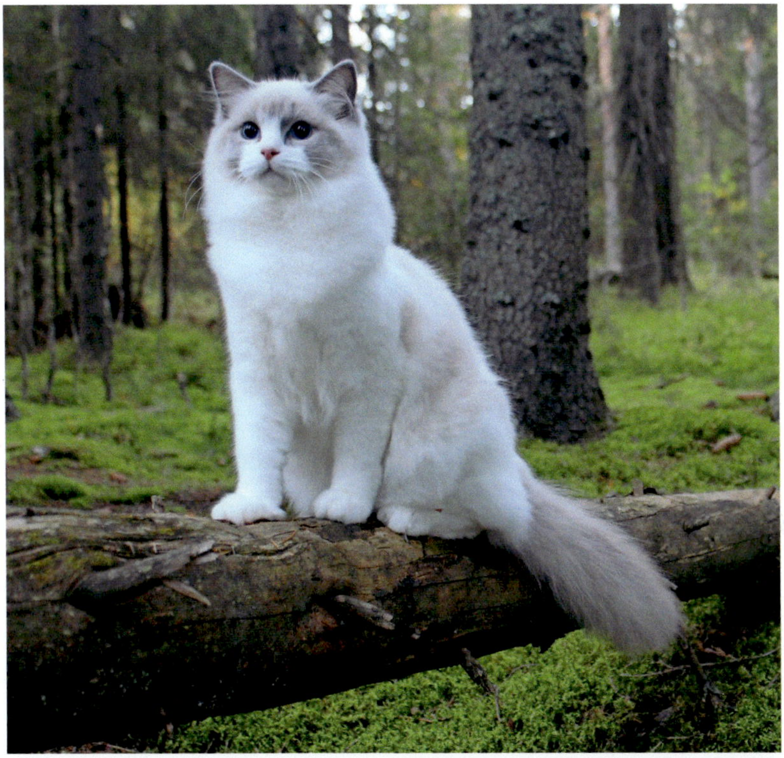

Fig. 1.11. The Ragdoll is usually kept as an indoor cat, though not always. (Photo: Aksel Ørbakk Knutsen, 2019)

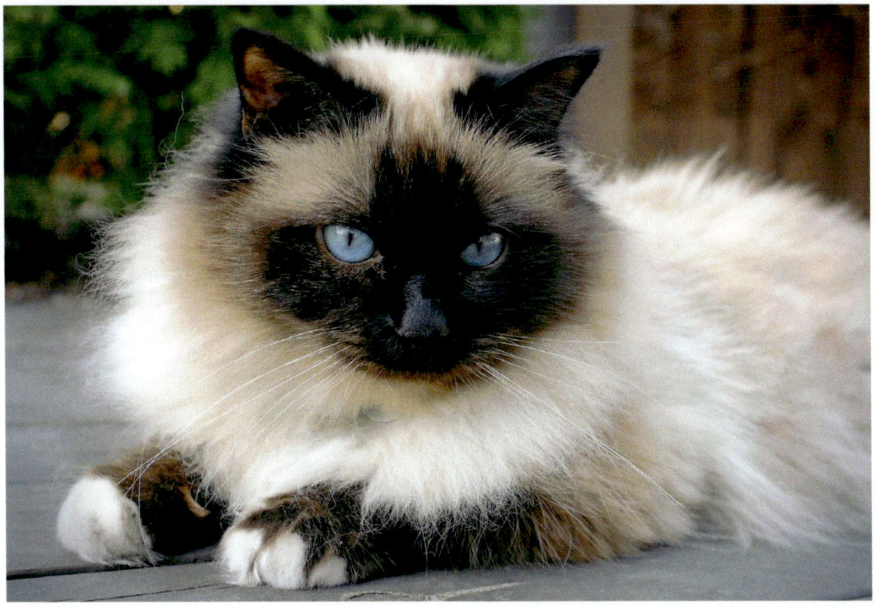

Fig. 1.12. The Sacred Birman is a very social cat. (Photo: Audun Braastad, 2019).

van is more closely related to random-bred cats found in Egypt. The Sokoke falls into the East African group, being closely related to random-bred cats in Kenya.

Cat breeds can differ from each other not only in appearance but also in behaviour, as we shall see in Chapter 3.

Further Reading

Driscoll, C.A., Clutton-Brock, J., Kitchener, A.C. and O'Brien, S.J. (2009) The taming of the cat: genetic and archaeological findings hint that wildcats became housecats earlier – and in a different place – than previously thought. *Scientific American* 300, 68–75.

FEDIAF (2021) Facts & figures 2021. European overview. Available at: https://europeanpetfood.org/about/statistics/ (accessed 23 September 2022).

Ottoni, C., Van Neer, W., De Cupere, B., Daligault, J., Guimaraes, S. *et al.* (2017) The palaeogenetics of cat dispersal in the ancient world. *Nature Ecology and Evolution* 1, 0139. DOI: 10.1038/s41559-017-0139.

Serpell, J.A. (2014) Domestication and history of the cat. In: Turner, D.C. and Bateson, P. (eds) *The Domestic Cat: The Biology of Its Behaviour*, 3rd edn. Cambridge University Press, Cambridge, pp. 83–100.

Vigne, J.-D., Guilaine, J., Debue, K., Haye, L. and Gérard, P. (2004) Early taming of the cat in Cyprus. *Science* 304 (5668), 259. DOI: 10.1126/science.1095335.

2 The Development of Kittens and Their Relationship with Their Mother and Siblings

The kitten's life during the first months will have a great impact on how it will function as an adult cat. This includes its experiences in the environment in which it lives, and its relationship with its mother, littermates and people. Therefore, the cat breeder has a great responsibility to ensure the kitten has a good start in life. The new owner must then continue to offer suitable experiences for the kitten's further development. For the cat to live in harmony with people, without behaviour problems, it is important to know how experiences of handling, socialization and play affect the kitten's future behaviour. In this chapter we examine how kittens develop. But we must begin before their birth; without heat, mating and a successful foetal period, there will be no kittens.

Heat, Mating and Gestation

Fertility of the cat

Female cats can be very fertile. A breeding female, called a queen, can potentially produce four litters a year, though two litters is more common. After a smaller first litter, three to five kittens per litter is typical up to six years of age, with a slow decline at higher ages. Litter sizes tend to be highest in short-haired, so-called oriental breeds such as the Burmese and Siamese, with one Burmese reported to have given birth to 15 liveborn kittens and four stillborn. Queens are most fertile from 1.5 to 7 years of age, but can have kittens until 8–10 years old, and occasionally after this. One mother even managed to produce two kittens when she was 30 years old. Queens can also become pregnant while nursing an existing litter, especially if the litter is small. All this goes to show that one queen has the potential to produce many kittens during her lifetime.

It is physiologically demanding for a queen to have frequent litters, especially if the litters are large, so best for her health to avoid more than two litters per year. To prevent unwanted pregnancies, contraceptive pills can be prescribed by a vet. However, these should not be given while a queen is nursing offspring, as they may reduce milk production or otherwise affect the kittens. The only solution then is to keep the queen away from males.

We must also consider that when more kittens are born than there are homes to take them, cat over-population quickly becomes a problem. Therefore, if we cannot be sure of finding good homes for all the kittens, a queen should not be allowed to have kittens. To ensure that she cannot become pregnant, it is safest to get her spayed. Owners of male cats must also take their share of responsibility in preventing the birth of unwanted kittens, not least among homeless female cats, by getting the males castrated.

Heat

Heat, or oestrus, means that a female is receptive to being mated (Fig. 2.1). Female kittens usually have their first heat at 6–10 months of age, but some come into heat by 4–5 months. Male (tom) cats usually reach puberty at 6–12 months but, like females, some may start breeding as early as four months of age. Except for the short-haired oriental breeds (e.g. Burmese), pedigree breeds typically become sexually mature a little later than non-pedigree cats. A general rule is that once a female reaches a weight of about 2.3–2.5 kg, we must expect her to come into heat. She will then cycle at roughly two- to three-week intervals, with the heat typically lasting 4–8 days.

Cats are considered seasonal breeders, being most likely to produce kittens during the spring and summer. If a queen gets less than 12 hours of daylight, she usually does not come into heat.

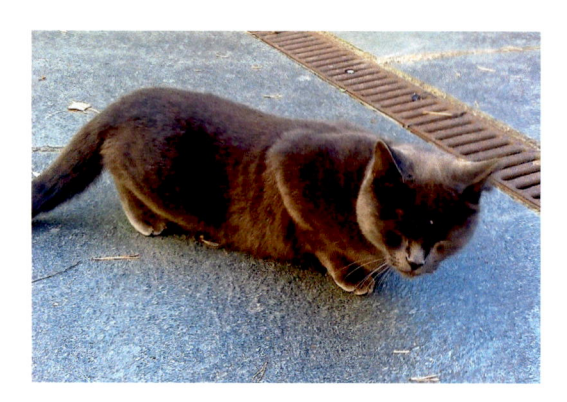

Fig. 2.1. Female cat in heat, soon ready to be mated. (Photo: Randi Oppermann Moe, 2019)

During long winter nights, her brain produces enough melatonin to suppress her cycles. But as the days get longer with the approach of spring, both males and females become restless indicating that the breeding season (or rut as it is termed for males) is on its way. Indoor cats can come into heat throughout the year if they get at least 12–14 hours of bright light. A heat is also more likely if there are fertile tomcats around, or other queens in heat. When living in social groups, queens can have synchronized heats and, if they then mate and become pregnant, their litters will arrive around the same time.

Normal heat cannot be mistaken. The queen shows clearly changed behaviour both towards the owner and towards male cats. She gets very cuddlesome, frequently brushing her body against our legs and the furniture. She rolls around on the floor and miaows loudly and deeply, attracting visits by the tomcats in the neighbourhood. She often urinates and may mark vertical structures in her territory by spraying urine on them. Unfortunately, this can include us and the furniture. Her urine contains chemical signals, called pheromones, which attract toms. She may suddenly become aggressive if someone pats her on the back. If she reacts similarly to a tom, this tells him that she is not yet willing to be mated. Eventually, she will stand with stiff legs and her tail upright or held to the side, treading with her front paws. This typically occurs about three to four days into the heat period and shows that she is becoming more receptive. If there is a tom nearby, her enticing heat behaviour may be even more pronounced.

However, if a female is young or has a low rank in her social group, she may have what is known as a silent heat, not showing the typical signs of being in heat. While it is not obvious that she is in heat, she can nevertheless still copulate and become pregnant.

Mating

The tomcat starts his courtship by sniffing the queen's head and hindquarters. If she is receptive, she will lie down on her chest, lift her pelvis and swing her tail aside. This posture, called *lordosis*, is an invitation to the tom to mate with her. He mounts her quickly and holds her by biting the scruff of her neck. The copulation itself may last for just a few seconds, and when the tom withdraws his penis, the female yowls. She then rushes forward or rapidly swings around towards the tom and hisses or snarls at him. The male pulls back quickly, while the female rolls around on the ground for a few minutes, licks her genitals and miaows. Mating usually occurs multiple times, and the male therefore waits nearby until the female is receptive to another mating – often after approximately 20 minutes.

It is possible for a queen to ovulate spontaneously without mating, especially if a tom is present but prevented from mating. However, most ovulations are triggered by copulation, with ovulation occurring around 24–48 hours later. This is called induced ovulation. The tom's penis is covered with tiny backward-pointing spines that play a role in stimulating ovulation (Fig. 2.2). It is the bit of pain the queen experiences as he withdraws that causes her to hiss at him. Multiple copulations increase the likelihood of ovulation. If there are other toms nearby, they can also mate with the queen. The consequence is that, in a single litter, different kittens can have different fathers. However, queens can be somewhat choosy about which males they will accept. They also show *inbreeding avoidance*, meaning that they are more likely to reject the advances of a closely related male if other males are available.

Gestation period

The gestation period of cats lasts about 63–66 days on average, but it may vary from about 52 to 71 days. Siamese cats tend to have a relatively long pregnancy. In general, gestation lengths and birthweights are lower in cats having larger litters. If you suspect that your cat is pregnant, a vet can check for this by examining the stomach (abdominal palpitation), or

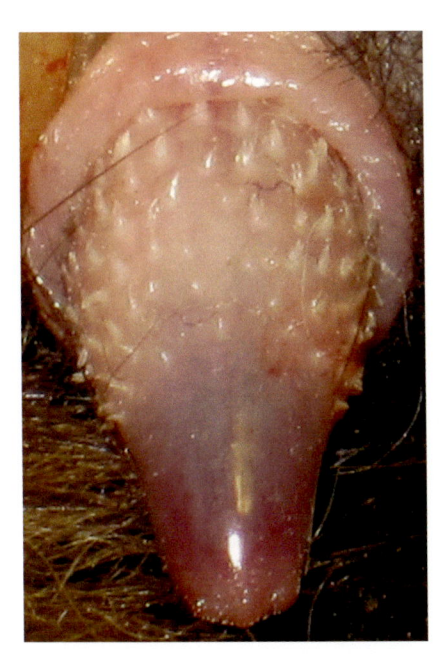

Fig. 2.2. A cat's penis is spiny. (Photo: Owe Gille; https://commons.wikimedia.org/wiki/File:Penisstacheln.jpg, CC BY-SA 3.0, https://creativecommons.org/licenses/by-sa/3.0/deed.en)

by ultrasound or X-ray. By about five weeks into the pregnancy, you will notice that your cat is getting a typical hanging belly. Pregnant cats can be as active as before, and they can catch mice. In the wild, a feral cat will be even more dependent on her hunting skills as her pregnancy proceeds and she needs more food. Only near the end of pregnancy does the queen become less active. She sleeps a lot and may hide away in places where she won't be disturbed.

Maternal Behaviour

Birthing den

When nearing term, the queen will start looking for a suitable place to give birth. She favours a dark and safe place, separate from the activities of people and other animals. It is not uncommon for her to find a place inside a closet, well hidden behind shoes and clothes – or under the duvet, as Bjarne experienced once. This is not so desirable for the cat owner, so it is better to offer her a birthing den that both parties can accept. It should be available a couple of weeks before the expected delivery, as the queen prefers to have this decided in good time.

The birthing den does not need to be a complicated construction, but must be a good hiding-place, well sheltered and with a roof to make it dark and secure. The mother seeks a place that she perceives to be safe from potential predators. Therefore, the opening of the den should be small enough for only the cat to enter, and not larger animals such as dogs. The cat owner can make a simple nest using a cardboard box of about A3 size (about 30 x 40 cm). Cut out a round opening approximately 15 cm in diameter near one end of the long wall and 5 cm up from the floor. Add newspaper to the bottom to capture the birth fluids, and place clean towels on top of the newspapers. Remember to close the lid, which should be set so it can easily be opened without creating a lot of disturbance. Put the box in a quiet place such as a bedroom or spare room where the door is always open. If the queen does not examine the box you offer, try putting it somewhere else. Keep all your cabinet doors and drawers closed if you do not want them to become the chosen nest site!

Behaviour around parturition

During the final days before parturition, the queen's behaviour will change. If she has not yet found a secluded den, she will look for one in all sorts of unthinkable places. She may become more aggressive towards both people and animals with whom she does not feel completely comfortable, especially dogs. But towards people with whom she is socially bonded, she can become more affectionate and social. Through this behaviour, she distances herself from potential threats to her offspring while remaining open to those she trusts who, under natural conditions, are close relatives such as sisters or her own mother.

When the delivery is underway, avoid disturbing the queen. Cats have the instinctive ability to give birth by themselves. Especially if your cat has a nervous disposition, disturbance may interfere with the natural behavioural sequences involved in giving birth. These include cleaning the newborns, biting through the umbilical cords, providing the first milk (colostrum) and bonding with the kittens. It is important that all the kittens get colostrum within the first hours after birth as it is rich in antibodies needed to protect them from disease. Nevertheless, you can quietly monitor the process from some distance, especially if this is the queen's first litter. A few mothers can 'forget' to bite the umbilical cord. While there is no rush for them to do this, if there are many kittens and the cords become tangled, then we may need to provide assistance. It is best to keep young children, dogs, and visitors away from the kittens for the first three weeks. If the mother perceives too much disturbance, she may carry her kittens to a new nest site.

Newborn kittens soon begin to crawl to find the mother's teats. They do not have to move much because the mother lies down beside them to nurse. If they become too scattered, she will gently retrieve them with her mouth. They just need to crawl a bit, and they will soon find the teats. However, if a kitten is very weak after birth and fails to find a teat, we can gently push it onto a teat to stimulate suckling behaviour. If the kitten does not manage to suck or if the mother has too little milk, we can feed it from a pipette and later, a bottle (Fig. 2.3). This must be done carefully; otherwise, we risk the kitten getting milk in its lungs. We must not use regular cow's milk as this is very different from cat's milk. Instead, buy a milk mix specifically made for cats and give the milk slowly. We need to see that the kitten is able to swallow it before giving more.

A queen will cannibalize stillborn kittens and those born very small and weak. It is rare for her to show infanticide towards healthy kittens, but the potential exists if she is highly stressed for some reason. It is safest to keep tomcats away from newborn kittens, as they can occasionally practise infanticide. This is most likely in the case of a non-resident male who is not a father of the kittens. With no kittens to nurse, the queen will return to heat sooner, giving him the chance to father her next litter of kittens.

Nursing period

The queen eats much more than usual in the last part of pregnancy. Her body stores fat for milk production after birth. Normally, the queen will not eat in the first day after giving birth, but after this she will eat a lot. A nursing mother with four kittens will usually eat two-and-a half times more than she did before becoming pregnant. Nevertheless, the nursing period will gradually deplete her body reserves. Studies show that she loses an average of 5–6 grams of bodyweight daily over the course of lactation, depending on the litter size.

The cat mother is active around the clock in the first couple of weeks. The kittens suckle on a regular basis, and the mother takes only brief

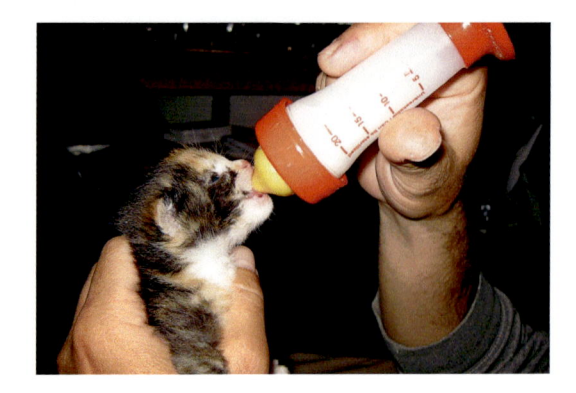

Fig. 2.3. If a mother does not have enough milk, the kittens must be given a specially made milk replacement for cats. (Photo: Linda Iren Jensen, 2019)

breaks to eat, drink and sleep. Already on the first day, nursing can occupy a total of 6–8 hours, and by the end of the first week, it is occupying about 70% of the 24-hour day. While nursing and resting with the kittens, the mother often spends time grooming them. This includes licking the area around the anus and genitals, which stimulates the kittens to eliminate urine and faeces. She consumes the waste that they eliminate. This behaviour, called *coprophagy*, is normal behaviour until the kittens are around 30 days old, helping to keep the kittens and nest clean.

Over the first three weeks, the mother takes the initiative to nurse her kittens by adopting a body posture that gives the kittens easy access to her teats. She mainly lies on her side but, as the kittens grow, she can also nurse in a sitting position. Over the next three weeks, this behaviour gradually declines as she spends more time lying on her belly or sitting in a manner that makes the teats inaccessible. In this way, she controls how much milk the kittens obtain and starts the gentle, slow process of weaning.

It is important to be aware that the kittens suckle eagerly during the first three weeks whether the mother has enough milk or not. Therefore, it is useful to check that the kittens are growing normally. A kitten weighs around 90–120 grams at birth depending on breed and litter size, with kittens in larger litters having lower birthweights than those in smaller litters. The most important thing is that each kitten grows steadily – a weight gain of 10–14 grams per day is typical. A digital kitchen scale with a flat surface, that shows the exact weight, can be used to weigh the kittens individually one or two times a week for the first few weeks. As a rough guide, kittens in litters of three to four weigh about 170 grams after one week, 230 grams at two weeks, 310 grams at three weeks, 400 grams at four weeks, 800 grams at eight weeks, 1200 grams at three months and 1600 grams at four months. However, growth rates vary and kittens in bigger litters tend to grow more slowly. By four months, we can see a clear difference in weight between females and males. While growth rates vary, as long as the kittens are continuing to grow, there is no need to worry. It is also normal for growth to spurt when the kittens begin eating solid food, especially in large litters.

From about three weeks of age, kittens play a more active role in initiating nursing sessions through begging for milk when they are hungry. After six weeks of age, if they don't beg for milk, they will not get any. Usually, kittens do not need milk after two months, but they enjoy suckling if allowed, and it does not harm kittens to continue suckling. The most important thing is that weaning from milk does not occur suddenly. A gradual weaning process leads to a natural end in suckling motivation. If weaning is abrupt, the kittens may remain motivated to suckle throughout life. This can result in a cat sucking on sweaters and other soft fabrics (see Chapter 11).

After the kittens are weaned, production of lactase stops. Lactase is an enzyme that breaks down lactose, the sugar found in milk. If they are later given milk again – for example because the owner gives the cat cow's milk – they may experience stomach pain because they cannot digest the lactose. Therefore, cats usually prefer to drink water after they are weaned from their mother's milk.

In nature, a cat mother will start bringing home mice to her kittens when they are around three-and-a-half weeks old. By then, the kittens are ready to start eating solid food. Cat owners can therefore start providing food for kittens from 3–4 weeks of age. Use wet food in the beginning, as it takes a while before the kittens can eat dry food pellets. When introducing pellets, you can mix them with wet food for the first days or weeks to provide a gradual introduction to pellets.

The queen must be able to get away from her kittens when she wants to. This becomes more important as the kittens grow older, so she can get enough rest. If the mother is not allowed to go outdoors or even leave the room, give her a shelf high enough off the floor so that she can be inaccessible to the kittens. Keep in mind that by two to three months of age, kittens can easily jump half a metre into the air.

Development of the Senses

Kittens are born quite helpless. Their most important tasks during the first three weeks are suckling and sleeping. To find the milk, they only need the senses of touch, smell and taste, and these senses are well developed at birth. They move their head from side to side as they crawl and when they smell milk, they know they are on the right track. If their nose touches a protrusion on the mother's abdomen, which is normally a teat, the kitten puts its mouth over it and begins to suck. The milk tastes good, causing the kitten to continue suckling – it has now learned where to find milk.

In the first few days, kittens cannot hear or see anything. The ear canals are closed and will not open until after about five days. Therefore, the mother cannot attract the kittens with sound even though the kittens miaow to attract her attention. Instead, she responds to the kittens' calls by licking them. The kittens' sense of hearing gradually improves after five days. Once developed, their hearing range is impressive. It extends from about 48 Hz, which we can also hear, to 85 kHz, which is in the ultrasound range and well above what we can hear. Later, when the kittens start to hunt, their large, flexible ears and ability to detect ultrasound will help them to pinpoint mice and other prey that communicate in ultrasound.

The eyes are also closed at birth (Fig. 2.4). After a few days, you can see small slits between the eyelids. The eyes open fully by nine days, on average, but there is great variation. Bjarne studied eye opening in 153 domestic kittens. On average, eye opening started at six-and-a-half days but ranged from one to eleven days. The time until complete eye opening ranged from four to thirteen days. Therefore, you cannot use the time of eye opening as a precise measure of a kitten's age. When Bjarne studied what could cause this big variation, he found that kittens who had a young mother up to two years of age opened their eyes earlier than kittens who had an older mother. Female kittens opened their eyes a little earlier than male kittens. If the cats were kept in a completely dark room, the kittens opened their eyes earlier than if there was bright light in the room. But the biggest effect was genetic; some tomcats had offspring that opened their eyes particularly early. In an Italian study, it was found that kittens of oriental cat breeds opened their eyes at five to six days, on average, while Norwegian forest cats did not have fully open eyes until they were nine to ten days old.

Nevertheless, it is not the case that kittens can see perfectly from nine days of age. The eye lens is present but there are still small blood vessels and connective tissue around the lens. This matrix of nutrient channels is involved in building the lens. Its presence causes kittens to have cloudy vision when the eyes first open, but it gradually disappears by about four weeks of age, after which kittens have clear vision. This is also why kittens appear to have blue eyes initially and their underlying true eye colour is revealed later.

Once their eyes are fully functional, cats are more near-sighted than people, but have much better night vision. This is due to a higher ratio of rods to cones in the retina, as well as the presence of a reflective *tapetum lucidum* behind the retina which causes their eyes to glow in the dark. The kittens' night vision will come in handy for future nocturnal hunting forays, as will their eyes' excellent motion-detecting ability. In the daytime, they can see the difference between blue and yellow-green colours but, like people with red–green colour blindness, cats cannot clearly discriminate red colours.

Behavioural Development

Behaviour during the first three weeks

The cat is a typical *altricial* species, having offspring that are born in an undeveloped state and who stay in the nest for a period after birth, rather than following their mother from day 1, as do the young of sheep and horses. During the first two to three weeks, kittens use their legs as paddles to crawl around. This restricts their movement to the nest area. Gradually, their ability to hold their legs beneath their body improves, allowing them to start walking. From three weeks of age, they can move quickly and efficiently, and they become much more active (Fig. 2.5). A new phase of development emerges, the socialization period.

The socialization period: 3–12 weeks

Play is important

Once the kittens become active, they will try out all kinds of movements – jumps, bounces, somersaults and short sprints. This is obviously fun for the kittens and is also an important part of their development. Through this *locomotory play,* they gradually gain better control of their muscles and develop well-co-ordinated movements. It is amazing how accurate their movements become as they grow up. For example, look at a cat deftly stepping around objects on a shelf without touching them, or elegantly jumping onto a shelf a metre above floor level without jumping a centimetre too high.

As the kittens' movements become stronger and more co-ordinated, their interest in *social play* (play-fighting) increases. People may participate in these games to some extent, but if a kitten becomes too rough, immediately stop playing, turn away and ignore the kitten. We don't want kittens to get in the habit of biting or scratching people. It is better to offer objects that encourage *object play*. All forms of play have a central place in the kitten's behavioural development and are fun for them just as play is fun for us. During play, the brain releases *dopamine*, which is a neurotransmitter secreted in situations when an animal is rewarded or experiences a positive expectation of a later reward (see Chapter 8).

Socialization to cats

Kittens neither experience enjoyment nor thrive if they are isolated from others of their own kind. If kittens are taken from their mother at two weeks of age and live just with people, they will develop emotional disorders. They grow up more aggressive, stubborn and frightened in novel situations. Such kittens are timid towards other cats. If they are taken from their mother and littermates between three and 12 weeks of age, they are also likely to have their psychological development negatively affected. This clearly shows how important it is for kittens to live with other cats during their first few months, and why it is strongly recommended that they stay with their mother and littermates until at least 12 weeks of age.

Just as in dogs, cats have a sensitive period for socialization, meaning that they need to learn basic social skills during this period if they are to behave appropriately in social situations later in life. The socialization period lasts from about three to 12 weeks of age, with social experience in the period between three and seven weeks of age being the most crucial for avoiding behavioural problems in

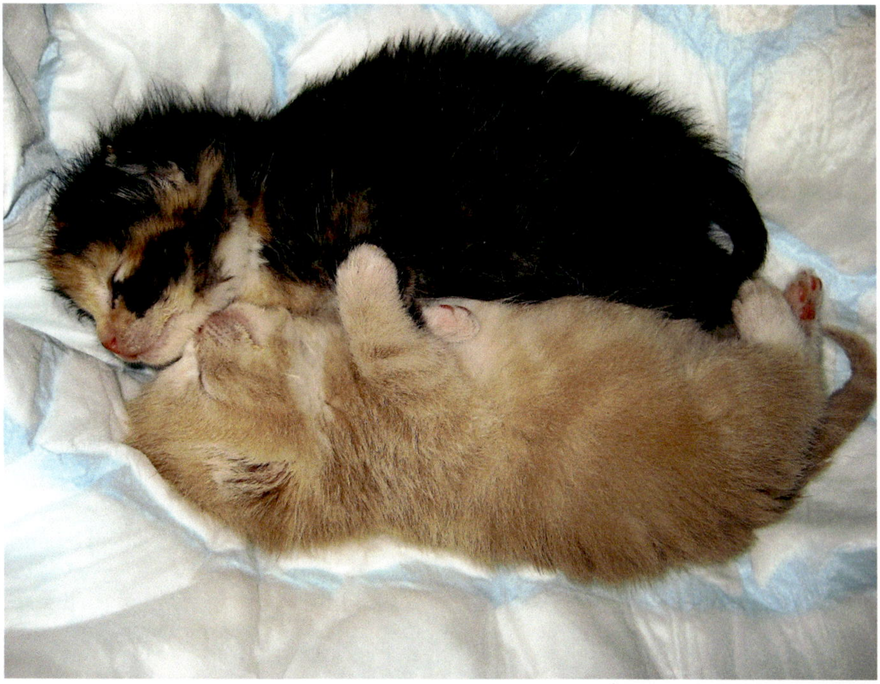

Fig. 2.4. Newborn kittens have closed eyes. (Photo: Linda Iren Jensen, 2019)

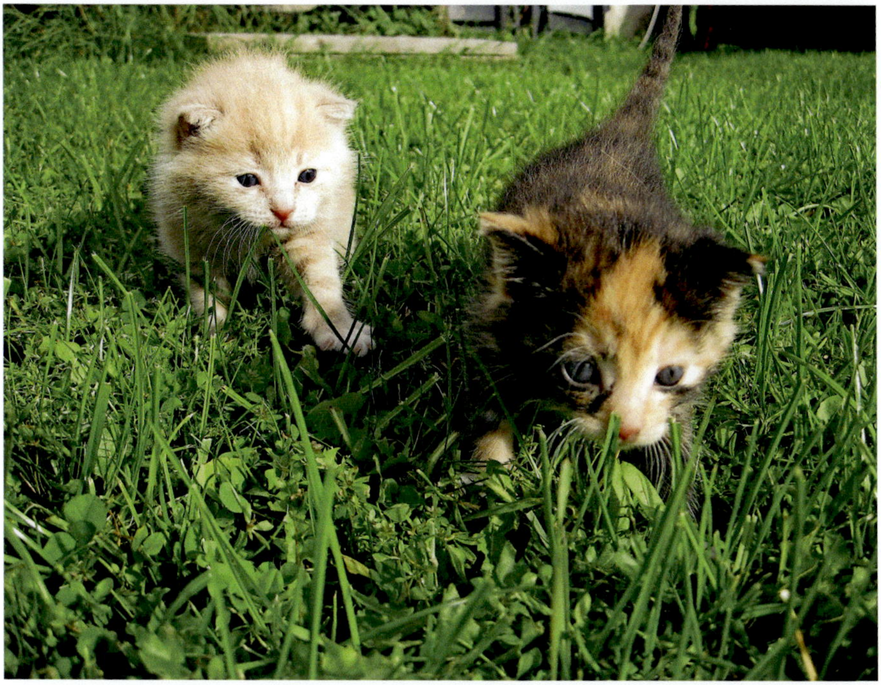

Fig. 2.5. Kittens on a tour of discovery. (Photo: Linda Iren Jensen, 2019)

adulthood. This experience is gained mainly through social play. Kittens begin to play with their mother and siblings at three weeks of age and their social play increases to its highest level between eight and 14 weeks of age. Through social play and general interaction in these weeks, they learn more and more details about cat social behaviour (Fig. 2.6). They become familiar with the characteristics of the different individuals with whom they interact. They learn to use their communication signals in the correct manner and context by finding out how others respond to them. For example, through social play, kittens learn to inhibit the strength of their bites and scratches because if they hurt their play partner, the play partner will not want to continue playing and the fun will stop.

Socialization to people

Socialization is important, not only with other cats but also with people. If kittens have no contact with a range of different people before three months of age, they will remain shy of people and be very difficult to tame later. The cat breeder has a great responsibility in this respect. The kittens must get experience of being lifted from the floor and held by humans. They also need to learn what different people look, sound and smell like, and how they behave. This experience can start from about two weeks of age through brief handling by the breeder. After three weeks of age, additional people can be involved, both in gentle handling and in playful activities.

Socialization activities should be enjoyable for the kittens and not forced, as the important goal is that the kittens learn to be comfortable around people and not afraid of them. We also want them to generalize from the positive experiences they have with known people to unfamiliar people who they will meet in the future. Such learning about people involves familiarization with a diversity of sensory stimuli, movements and activities of different people as well as socialization so the kittens learn to behave appropriately around people. Socialization includes learning to inhibit scratching and biting of people, learning to recognize when people are open to friendly interactions such as play, social grooming and resting together, learning to avoid being accidentally stepped on or bumped into by people, and learning from positively reinforced training exercises conducted by people. You can read more about learning and training of cats in Chapter 10.

Experiments show that the most effective socialization is achieved if the kittens have positive exposure to people for 30–60 minutes each day, especially during the period from three to seven weeks. Contact beyond one hour daily gives no added effect. It is easier to socialize kittens if the mother is present and she shows friendly behaviour

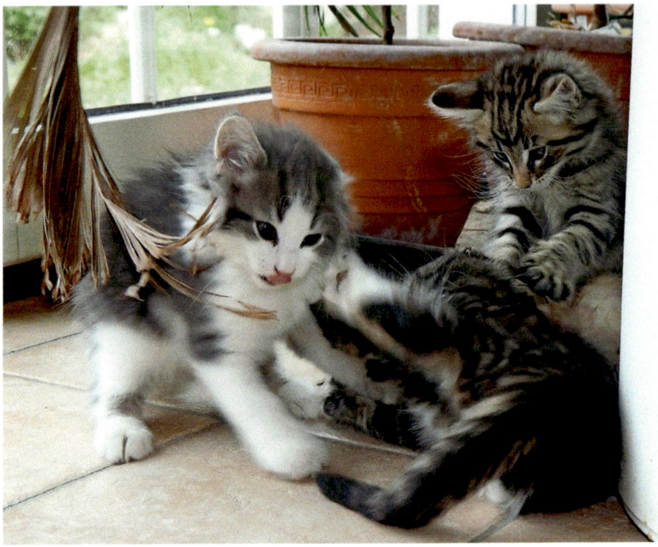

Fig. 2.6. Play-fighting is important for the kittens' social development. (Photo: Maria Myrland, 2019)

towards people. If the mother is not friendly, then it is better to socialize the kittens in a different room, but with all their littermates so they provide social support to each other. Kittens that are well socialized to one person will more quickly accept new people, too. Therefore, their social experience can be gradually expanded over the period from three to 12 weeks, so they get to know different types of people, both women and men, children and adults. The kittens will then get a more general understanding of humans. Many cats that have only ever lived with a woman fear men, particularly when they hear the deeper sound of a man's voice. If you are a single cat breeder, please include people of the opposite sex in your socialization programme. If you do not have children, you can invite neighbours to bring their children to socialize with the kittens. Of course, you can also dress up to change your appearance to look different.

Socialization to dogs

The above guidelines for socialization also apply to different kinds of animals with which we want the kittens to be social as adults, such as dogs. As this is to teach the kittens about dogs, it is important that the right dogs are used so they do not frighten the kittens by barking at them or attempting to chase them. It is safest to restrict this socialization experience to dogs that have themselves been socialized to cats when they were puppies, and are trained to be calm and to look away from the kitten to the owner when asked. Initially, dogs should be on a leash or separated by a fence when introduced to kittens and they must be supervised. If kittens are going to a home that has a dog, it is important that the owners have prepared and planned for the introduction and continue to supervise the relationship as the kitten gets older and more active so all the good work by the breeder is not undone by the kitten being chased by the family dog. They may need to ask a dog trainer or behaviourist for advice (see Chapter 11).

Care should also be taken to avoid introducing diseases to the kittens through exposure to other animals such as cats and dogs from outside the household. Follow your veterinarian's advice regarding vaccinations.

Object play and hunting training

Kittens and many adult cats love running after and catching small, moving objects. Table tennis balls, yarn balls and strings are excellent objects for stimulating object play. Such play occurs from around four weeks of age, but the most active period for object play is from 18–21 weeks. Object play develops hunting skills and is sometimes referred to as predatory play. The kitten learns to intercept the movements of objects and capture them while in motion. For wild-living cats, it is essential that they become competent at this if they are going to eat.

When the kittens are around five weeks old, the mother may bring a live mouse home and drop it in front of the kittens. Their attempts to catch it give them valuable training in catching prey. If the mother is an indoor cat or does not have access to mice where she lives, the kittens will miss out on this early training. This practice in catching prey is continued throughout life, especially when cats are not very hungry. That is why they often do not kill the prey they catch right away but take opportunities to catch and release the same mouse several times. This does not look pleasant to humans (or the mouse), but it is important, if the cat will have to be dependent on catching live prey for its survival.

Object play is the play best suited for people to participate in (Fig. 2.7). Be sure to have appropriate objects, small enough for the cat to move and lift easily. The simplest things we can use are a table tennis ball or the traditional string with a piece of paper or cardboard tied to the end. When you move the string near the cat, be patient. Do not expect the cat to run after it immediately. As we shall see in Chapter 6 on hunting behaviour, cats often prefer to lie in ambush until they suddenly pounce with lightning speed. Part of the fun of play is the surprise element, which you can contribute to by moving objects suddenly in different directions. A string by itself is also an attractive play item. Cats have an instinctive urge to catch long, narrow objects. In nature, they could be small snakes, which cats can be highly skilled at catching, the instinctive urge perhaps being evolved to kill a predator that may be a threat to their kittens.

When can kittens go to new owners?

To ensure that kittens learn what they need to learn about social behaviour, you should not take them away from their mother and littermates until they are at least 12 weeks old. It is a legal requirement in some countries (e.g. Norway) not to separate kittens before 12 weeks of age, and it is also a requirement of some pedigree cat clubs. The FIFe

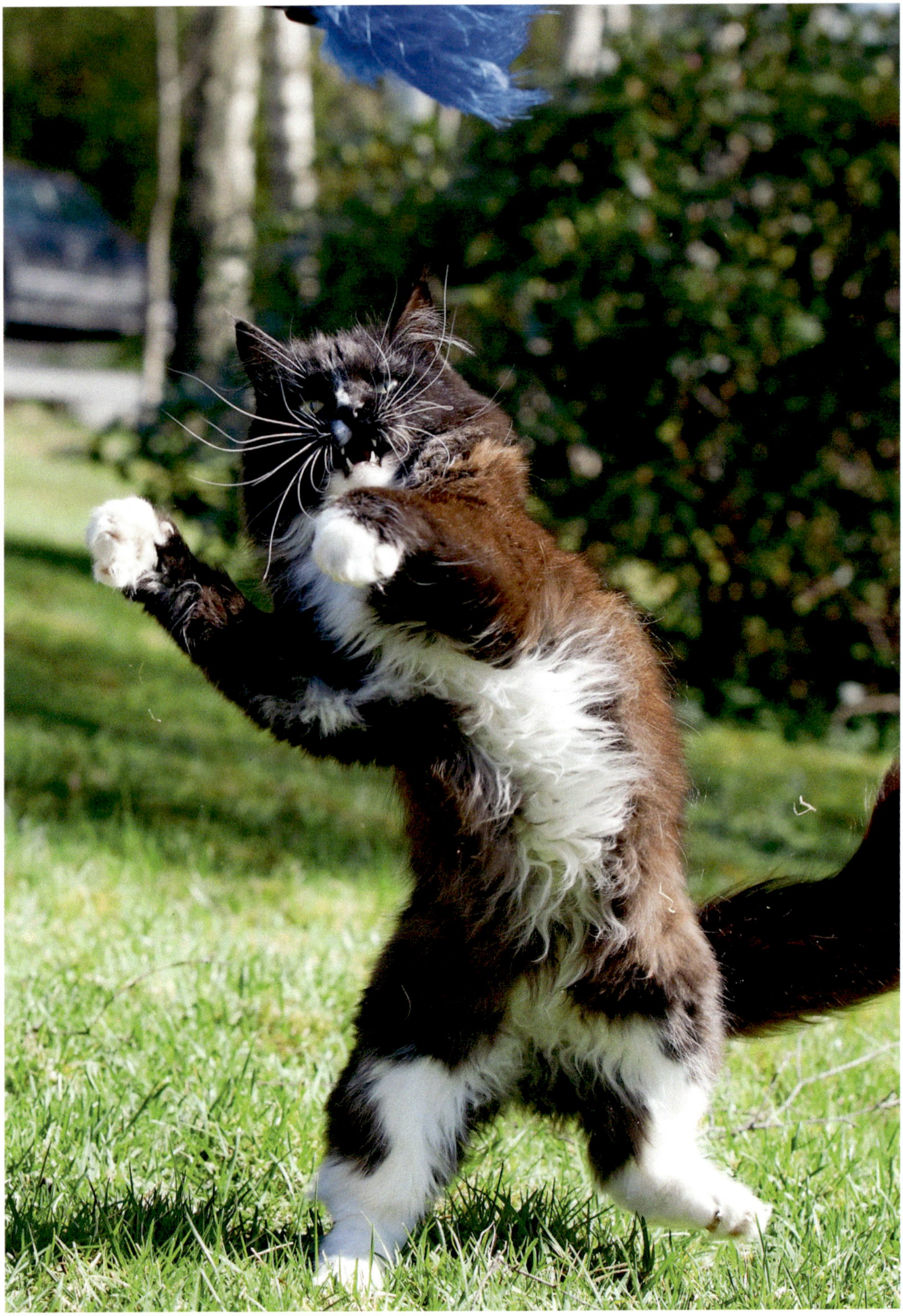

Fig. 2.7. Object play with a feather stick can give cats good hunt training. (Photo: Audun Braastad, 2019)

(Fédération Internationale Féline, an international cat fancier society covering 39 countries) has decided to extend this to 14 weeks, effective from 2023. Remember that the third month of life is the peak period for social play between kittens. It is a great advantage if the new owners can make some visits to develop familiarity with a kitten before it comes home with them. This will make the transition to the new home less alarming for the kitten. Some breeds, such as the oriental breeds, may develop more slowly than others, and many cat experts suggest kittens of these breeds should wait until they are 14 weeks old before they are sold. Also, consider the development of the individual kitten. If growing more slowly than average, you may wish to wait a few more weeks. A recent large survey in Finland shows that kittens transferred to new owners at eight weeks of age are more likely to show aggression towards people and cats as well as other behavioural problems. The fewest behaviour problems were reported in kittens that moved to their new home after 14 weeks of age.

New Home from 12 Weeks of Age – How to Achieve a Good Start

Choosing a kitten – the choir of choice

There is little gender difference in behavioural development before the kittens reach 12–16 weeks. From around 12 weeks, one can observe that male kittens play somewhat more actively than females. Therefore, potential owners who come to inspect a three- to four-month-old litter are easily attracted to male kittens when comparing the littermates. But you should not just note the activity level; think about what kind of relationship you would like to have with the cat. If you want a pet, choose a kitten that comes to you and does not object to being picked up and petted. An active male cat may become too independent, but at the same time may be fun to play with. Be somewhat sceptical about the smallest kitten in the litter. Is it completely healthy? If the eyes show secretions, it may indicate an eye infection or, in some Persian cats, improperly formed tear ducts. Is the kitten shy of its littermates? If you want just one indoor cat, this kitten can still be a good choice. If there are dominant cats in your neighbourhood, or you already have another cat, you could be more sceptical about this kitten.

If you are unsure how a new kitten will adapt to your cats at home, you may ask the breeder if you can try it out for a couple of weeks with return rights. During these weeks, you will get a good indication of whether the cats will get along, although they will hardly become best friends in only two weeks. Some breeders agree to such a test arrangement, as they really want their kittens to thrive well in their new home, while others are unwilling due to concerns about introducing diseases to their cattery with a returned kitten.

Knowledge is required

To ensure the proper care of cats, new cat owners are obliged to acquire the knowledge needed to understand their needs. The official owner should be at least 16 years old and have the maturity and competence to be responsible for the cat. Feel free to give children co-responsibility, but parents should not delegate the main responsibility for the animal to a child. This book aims to give you the necessary knowledge to be a responsible cat owner.

Cat breeders, or anyone else who sells or gives away a cat, are responsible for ensuring that the new owner has the necessary information to take care of the cat. This includes telling you about the food the cat is used to, what kind of cat toilet and cat litter it uses, typical places where it is used to finding water, any health issues of the cat or its parents, the vaccinations and medications it has received, and particular aspects of the cat's personality and history you should know about. If the cat has been exposed to any unusual situations, new owners should be told about them as this information can provide an important background for understanding behavioural problems that may occur later on. If you receive no such information, ask for it. Ideally, all animals would come with a manual, like the technical equipment you purchase. The new owner must at least note the address, telephone number and e-mail address of the person supplying the cat and be able to contact him or her if any questions arise, especially if they may be related to the previous experience of the cat.

Be sure to meet the cat in its current residence before buying it, and look at the conditions in which it has been kept. Avoid buying a cat without directly seeing where it has been living. Beware of 'cheap' purebred cats – get them only from reputable breeders.

Anyone selling or giving away a cat must be able to assess potential owners and check that they have the necessary knowledge, attitude and time to look after a cat, and provide them with appropriate advice. If you

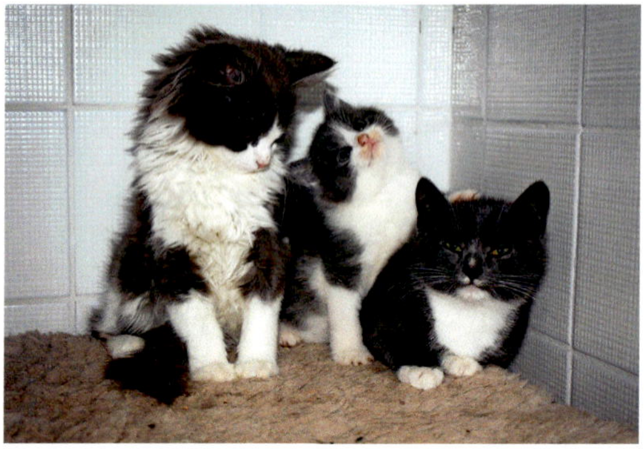

Fig. 2.8. Kittens should stay with their mother and littermates until they are at least 12 weeks old. (Photo: Janne Helen Lorentzsen, 2019)

are in doubt as to whether your cat will do well in its new home, find someone else to be the new owner.

Vaccination, ID marking and neutering

When a kitten is sold or given away at three months of age, it should have already been vaccinated for the first time and labelled with a microchip for identification. Cats should be given vaccines according to recommendations of the veterinary authorities in your home country. The most critical ones give protection against feline distemper (feline panleukopenia virus), feline viral rhinotracheitis or cat flu (feline herpesvirus 1), feline calicivirus, and rabies, but there are several others that could also be relevant. A new owner must, of course, receive a certificate of vaccination and proof that the kitten is ID-marked. They must also follow up with booster shots and regular re-vaccinations. Cats are usually quite healthy animals, but your cat may suddenly catch a serious infection. Cat distemper is common and is highly contagious. The owner can bring an infection from outside to indoor cats, so no cat is safe without vaccination.

Some veterinarians propose six months or a bodyweight of 2.5 kg as a general rule for the age to neuter or spay a kitten. Other veterinarians recommend that this be done earlier, at three to four months of age, to avoid unwanted kittens. There appear to be no medical or physiological arguments that speak against this. It is currently unclear whether early neutering weakens a cat's ability to cope with social competition from other cats or increases the risk of behaviour problems.

At the new home

When you are ready to bring a new kitten home, it can be a good idea to bring the carrying basket from your home and leave it in the room with the kitten overnight or for a few hours on the day of collection so that the kitten can start getting used to new smells from your house while still in a familiar place. You can also wipe a cloth or towel over the kitten's mother or let her rest on one that you then place in the carrying basket so you can bring home her familiar scent.

Once you have brought your new kitten home, open the carrying basket but leave it in the room as a safe retreat for several days, after which it can be gradually moved to its final location where it will remain as one of the cat's resting places (Chapters 10 and 11). Allow the kitten to decide when to come out of the carrying basket – do not force it. Let it sniff and check all the nooks and crannies in any rooms it is allowed into. The kitten will not feel safe until it becomes familiar with all parts of its new home. It must learn where it can sleep, where to find food and water, where the cat toilet is and, not least, possible hiding-places. If the kitten is scared of something, it must know immediately to where it can run and hide. Make sure it cannot get outdoors. In a big house, restricting the kitten to one or two rooms initially will help it to establish a home base. Along with the carrying basket, you may provide a cardboard box as an extra hiding-place. Give the kitten the same type of food and cat litter that it is used to. After a few days, you can allow access to additional rooms, perhaps one at a time.

As important as getting to know the new home is getting to know individuals with whom the kitten will have social contact, both people and other animals. This must be done in a gentle, unforced manner. Do not chase after the kitten trying to catch it, and be careful that children do not do so. Make contact in the kitten's premises and at the kitten's pace – you need to work in 'kitten time'.

Sit down on the floor and wait for the kitten to come to you, but have great patience. The kitten will come only when it feels safe. How long this takes can vary enormously, depending on the personality of the cat, hereditary characteristics and past experiences with strangers. If you have already been visiting the kitten before bringing it home, you have made a good start, but remember that this occurred in the kitten's home environment and probably in the presence of the mother and littermates.

Now everything is new, and some adjustment time is needed.

Keep other animals in the household, both cats and dogs, at a good distance in the beginning. The best thing is to let the new kitten get to know its new home well before it starts meeting other animals; then it will feel safer when it meets them, as it already knows where to find hiding-places and there is less risk that the kitten will panic. Be present in the room when the animals meet for the first few times. Be careful not to allow older cats to attack the new arrival. At the same time, avoid jealousy; give your older cats plenty of play and petting. They must not get the impression that you will replace them with the new cat. If they regard the new one as an intruder who will compete with them for resources, the relationship between the cats can be difficult for a long time. Give all the cats food at the same time, but in individual food bowls placed a good distance apart. It is a good idea to give the kitten its own litter tray, as it may be afraid to enter one that smells of unfamiliar cats.

Once your kitten has become familiar with its new home, you can start some basic training (see Chapter 10). One of the first things to teach the kitten is for it to come to you when you give it a specific signal such as a whistle or calling its name. When it comes to you, reward it with a treat or gentle stroking. It is also useful to train the kitten to walk on a leash.

Many owners will keep their cat indoors, or give them access to a safe, enclosed outdoor area, a catio. Others will want to take their cat out for walks on a leash or let it roam the neighbourhood. There are advantages and disadvantages to both these choices (see Chapter 11).

A new cat must not be let outdoors before it is familiar with its new home – this may take two to three weeks. It must also have been well socialized to people. This is equally important whether the new cat is a kitten or an adult cat. Nevertheless, a kitten should not go outdoors until it is four to five months old and is fully vaccinated. You must wait longer if there is a lot of traffic or other hazards where you live.

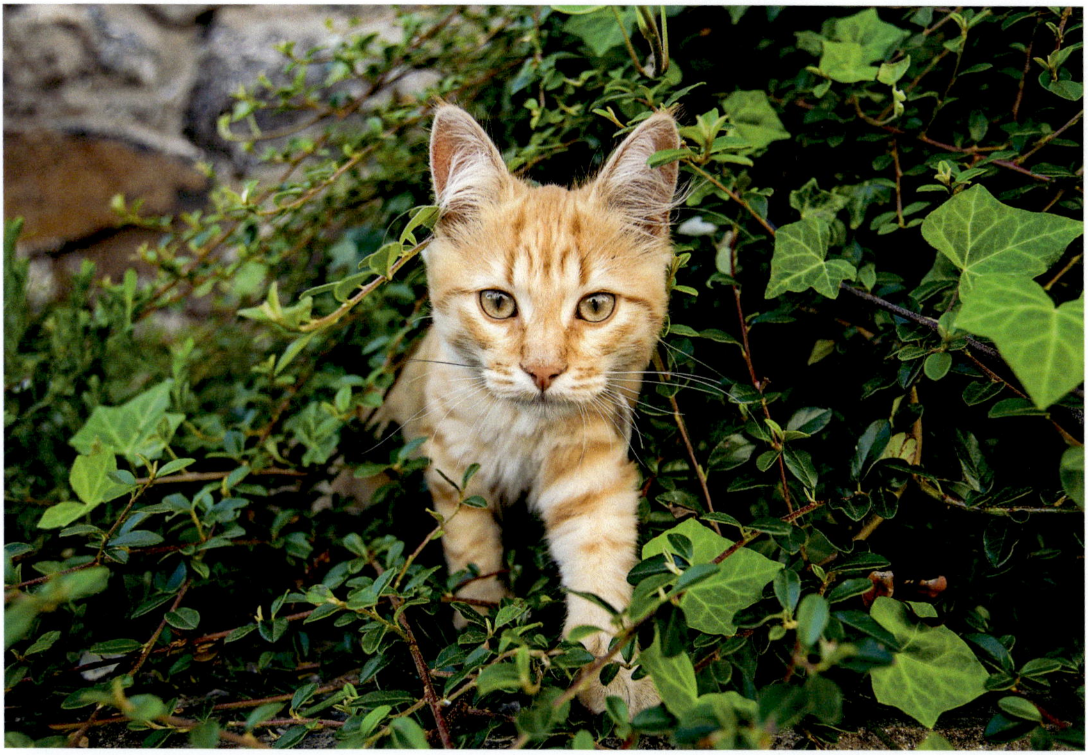

Fig. 2.9. After the kitten has become well acquainted indoors, it can be released and gradually gain more outdoor experience. (Photo: Audun Braastad, 2019)

The first few times the new cat goes out, you must go out with it. If you have trained the cat to walk on a leash, you can easily take it out and go for a walk around the house or in the garden (see below for a link to a short video clip showing Ruth's kitten making an early foray on a leash). Otherwise, stay outside the house and let the cat see you while it gradually inspects the surroundings and gets familiar with them (Fig. 2.9). Then the cat learns that the area around the house is your territory, and eventually it will consider this as its own territory, too. If possible, leave a door open so the cat knows that it can escape indoors if it is scared by something. Give your call signal a few times while the cat is outdoors, so it learns where the door is and knows that it is welcome indoors.

The sense of place does not come by itself. The cat will develop good orientation ability as it becomes more familiar with the area and walks further away from home, and then finds its way home again. Therefore, you can gradually give the cat greater freedom, but be sure to stay close by in the beginning so the cat can come in whenever it wants to. Look and listen so you know when it wants to come in, or signal for it to come home if it is getting late. If you have a cat flap in a door, you can now teach the cat to use it. This training should also be done gradually. First, teach the cat to go through the cat flap with the flap taped open. When the cat easily enters through the hatch, close it almost completely and let the cat learn to push the flap up with its head. Once this has been learned, you can close the flap completely. You can read more about the cat's orientation and navigation capabilities in Chapter 7.

When the cat is fully familiar with coming and going and wants to be out for extended periods of the day, it can be out alone during the day while you are at work. Then it will soon learn that you usually come home at a certain time and will be ready to enter the house with you when you arrive home. That does not mean that the cat has been waiting for you all day; cats quickly learn regular routines and while you are at work, the cat is on reconnaissance trips, hunting or resting under a bush. If you approach this stage gradually, the cat will feel secure while learning to master new challenges outdoors.

Further Reading

Ahola, M.K., Vapalahti, K. and Lohi, H. (2017) Early weaning increases aggression and stereotypic behaviour in cats. *Scientific Reports* 7, 10412. DOI: 10.1038/s41598-017-11173-5.

Braastad, B.O. and Heggelund, P. (1984) Eye-opening in kittens: effects of light and some biological factors. *Developmental Psychobiology* 17, 675–681.

Casey, R.A. and Bradshaw, J.W.S. (2008) The effects of additional socialization for kittens in a rescue centre on their behaviour and suitability as a pet. *Applied Animal Behaviour Science* 114, 196–205.

Little, S.E. (2012) Female reproduction. *The Cat*, 1195–1227. DOI: 10.1016/B978-1-4377-0660-4.00040-5.

Seitz, P.F.D. (1959) Infantile experience and adult behaviour in animal subjects. II. Age of separation from the mother and adult behaviour in the cat. *Psychosomatic Medicine* 21, 353–378.

Supplementary materials entitled 'The kitten's senses', 'Birth and the kitten-mother relationship', 'The kitten's development from 3 to 12 weeks of age' and 'The kitten's first period in its new home' can be accessed at: www.cabi.org/the-cat-behaviour-and-welfare/

Video

Ruth's kitten explores the garden on a leash.

video.cabi.org/KSSTW

3 The Cat's Personality – Individual Variation and Breed Characteristics

Experienced cat owners know very well that you will not find two cats with exactly the same personality or behavioural traits. Cats can be as different as people, and this is one reason why cats are so fascinating. Some characteristics may change with age and there may be gender-based differences in behaviour. There are also marked differences in typical behaviour between cat breeds. As with other animals, and people, cats develop different individual characteristics due to their inheritance (genes), environment and personal experiences. This chapter looks at various factors that lead to the individual characteristics of cats.

What Is the Typical Behaviour of Cats?

In 2014, a survey of cat behaviour was conducted by Silja Eriksen for her Master's thesis in ethology (animal behaviour) at the Norwegian University of Life Sciences. Cat owners answered 99 questions about the behaviour of their cats (the Fe-BARQ survey). The owners scored their cat on a scale from 1 (never occurs) to 5 (always occurs) for each question. Results were received on 1204 cats and the answers were grouped into 22 more general traits.

From the results, we can conclude that most of the cats were quite sociable towards people, seeking contact and vocalizing to attract attention. They were moderately active and playful, and liked to hunt for prey if the opportunity arose, but also rested and slept a lot, as expected for carnivores. Most cats were considered easy to train. They learned to come when called, though did not always do so when motivated to do something else. Some cats had separation problems that were apparent when the owner was getting ready to go out, but few cats had toileting or other behavioural problems. Aggression towards unfamiliar people, or dogs and cats in the household, was quite rare. Aggression when touched or being held was not common if the cat and owner had a good social bond. The graphs in Fig. 3.1 show the response distribution for these behavioural traits. You can see what was typical across the cats in general, but at the same time note that there were big differences between individuals.

Differences in Personality

If two cats show consistent, long-lasting individual differences of behaviour, they can be said to differ in personality. Certain traits tend to occur together, allowing them to be grouped into major personality types. In Austria, the behavioural scientist Kurt Kotrschal and his colleagues have described four main personality axes in domestic cats: active/playful; anxious; sociable; and feeding style. The latter concerns whether the cat shows gluttony, which is most common in male cats, or carefully examines its food before deciding whether it is safe to eat, which is more typical of females. Another typical personality difference is whether a cat is calm, not showing much response to things around it, or alert, quickly exploring new things in the environment and paying close attention to what other cats are doing. You can also talk about personality types like *nervous*, *aggressive* and *self-confident*. All cats will be somewhere on a scale for each of these personality types, from very low to very high.

The owner's personality affects their cat

Kotrschal and colleagues have also investigated the relationship between the personality of the cat and the personality of the owner, measured across the five domains of human personality (see Chapter 12). *Neurotic* owners have intense social interactions with their cats. They often kiss their cats and are typically very particular about the type of food they give. At the same time, they tend to engage in less object play with their cats compared to more *extrovert* owners. For neurotic owners, the cat is important to them for social support. Cat owners

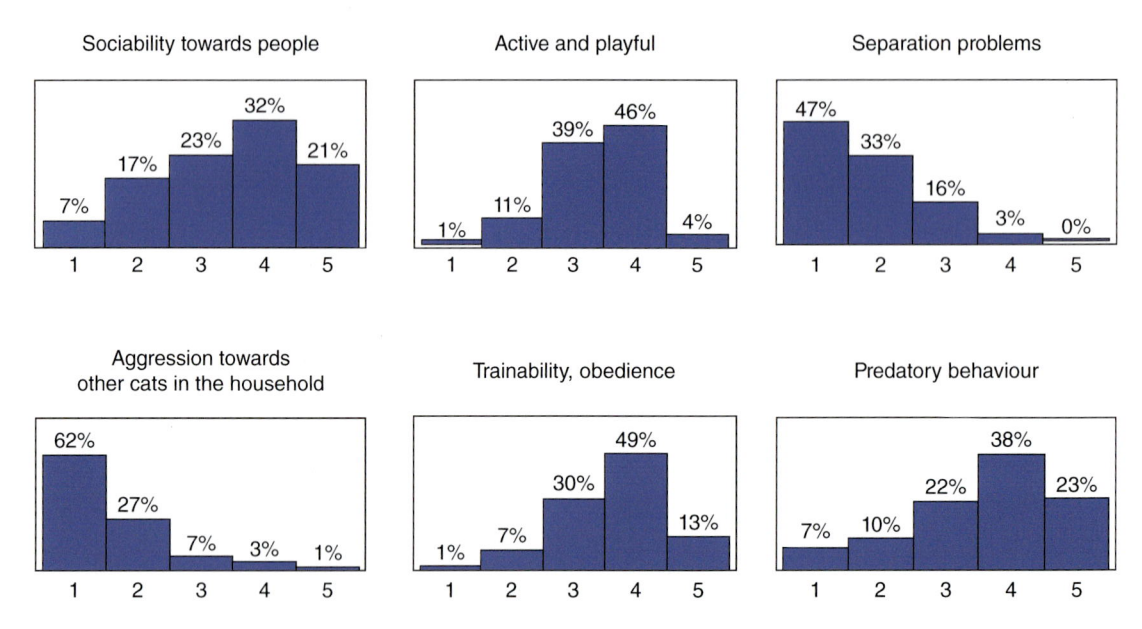

Fig. 3.1. Individual variation in the occurrence of six behavioural traits in 1204 Norwegian cats. 1: Never, 2: Seldom, 3: Now and then, 4: Often, 5: Always. (From Silja C.B. Eriksen, 2014)

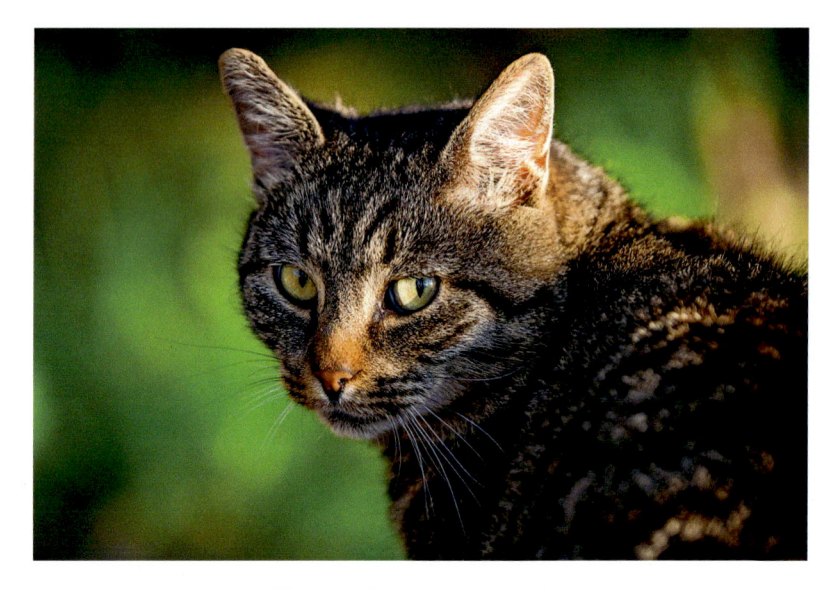

Fig. 3.2. Each cat has its own personality. (Photo: Audun Braastad, 2019)

who score high on *openness* participate in more object play with their cat. Their cats tend to have lower levels of fear and tension. They are also likely to be more self-confident and to spend less time exploring new things before deciding if they are safe. To cat owners scoring high on openness, the cat is also a source of social support, especially in the role of a playmate.

Age Differences

Some behaviour traits tend to increase or decrease with age. Older and geriatric cats may become more aggressive towards other cats in the household, and miaow more to obtain something from the owner. They can become less interactive and show more reluctance to be held. They can also become generally less active and playful, less social towards people and unfamiliar cats, and catch less prey.

Old cats may get dementia

Older cats do not generally have more behavioural problems than younger cats, but when they reach 12–15 years of age, some may develop new problems; they may nag their owner more about something, wake up the owner more frequently at night, show anxiety, or start urinating or defecating outside the litterbox. Some may also become disoriented, wander off, stare straight ahead or become more restless. They may show repetition of a behaviour, termed a *behavioural stereotypy*.

Many such behavioural problems can be due to physical illness. Arthritis gives a stiff gait, and the cat typically becomes cautious when jumping from heights due to aching joints. Toileting problems may be due to urinary tract disorders or finding it difficult to get into the litter tray. Other problems may be due to diabetes, cardiovascular disease, high blood pressure or impaired vision or hearing. If your cat suddenly changes its behaviour, take it to the vet for a health check (see Chapter 11).

Several behavioural changes may be associated with *cognitive impairment*. Cats and dogs can develop dementia, similar to Alzheimer's disease in humans. The same changes can occur in the brain, with disturbed nerve function and, eventually, shrinking of the cerebral cortex. Gary Landsberg from Canada has found signs of cognitive impairment in 28% of cats aged 11–14 and 50% of cats over 15 years of age. If the vet can rule out other illnesses or injuries, or an unsuitable environment, dementia may be the cause. On the other hand, old cats may have dementia along with other health conditions.

How can we prevent dementia? Today, there is no effective medicine against dementia, although some preparations may slow down its progress. Instead, we must try to prevent cognitive impairment and dementia through providing mental stimulation and environmental enrichment throughout the cat's life, even when elderly. Give your cat tasks that stimulate the intellect. There are cat puzzles and feeders where the cat has to work to get toys or dry pellets. Engage your cat in object play to stimulate the senses and encourage movement. This is particularly important for indoor cats. If you suspect that your cat has dementia, avoid big changes. Introduce one new thing at a time. The cat may become stressed if exposed to novel objects or situations too frequently.

Sex Differences

At 12–16 weeks of age, male kittens become more active than female kittens. In adult cats, apart from behaviour associated with mating and reproduction, the clearest sex difference found in the study by Eriksen was in sociability towards unfamiliar cats. Here the males scored higher than the females. On average, males also sought more attention and purred more when in contact with their owner, whereas females were more reluctant to be held. This may be part of the reason why people tend to develop a stronger social bond with male than female cats (see Chapter 12). Female cats were more likely to show aggression towards other cats in the household and had a clearer preference for specific rest areas.

Genes and Behaviour

People sometimes ask whether a particular type of behaviour is determined by inheritance or environment. In practice, it is invariably both. All behaviours have a certain genetic basis and are influenced by the conditions in which the cat lives. The genes make it possible for the brain to control the muscles and hormones so a certain behaviour can be performed. Genes also vary in their activity over time and influence the sequence of changes in behaviour as a kitten matures. However, when responding to particular stimuli, the cat's current needs and learning from past experiences influence decisions about when and where to perform particular behaviour patterns. Experience tells the cat in which situations it is wise to perform a certain behaviour.

Some behaviour patterns are strongly influenced by genes, such as how the cat eats, drinks and grooms, and how it mates, gives birth and nurses offspring. There is little individual variation in how cats perform these behaviours. Most other behaviour patterns show pronounced individual differences between cats. These differences are more influenced by specific environmental conditions or experiences. Environmental conditions during the mother's pregnancy can even affect kittens before they are born by altering the expression of their genes. Variation between individuals in the way they are affected by the environment explains why cloned cats with identical genes will not grow up behaving exactly the same way.

In England, Sandra McCune found that the cats that were most friendly to people were more likely to have a father with the same trait, even though they never had contact with their father. This shows that this trait is related to a specific genetic make-up. Cats with fathers that were more sociable towards people were also less reluctant to explore novel objects. Such studies indicate that there is a relationship between the cat's confidence or boldness and its inclination to be sociable. Socializing involves some risk, and more timid cats usually prefer to be alone.

Several interesting studies indicate that the cat's hair colour is related to its behaviour. This is linked to the genes behind the different colour pigments, which also affect the production of hormones affecting behaviour. Black cats tend to be tolerant of other cats whereas cats that have the red/orange gene variant, such as orange, cream-coloured and tortoiseshell cats, may show a more offensive attitude. These cats are more likely to be aggressive than black cats and may struggle to escape if handled by strangers. In Italy, the ethologist Eugenia Natoli and her co-workers have investigated how cats with different coat colours behave during the mating season. Where there is a high population density of cats, such as in Rome, black males are more successful in obtaining copulations with females than are orange males. While the orange males spend time arguing with each other, the black males are busy courting and mating the females. In rural areas, on the other hand, where cats are spread further apart, an orange male can focus on keeping black ones away from females in heat. This can explain why black cats are more common in places with a high cat population. An aggressive attitude places the orange males at a disadvantage, so they father fewer offspring and orange males become rarer. However, this behavioural difference between orange and black cats is not pronounced and has not been found in all studies (Fig. 3.3).

A relationship between colour and aggression is not only found in cats; something similar is seen when comparing red cocker spaniels with black and other spaniel colour variants, and when comparing farmed salmon with many pigment spots to those with few. An old myth says that red-haired Scottish people are particularly aggressive. Anyway, such tendencies may show up only when we observe many individuals. Orange cats are not always aggressive; many are very pleasant cats, including famous ones such as the streetcat Bob, in England; the library cat Dewey, who lived in Iowa, USA; the tomcat Bolle, in Lübeck, Germany; and the Norwegian cats Jesperpus, famous for accompanying his owner on cross-country skiing tours, and

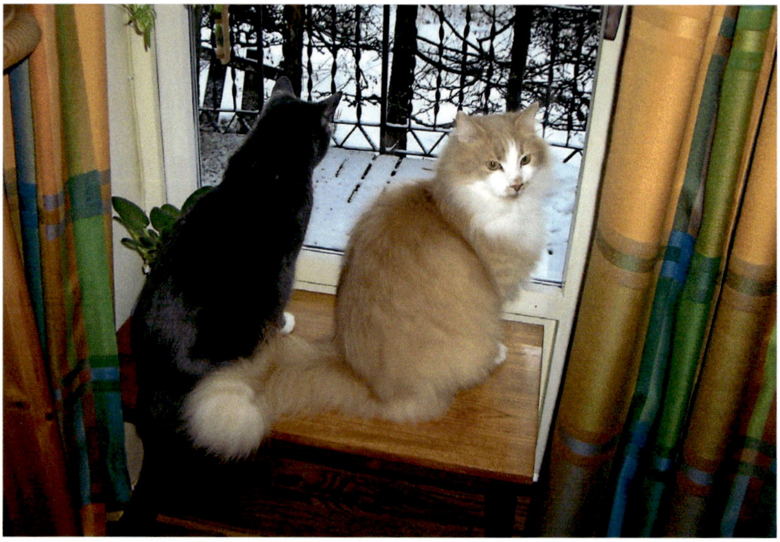

Fig. 3.3. Orange cats tend to be more aggressive than black cats, though this does not apply to all. (Photo: Leif Aslaksen, 2019)

Pusur, a Facebook favourite. There might be a connection here. These famous cats are obviously very self-confident. This self-confidence may form the basis for the competitive ability of orange males in social contests.

Inheritance of behavioural traits

In another Master's thesis from the Norwegian University of Life Sciences, Ingrid Westbye examined hereditary differences in behavioural traits among Siamese and Persian cats. She examined the effect of paternity by having 20 males of each breed each father five litters. The highest heritability was found for the degree of activity and playfulness. The cat's tendency to approach unfamiliar adults or children visiting the family also had high heritability. Among behavioural problems, Westbye found the highest heritability for anxiety or fearfulness when exposed to loud sounds or unfamiliar people. These results are probably applicable to other cat breeds.

Behavioural traits that are desirable for the cat owner and improve the cat's welfare must be considered when selecting breeding males and females. This will have positive ripple-down effects. Behavioural problems will diminish, and cat owners will be more pleased with the behaviour of their cat. The behaviour will also be more in line with owner expectations.

The international breed standards for cats should also consider cat behaviour. The standards should encourage the selection of cats with lower fearfulness of people and novel environments, higher sociability towards unfamiliar people, and lower likelihood of aggressive behaviour. The latter has already been achieved to some extent, as judges at cat shows may refuse to judge aggressive cats. Because both parents contribute to the temperament of their offspring, cat breeders must carefully consider the behaviour of both males and females to be used as breeding animals.

Breed Differences in Behaviour

In her Master's research, Westbye also described behavioural differences between Siamese and Persian cats and non-pedigree house cats. She found several consistent differences in behaviour between them which are summarized here, but keep in mind that there is marked individual variation within each breed.

The Persian cats were calm, showing little fear or anxiety towards unfamiliar people or when hearing loud sounds (Fig. 3.4). Aggressiveness towards people and other cats was rare, and Persians rarely engaged in social conflicts with other animals in the household. Persians often approached familiar and unfamiliar people, though not as frequently as the Siamese cats.

Cats of the Siamese breed were active and outgoing (Fig. 3.5). They frequently approached both adults

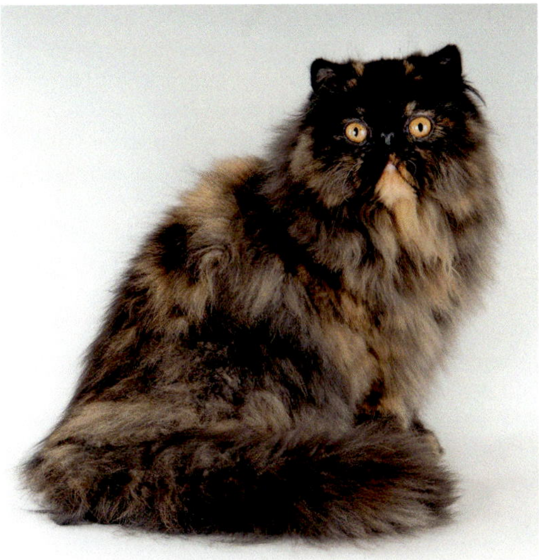

Fig. 3.4. Tortoiseshell Persian cat. (Photo: Maria Myrland, 2019)

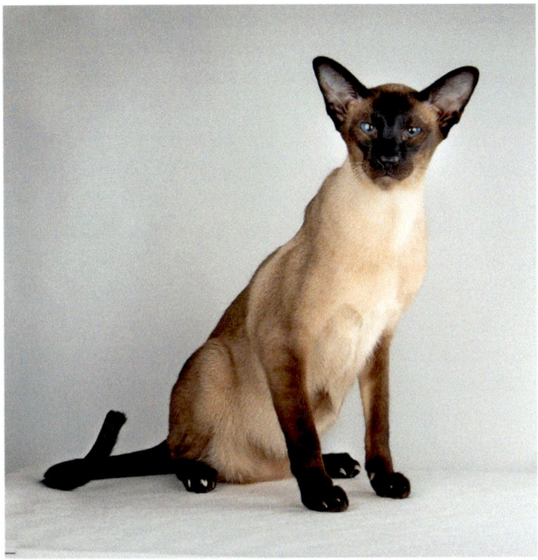

Fig. 3.5. Sealpoint Siamese cat. (Photo: Maria Myrland, 2019)

and children, and they showed little fear or anxiety towards unfamiliar people. They vocalized often when communicating with their owner, greeted the owner often, and frequently visited the owner's lap to be stroked or to rest for extended periods. On the other hand, if there were other animals in the household, they could have social conflicts with them – the Siamese cats demanded attention by their owner and would rather have the owner all to themselves. The Siamese could be somewhat more difficult to housetrain; they were more prone to urinate outside the litterbox than house cats, and they did the most frequent urine marking.

Of the three breed types, the non-pedigree house cats were most likely to go outside when allowed to and roamed the most widely. They were the most likely to encounter other cats in the neighbourhood, which could trigger aggression and social conflicts. They were also the most likely to show aggression towards other animals in the household. They showed the most fear or anxiety towards other cats, loud noises and unfamiliar people, and were the most reluctant to approach unfamiliar adults and children. Their tendency to be more fearful also increased the risk of aggressive scratching and biting. Overall, as might be expected, their behaviour was more reminiscent of that of wild ancestral cats.

In Italy, scientists compared behavioural development of the Norwegian forest cat with the oriental breeds (mainly the Oriental and Siamese). When kittens were placed in an unfamiliar environment, the kittens of oriental breeds were more passive and had a higher heart rate than the forest cats, who were more eager to explore the new surroundings (Fig. 3.6).

In her Master's study, Eriksen used the owner reports to examine differences in the behaviour of the most common breeds found in Norway. Table 3.1 shows which breeds scored the highest and the lowest for each of 13 important behavioural traits. As can be seen, the Burmese was ranked the most sociable and contact-seeking, while the Persian, Norwegian forest cat and Egyptian mau were the most sociable towards unfamiliar cats. The most active and playful breeds were the Bengal, Abyssinian, Oriental, Burmese and Siamese. The Abyssinian ranked highest for aggressiveness, whether towards other cats in the household or unfamiliar people. The Bengal showed the most separation problems and the most fear of novelty, probably because this is a new breed formed by crossing domestic cats with a wild species, the mainland leopard cat, for whom being cautious of novelty is an important survival trait. Scores from an American survey by Benjamin Hart suggest that American Bengal cats may exhibit a wilder nature than those found in Norway, possibly due to strong selection for tameness by Norwegian breeders.

Although Eriksen's survey indicated statistically significant breed differences, the differences were not dramatically large. Is your pedigree cat unlike the breed averages shown in the table? It may well be so, as there is great individual variation within each breed. Therefore, when picking a kitten, watch the behaviour of each kitten in the litter closely. Find one that you think will suit you and your lifestyle. Do you prefer an active, independent cat, or a highly social cat that wants to stay near you? In Figs 3.7 and 3.8 you can see how the most common breeds varied in sociability towards people and in activity/playfulness, with scores from 1 (never) to 5 (always).

On average, the non-pedigree house cats were more reluctant than the pedigree cats to be held by people, and they were more likely to exhibit fearfulness towards unfamiliar cats and dogs. Several studies indicate that these cats, which are more often allowed outdoors than are pedigree cats, may be stressed by things that happen when roaming outdoors and bring some of this stress into the house, resulting in some behavioural problems.

Intensive cat breeding has not been practised for long (only about 60–150 years for many breeds), and it has been directed to selecting for different physical looks rather than behavioural traits. Breed differences in behaviour are likely to increase as systematic selective breeding continues across many generations. Pedigree cat breeders have a responsibility to contribute to the selection of more healthy cats in terms of both physical and psychological health, by reducing breed-specific diseases and anatomical defects and promoting favourable behavioural traits that result in satisfied cat owners.

Environment and Experience

Although genes are important for behaviour, you cannot always blame your cat's parents if the cat has behavioural problems. We have previously considered how important it is that a kitten develops a good relationship with its mother and the people in the household. But the environmental impact already begins at the foetal stage. Research

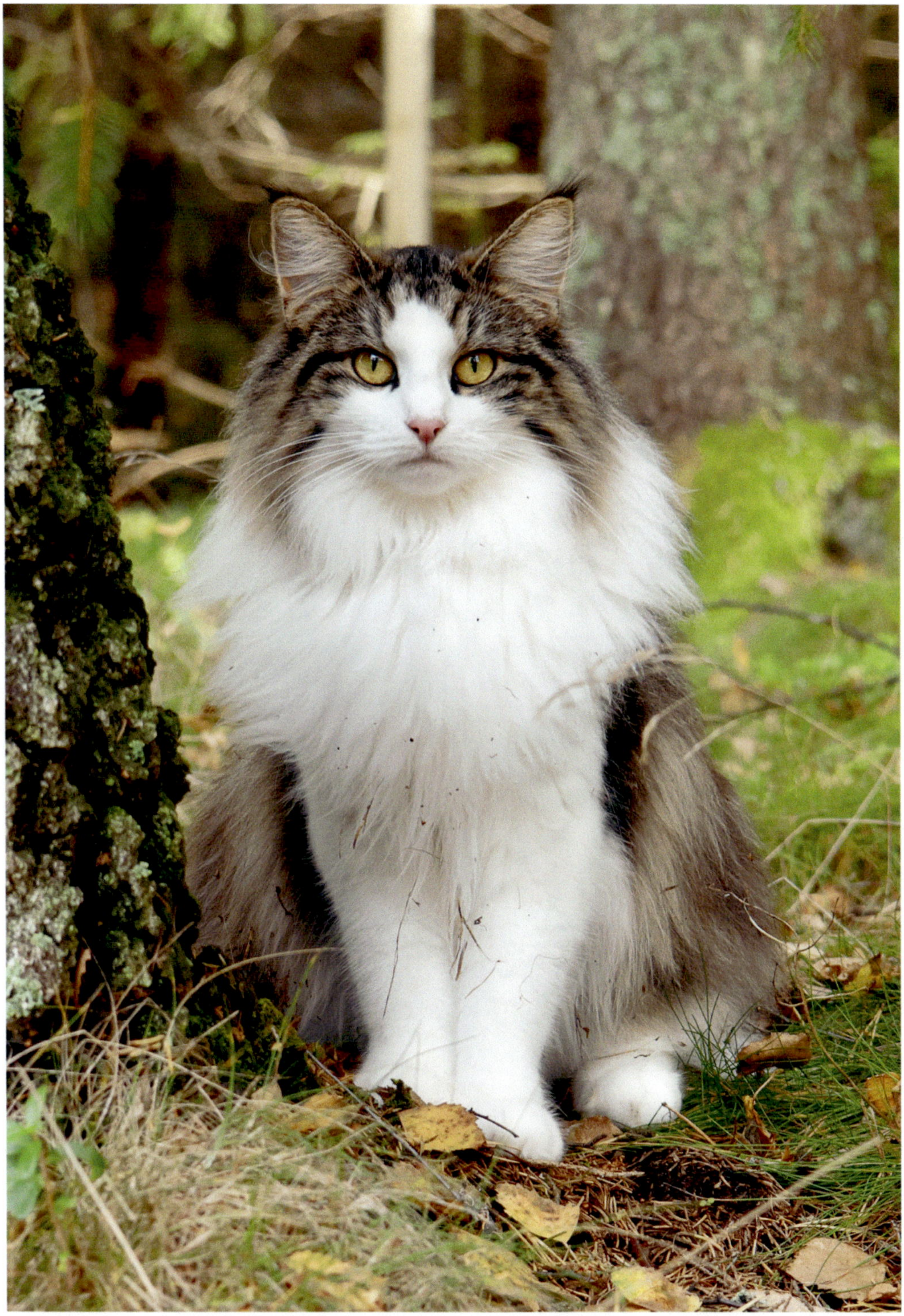

Fig. 3.6. Norwegian forest cat in its element. (Photo: Maria Myrland, 2019)

Table 3.1. Breeds scoring the highest and the lowest for each major behavioural trait, on a scale from 1 (never) to 5 (always). The breeds are ranked, so the one with the highest score is presented first in the middle column and the one with the lowest score is presented first in the right-hand column. Non-pedigree cats are termed 'house cats' for simplicity. (From Silja C.B. Eriksen, 2014)

Behavioural traits	Highest scores	Lowest scores
Sociability towards people	Burmese	House cat
Active and playful	Bengal, Abyssinian, Oriental, Burmese, Siamese	Persian
Separation problems	Bengal, Burmese	Persian
Aggressive towards other cats in the household	Abyssinian, House cat	Egyptian mau, Persian, British shorthair
Aggressive towards unfamiliar people	Abyssinian, Egyptian mau	Persian, Sacred Birman, Siamese, Ragdoll
Sociability towards unfamiliar cats	Persian, Norwegian forest cat, Egyptian mau, Oriental	Abyssinian, British shorthair
Resisting restraint	House cat, Siberian cat	Oriental, Egyptian mau, Burmese, Siamese
Aggressive when touched	House cat, Maine coon, Siberian cat	Egyptian mau, Oriental, Abyssinian, Siamese, Persian, Burmese
Contact-seeking	Burmese, Oriental	Persian, Ragdoll
Fear of novelty	Bengal	Persian, Oriental
Vocalization (calling to people)	Burmese, House cat, Maine coon	Persian, Sacred Birman, Oriental
Fear of unfamiliar cats and dogs	House cat, Bengal, Sacred Birman	Oriental, Egyptian mau, Burmese
Crepuscular activity	Egyptian mau, Burmese, Abyssinian, Norwegian forest cat	Persian, Bengal, Maine coon

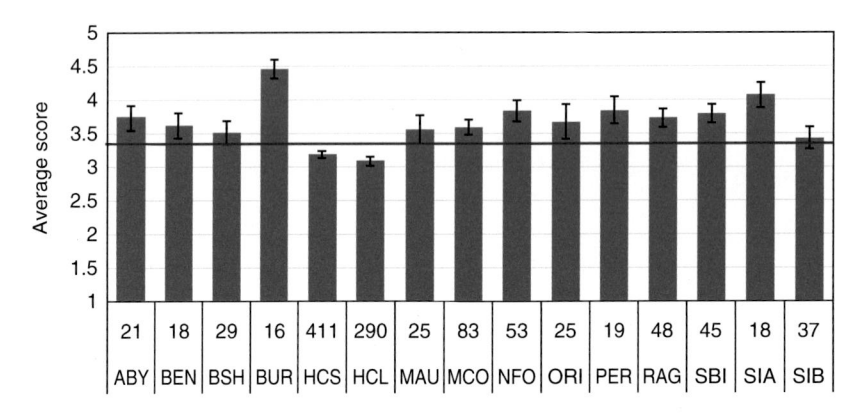

Fig. 3.7. Breed differences in the degree of sociability towards people. The scale goes from 1 (not at all) to 5 (very much). The breed codes follow the Easy Mind System (EMS code): ABY = Abyssinian, BEN = Bengal, BSH = British shorthair, BUR = Burmese, HCS = House cat shorthair, HCL = House cat longhair, MAU = Egyptian mau, MCO = Maine coon, NFO = Norwegian forest cat, ORI = Oriental, PER = Persian, RAG = Ragdoll, SBI = Sacred Birman, SIA = Siamese, SIB = Siberian cat. The bars show the average score and standard error. The number above the breed code shows the number of cats within the breed, based on survey responses from owners. The red line marks the average across all the cats. (From Silja C.B. Eriksen, 2014)

on many species – such as mice, rats, foxes, sheep, goats, chickens, salmon and humans – shows that if a pregnant female experiences severe stress during the last third of a pregnancy, this can have lasting consequences for hormonal regulation and behaviour of her offspring. This is called *prenatal stress* and it can cause the offspring to be more anxious, reacting more strongly and for longer to stressful

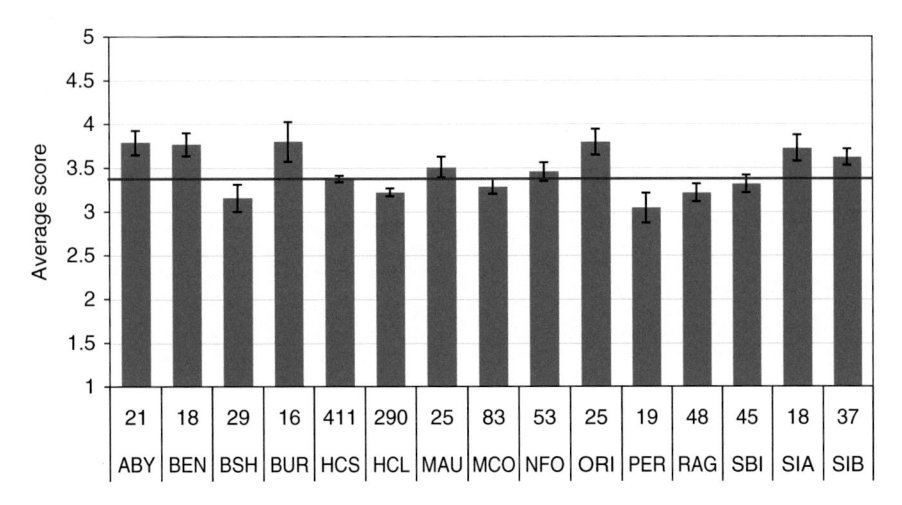

Fig. 3.8. Breed differences in the level of activity and playfulness. For explanation see Fig. 3.7. (From Silja C.B. Eriksen, 2014)

situations. Learning ability and sociability may be impaired, and the animal may be more nervous in general. In females, this anxiety may also impair the ability to provide consistent care for babies. Thus, stress in a mother can have long-term consequences, not only for offspring but for grandchildren as well.

Research in mice shows that when a pregnant mother is severely stressed, this can cause chemical changes in the brain of the foetuses that block parts of their DNA code from being read. This so-called *epigenetic* effect can reduce the production of specific proteins that bind *cortisol*, an important stress hormone, to brain cells in the hippocampus. The hippocampus is a structure in the *limbic system* of the brain that plays an important role in learning, memory and regulation of emotions. The consequence is that, later, when the offspring are stressed and their body produces cortisol, there are fewer cortisol receptors in the hippocampus to mop up the cortisol and switch off the stress response. This results in over-reaction to stressful events, which may be a lifelong trait. Such research is not currently available for cats, but there is no reason to believe that the same mechanism does not apply to them also. The moral is to take good care of pregnant mothers!

Research on mice and rats during the last two decades suggests that we can, to some extent, remedy the effect of prenatal stress if we suspect that it has occurred. If we ensure that the kittens get plenty of opportunities for socialization with other cats and people during the socialization period, and continue with this training as they get older, this should affect their behavioural development in a favourable direction. An enriched environment with plenty of interesting things to do should also help, by enticing them to voluntarily come out of their hiding-places to explore and play. While much remains unclear about how this works at neuronal level, we do know that during the socialization period the brain continues to develop rapidly, hence its importance.

As cats grow older, they are affected by their own experiences, but there is variation in the age when different behaviours are most affected by experience. For example, hunting skills can differ between kittens at two to three months of age, but such differences diminish when they all get more experience. The opposite can occur for social characteristics in a litter where the kittens have different fathers. If a queen mates with two or three tomcats, each of the males may father some of the kittens. Around eight weeks of age, all the kittens may be similarly friendly towards unfamiliar people, especially if their mother is friendly to strangers. However, by 20 weeks of age, the genetic influence of paternity appears, resulting in differences between the kittens in how they respond to strangers.

Sometimes it is important not to judge cats too soon. For example, cats that have stayed in quarantine for some months can be more tame and friendly when they finally arrive at their new home. But if the separation from their owner while in quarantine was a traumatic experience, then after three months in their new home, some of them may start showing nervousness and miaowing when they feel alone. For other traits, differences seen between kittens at an early age do not change so easily. This applies, for example, to activity level, curiosity, boldness and competitiveness, indicating stronger genetic influences on such traits.

Further Reading

Duffy, D.L., Diniz de Moura, R.T. and Serpell, J.A. (2017) Development and evaluation of the Fe-BARQ: A new survey instrument for measuring behavior in domestic cats (*Felis s. catus*). *Behavioural Processes* 141, 329–341. DOI: 10.1016/j.beproc.2017.02.010.

Hart, B.L. and Hart, L.A. (2013) *Your Ideal Cat: Insights into Breed and Gender Differences in Cat Behavior*. Purdue University Press, West Lafayette, Indiana.

Kotrschal, K., Day, J., McCune, S. and Wedl, M. (2014) Human and cat personalities: building the bond from both sides. In: Turner, D.C. and Bateson, P. (eds) *The Domestic Cat: The Biology of Its Behaviour*, 3rd edn. Cambridge University Press, Cambridge, pp. 113–127.

Landsberg, G.M. and Denenberg, S. (2009) Behaviour problems in the senior pet. In: Horwitz, D.F. and Mills, D.S. (eds) *BSAVA Manual of Canine and Feline Behavioural Medicine*, 2nd edn. British Small Animal Veterinary Association, Quedgeley, UK, pp. 127–135.

Litchfield, C.A., Quinton, G., Tindle H., Chiera, B., Kikillus, K.H. and Roetman, P. (2017) The `Feline Five': An exploration of personality in pet cats (*Felis catus*). *PLoS ONE* 12(8): e0183455. DOI: 10.1371/journal.pone.0183455

Marchei, P., Diverio, S., Falocci, N., Fatjó, J., Ruiz de la Torre, J.L. *et al.* (2009) Breed differences in behavioural development in kittens. *Physiology and Behaviour* 96, 522–531.

McCune, S. (1995) The impact of paternity and early socialisation on the development of cats' behaviour to people and novel objects. *Applied Animal Behaviour Science* 45, 109–124.

Mendl, M. and Harcourt, R. (2000) Individuality in the domestic cat: origins, development and stability. In: Turner, D.C. and Bateson, P. (eds) *The Domestic Cat: The Biology of Its Behaviour*, 2nd edn. Cambridge University Press, Cambridge, pp. 47–64.

Natoli, E. and De Vito, E. (1991) Agonistic behaviour, dominance rank and copulatory success in a large multi-male feral cat, *Felis catus* L., colony in central Rome. *Animal Behaviour* 42, 227–241.

Turner, D.C., Feaver, J., Mendl, M. and Bateson, P.P.G. (1986) Variation in domestic cat behaviour towards humans – a paternal effect. *Animal Behaviour* 34, 1890–1901.

Supplementary materials entitled 'Why cats are so different - individual variation' can be accessed at: www.cabi.org/the-cat-behaviour-and-welfare/

4 The Cat's Language – Communication

The cat's language signals may be the most important aspect of the cat's behaviour, which you must understand in order to develop a harmonious relationship with your cat. Cats expect that we understand the signals they send, and if we misinterpret them we may risk the cat becoming severely frustrated resulting in bites and scratches. Interpreting the cat's language is not as difficult as many think; it is just a matter of knowing what to look for. The signals are made up of many elements and each of them may represent a whole sentence in human language. Understanding your cat is easier if you have some general knowledge about how animals communicate.

How Animals Communicate

Cats and other animals do not communicate in the way that humans do, in that they do not use words. Nevertheless, cats have many ways to communicate so that other cats can understand what they mean at that moment. They communicate the way they are feeling – their emotions and their intentions – what they want to do and what they want from other individuals. In this way, they can influence the behaviour of others in a preferable direction.

The *signal* is the basic unit of communication. A signal is a stimulus sent from one animal and perceived by another that can alter the behaviour of the recipient in a manner that benefits the signaller. It could be a particular vocalization, a tail movement or a urine mark. If the signal is not perceived by the other party, no communication has occurred. Therefore, during evolution, animal signals have evolved to become simple and distinct, so they stand out from ordinary behaviour.

Cat signals are used in communication between a queen and her kittens, regulation of social relationships, competition for resources and courtship. Signals are used when one cat is uncomfortable being close to another cat. We call such signals *agonistic* signals. They can either be part of *offensive aggression*, where the animal is threatening that 'If you do not leave, I shall attack you', or *defensive aggression*, where the animal is instead threatening that 'Although I don't want to fight, if you attack me, I can defend myself with teeth and claws' (see Fig. 4.1). Defensive signals imply that the animal is experiencing fear for its safety. As the subordinate cat displays its defence weapons, these are not signals of submission but of readiness to fight if provoked. If a subordinate cat finds a dominant cat too troublesome, it will run away or even emigrate to another area, as we shall see in Chapter 6. *Flight* is a component of agonistic behaviour, but it is usually not necessary to escape that far to get away from the threat.

Offensive signals are typically given by cats with high social status due to their strong competitive ability, while low-status individuals more often display defensive signals. Such signals minimize serious fights. Giving defensive signals counteracts attacks by the opponent. There would be no point in attacking the subordinate individual, as such attacks would unnecessarily risk getting hurt. By using offensive signals, a high-status cat can also prevent an attack by a young upstart with little chance of winning a fight. Fights occur most frequently between individuals who have comparable competitive ability, where neither party manages to repel the other with threat signals.

The African wildcat, the ancestor of domestic cats, defends a territory against neighbouring wildcats using agonistic signals. The domestic cat has more flexible social behaviour, as described in Chapter 5, involving more varied use of communication signals. Domestic cats miaow more to other cats than the wildcats, and towards people after separation from their mother. They use signals in adulthood that wildcats only use as kittens towards their mother. The domestic kitten thus transfers its use of communication from the mother to people. Therefore, it is no surprise that cats miaow to communicate their needs. Continuing to perform juvenile behaviour in

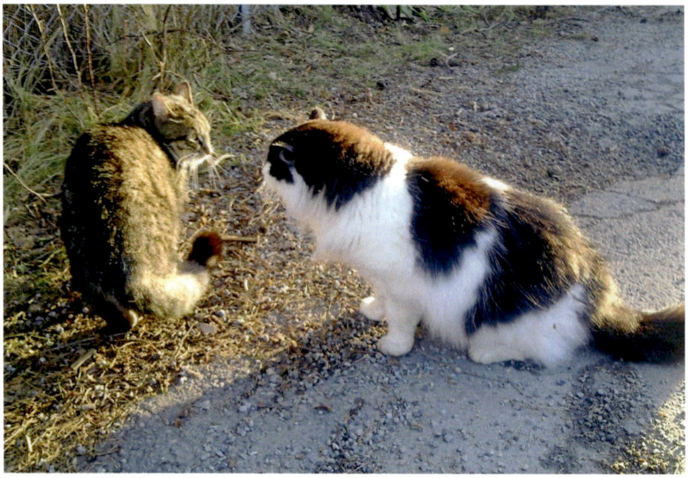

Fig. 4.1. When two unfamiliar cats meet, they will often send offensive or defensive signals. (Photo: Agnethe-Irén Sandem, 2019)

adulthood is a common phenomenon in domesticated animals called *neoteny*.

It is useful to be aware of what animals usually *do not* communicate. Animals are not likely to signal that they are sick or injured. In nature, this would reveal a vulnerability that could attract predators. Instead, they try to hide such disabilities. We must look for signs of illness or injury in another way. If the animal is unusually passive and there is a change in how much it eats or drinks (less or more) than before, this may indicate a disease. If the animal reacts with aggression or withdrawal when we touch a certain part of its body, this may indicate that the animal has an injury or disease that hurts at this spot. If you notice this more than once, you should take the cat to a vet.

Cats can use sounds, body postures, facial expressions, movements, scents, and touch to make themselves understood. They often use several types of communication signals simultaneously, making their intentions clearer. It is therefore important for the cat owner to listen carefully to the vocalizations and at the same time note the visual signals. We are not able to detect all the different scent signals used by cats, but the odour of urine marking by an intact male will be unmistakable. Some cats are more communicative than others. We must therefore get to know that individual to interpret its intention or emotion correctly. Some may be more vocal and miaow at all hours. For cats who are less vocal in general, even their weak signals may be informative.

Sound Signals – Acoustic Communication

Cats use many types of sounds in their communication with others – purring, miaowing, yowling, growling and hissing. These sounds vary depending on the situation and the individual cat. Most sounds are made using the vocal cords. But cats do not shape the sound with the tongue tip like humans do. Instead, they produce different 'vowel' sounds by varying the muscle tension of their larynx, mouth, lips and face. They produce 'consonants' by closing or shaping the mouth in different ways that change the resonance. Muscle tensions and the shape of the mouth can be varied on a continuous scale. In this way, they can fine-tune a signal and how strongly it is expressed, whereas people choose different words or stronger adjectives to adjust their meaning.

Purring

Soundtrack no. 1: purring

video.cabi.org/abcde

For cat lovers, a cat's purring is usually a relaxing sound. You are happy when you relax on the sofa with a purring cat against your chest. But what is purring really, and why does the cat purr?

Purring is a deep sound produced by muscles of the larynx and diaphragm. The entire chest region of the cat vibrates at low frequency with fundamental frequencies of about 25 and 50 Hz but including vibrations up to 150 Hz. It is thought that a neural oscillator controls these muscle vibrations, allowing purring to continue during both inhalation and exhalation.

Purring is a sound that kittens give when suckling their mother's milk. It signals the mother to keep calm and provide care, which includes giving milk, grooming, warmth and protection. Purring helps to maintain the bond with the mother and is usually associated with comfort and relaxed pleasure. Mother cats also purr when providing care to their kittens in the nest. When very young, the kittens feel the vibrations from the purring and stay close to her even though they don't hear them, as their ears are not yet open. The mother is signalling her desire to give them care.

When kittens and adult cats purr towards people, the meaning is usually the same. The cat expresses that it wishes to relax in close contact with us, whether in our lap or on the sofa next to us. 'Here I shall remain for some time, so keep calm and show me you care,' the cat says. While we don't produce milk, lick the cat or purr, we can provide a safe haven for resting, share our warmth, groom the cat and whisper sweet nothings. The cat has learned to accept our gentle strokes as the equivalent of being licked and our gentle words as the equivalent of purring. The relationship is mutually rewarding. It is not just about taking care from us but also giving care. The cat shows its care for us by purring, presenting its warm belly, and grooming us with its raspy tongue if allowed. The stronger the purring, the more intense is the cat's pleasure. You can notice this while you gently stroke a resting cat.

Although purring is usually associated with pleasurable situations, there is another form of purring that is louder and higher-pitched. Air is pressed through the vocal cords resulting in a higher sound frequency, creating strong sounds around 200–500 Hz. This more demanding purring is not relaxing to humans, but rather to the contrary – it sounds a bit annoying and cannot be ignored. It is a begging vocalization expressed when the cat is frustrated because it wants something it can't get by itself, or feels a more urgent need for care. Some cats direct these 'solicitation' purrs towards us when they have sniffed that there is inaccessible food nearby, or when we have slept in and they want us to wake up and feed them. They usually have the desired effect of cajoling us into action.

Solicitation purrs can also occur when cats are frightened, ill or in pain. Occasionally, vets experience this. In such situations, purring is not an indication of well-being, but instead indicates that the cat seeks help. Cats that purr in a veterinary clinic are familiar with people and use the purring as needy kittens would when begging for care from their mother. So such purring means 'I need care'. If your cat has been ill and starts purring like this, don't be fooled into thinking that the cat has recovered.

Interestingly, regular purring corresponds to the vibration frequency of medical instruments used for healing injuries and promoting bone density. Since purring is also associated with the release of endorphins – the body's natural soothing, pain-relieving hormones – it has been suggested that purring may aid cats in self-recovery from injuries. This may be a positive side-effect, though it is hardly the primary function of purring given that purring is a communication signal used in social contexts and cats rarely purr when alone. Gentle purring by the mother and littermates may contribute to kitten growth and bone density, though this has not been studied.

Miaowing

The cat's miaow is another well-known vocalization of cats. It mainly occurs in kittenhood, in the communication between kittens and their mother. The miaow can be expressed in an incredible variety of ways. Research shows that people who are familiar with cats recognize the meaning of different miaows better than those lacking experience with cats. To understand miaows, we must listen carefully to how they are pronounced by each individual. Fortunately, there are some general rules that can guide us. The American behaviourist Mildred Moelk has contributed to this knowledge through her extensive study of cat vocalizations.

M-I-A-OW – the miaow consists of four syllables. To interpret the miaow, we must listen to which of the four syllables the cat emphasizes – which one is loudest or the most long-lasting – and note if any are missing. Some of these differences are shown in Fig. 4.2.

Mrrr, trill

Soundtrack no. 2: mrrr

video.cabi.org/abcde

The trill, or chirrup, is mainly an *m* sound, the first letter of the M-I-A-O, often without any of the following vocals. This may sound like *mrrr* or *mhrn* and may vary in duration from a short *mr* to a *mhrrrrrn*. It is given with closed mouth. If it starts abruptly, a phoneticist will write it like this: '*mhrn*. This sound can be heard from a distance of about 12 metres and is much more powerful than regular purring. It is used by confident cats when initiating contact with a social partner. It simply means 'hello'. When the cat wakes up from its chair and approaches us, it can greet us with a *mhrn*. When returning to her kittens, a cat mother uses this sound to announce her presence.

When the sound starts more abruptly and vigorously, '*mhrn*', it is a short-distance call sound. Then it is often repeated. Not only 'Hello, here I am' but 'Hello, I want contact with you'. The same applies if the *mhrn* sound goes up in pitch at the end. We can indicate this by writing the raised notes as superscripts: *mhr^{rnn}*. If a cat mother gives this

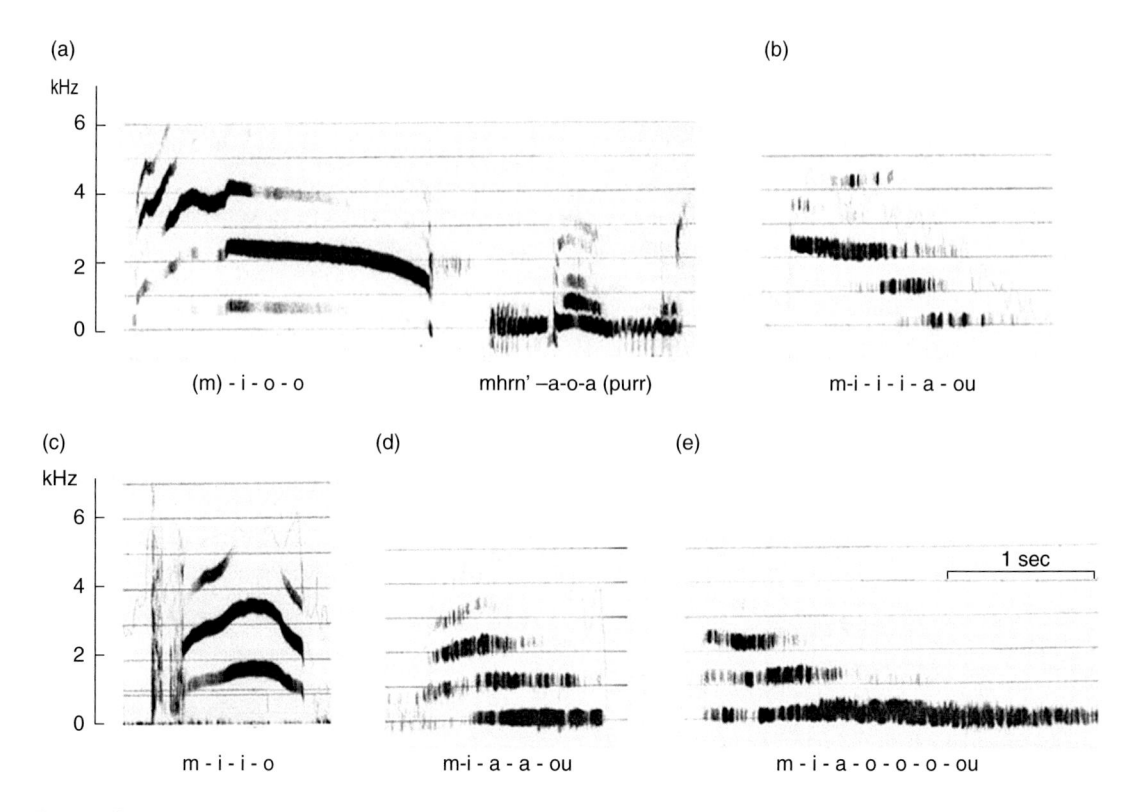

(a) kHz
(b)

(m) - i - o - o   mhrn' –a-o-a (purr)   m - i - i - i - a - ou

(c) kHz
(d)
(e)

1 sec

m - i - i - o   m - i - a - a - ou   m - i - a - o - o - o - ou

Fig. 4.2. Spectrographic images of different miaow types. (a) a mioo or meoo from a lonely, worried kitten, followed by the reassuring response of its mother, a mhrn'-aoa and purring. This is like the mother saying 'Hello, I'm back again; now we can have a nice time together'; (b) a miiiaou or meeeaow from a cat experiencing an unpleasant or painful situation; (c) a miio or meeo from lonely or otherwise distressed kitten; (d) a miaaou or meaaow from a demanding cat; and (e) a miaooou or meaooow from a frustrated cat. The horizontal axis denotes time (the length of *one* second is illustrated) while the vertical axis shows the pitch tone in kilohertz (kHz). Note that miaowing sounds occur in several harmonic series, one octave apart, and can reach a pitch of 50–60 kHz in the ultrasonic range beyond human hearing.

sound to her kittens, she may be inviting them to suckle from her.

The cat can also give a stronger 'Hello!!!' by adding vowels to the *mrr* sound. Then it sounds like *mhrraow*. In Fig. 4.2a we can see an example of such use at the beginning of the mother's response; a *mhrn-ao* where the mother responds to reassure a lonely, worried kitten. Exactly what the cat aims to express in addition to 'Hello!' depends on whether the cat uses a long *a* or *ow* sound (see *miaaao*, *miaoow* and call sounds below).

Miiiao

Soundtrack no. 3: miiiao
video.cabi.org/abcde

A long *e* syllable in the miaow, *miiiao* or *meeeao*, gives a whining sound. It can indicate that the cat is experiencing discomfort or pain, meaning 'Ouch! Help me!'. If we accidentally step on the cat's tail, or the cat gets stuck, we may hear this sound. The longer or stronger the sound, the stronger is the discomfort. See an example in Fig. 4.2b.

Young kittens, only a few weeks of age, do not manage to miaow with a diphthong, the *ouw* part of the sound. Instead, they say *miiy*, *miio* or *meeeo*. This is not necessarily a pain signal. The small kitten can also give a marked *e* sound in situations when a juvenile or adult cat would use a marked *a* sound (see below). You can see an example of this in Fig. 4.2c, where a kitten has been briefly separated from its mother and seeks contact with her.

Miaaao

Soundtrack no. 4: miaaao
video.cabi.org/abcde

A long *a* sound in the miaow is probably the most typical miaow sound, *miaaao*. See an example in Fig. 4.2d. A long-lasting miaow with a marked *a* sound indicates that the cat desires something. It is saying, 'I want something now!'. The miaow does not tell us what the cat wants. We must infer this from the context in which the sound is given. If a cat is sitting by the food bowl expressing a *miaaao*, we can understand that it is begging for food – even if there is food in the bowl, it may want something better. Perhaps the canned food is starting to spoil. Cats will naturally avoid food that does not smell fresh. This is a mechanism that prevents them from ingesting harmful bacteria.

In other cases, the cat may *miaaao* at the front door indicating that it wants to be let out, or in front of us when we sit on the sofa, asking to sit on our lap. It may *miaaao* while standing by the litterbox, indicating that it wants it cleaned. The longer the *a* syllable in the miaow, the stronger the request. The cat typically starts with a short *miaow*, then *miaaow* and eventually *miaaaow* if the desired goal is not yet reached. If your cat is miaowing with a long *a* sound quite often, and you are sure that it has everything it really needs, this could be because your cat has learned that this is an effective way of getting you to respond to its slightest whims. For example, if you find yourself frequently giving treats or opening the door several times in short succession, you may be pandering to your cat's demands too much, an issue to which we shall return in Chapter 11.

Miaooww

Soundtrack no. 5: miaooww
video.cabi.org/abcde

If your cat begins to lose faith that its wishes will be fulfilled, it will start getting frustrated. The cat signals this by dragging out the closing end of the miaow and we can hear a *miaooww*, as shown in Fig. 4.2e. This usually drops in pitch – *miao$_{ouw}$*. The longer the *ow*-sound, the stronger the frustration. The cat may have begged for food with a *miaaao* without success and now becomes more and more frustrated, and we can hear that the miaow transforms from *miaao* to *miaaaao*, *miaoww*, and finally a long *miaoouuu* – 'I was expecting food, but it seems that I won't get any this time'. Kittens extend their isolation cries when worried that their mother has not returned, as seen in Fig. 4.2a.

Mngaow

Occasionally, we can hear that the cat puts a *ng* element into the miaow, which then sounds like *mngaow*. This signals a protest over a result the cat is not satisfied with. For example, perhaps the cat has been begging for food and we put down a bowl of freshly boiled fish. We quickly remember that the cat cannot eat scorching hot food and remove the bowl to allow the food to cool down. The cat does not understand this and expresses its *mngaow*. 'Hello, put the food down again immediately. It's mine!'

Calling miaows

Calling vocalizations typically increase in pitch at the end in an invigorating, expectant way. Such calling miaows can have both short and long *a* sounds, depending on the strength of the cat's motivation to attract another. Male cats use such miaows when they call females in heat, sounding more like a *mowl*. If they have difficulty finding females, they may add a *mrr* sound and make the *a* sound long and deep, yet with an increase in pitch at the end like the typical male mating call. We can write this as $mhrr_{aaa}^{ou}$. Also, females can use such a sound when calling others, such as calling males when they are in heat. All cats can use a calling miaow when calling social partners, whether cats or humans. In both wild and domestic cats, cat mothers use a calling miaow when attracting kittens who have got lost. At short distances, a *mhrn* (greeting) that goes up at the end, *mhr^rn*, can also indicate a desire for contact – 'I would love to see you, but where are you?'.

Yowling

Soundtrack no. 6: yowling
video.cabi.org/abcde

Whilst both male and female cats yowl as part of their communication with an opponent, there is not much that causes more complaints about cats than the yowling of tomcats during the mating season (Fig. 4.3). If accidentally coming too close to another male opponent, a tomcat may make a short howl starting with a loud *a* sound followed by a brief closed-mouth murmur. If finding himself facing another intact male of similar size – and visual threat signals do not have the desired effect – a yowling competition will start. It's all about who can make the longest, most powerful yowl. Since the yowl is energy-intensive, it displays the strength and vigour of each cat. The yowl is a type of miaow, where the *a* and *ouw* syllables are drawn out to the extreme and can last for many seconds. The yowl sounds like *miaaaaaaaaooooaaaaaaaooouw*. The extended *a* sounds in the yowl mark a strong desire for something, namely that the opposing party will go away. The *ouw* sound in the yowl shows frustration when the other does not comply.

If the yowling becomes very strong, the competition may escalate into a fight resulting in scratches or damage to the ears and paws, so this is clearly a type of offensive aggression. Fighting is always a last resort, but this can happen if neither visual signals nor yowling identify a winner. During yowling, the cats can approach and keep their heads just a few centimetres apart. Great courage is needed to tolerate such close-up yowling, but the males are competing for access to females in heat. Mating is a priority for a fertile tomcat, so he will not give up until his health and safety are seriously threatened.

Growling

A cat can growl almost like a dog, with a deep murmur with almost closed mouth. Growling

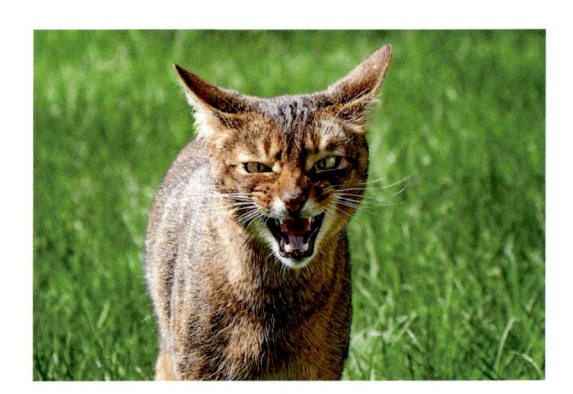

Fig. 4.3. A tomcat expresses his offensive attitude by vigorous yowling while holding his ears slightly backwards. (Photo: Audun Braastad, 2019)

implies a warning, and can be directed to cats, other animal species and people. It happens when a cat has a resource to defend, such as its food, or wants to be left in peace for other reasons. It is therefore a type of defensive aggression. The cat says 'Stay away, this is mine' or 'Stay away, I feel uncomfortable when you are so close'. If the cat needs to make this point even stronger, the growling can grow into a powerful miaow: *grrrraaao*. If the recipient does not respect this growl, the cat may attack as a defensive response. People can only blame themselves if they get bitten when not respecting the cat's desire to be left in peace.

Hissing and spitting

Hissing consists of air pressed out of an open mouth without use of the vocal cords. It is typical of snakes and cats. Hissing is used as a defensive signal, especially among cats that are cornered and cannot escape. Never touch a cat that is howling, growling or hissing. If you do, you can experience powerful bites and scratches as the cat tries to defend itself. The cat has warned you and you are responsible if you do not heed the warning. Slight hissing can already be seen in newborn kittens when picked up by people. They open their mouth abruptly and repeatedly, as is the case in hissing by adult cats, but are unable to blow out any air.

Spitting occurs when a cat suddenly opens its mouth and blows a loud noise, again without using the vocal cords. It may sound like an abrupt *the*. It is a quick defensive warning that the cat gives if startled by the sudden appearance of an unexpected opponent. The intruder may also be startled by this abrupt sound.

Chatters and chirps

The chatter is a staccato, rattling sound, like a rapidly repeated *ke-ke-ke*. Cats make this sound by clacking their teeth, but chatters can be accompanied by voiced elements as well, such as chirps. Cats occasionally chatter and chirp when they see prey at a rather short distance. The most typical situation is a cat who sees a bird sitting on the other side of the window. It appears that these sounds may lure prey by mimicking their sounds, or that of insects the birds eat. Perhaps the cat thinks if the bird came even closer, it would be able to catch it. Outdoors, these sounds may be given as a 'Come hither!' when a potential prey is just out of reach. If the sound attracts a bird to hop a little closer or, at least, relax its vigilance and wander closer, the waiting cat could launch a successful attack. A cat does not vocalize to other cats when hunting. Hearing those types of sounds would alert prey to the danger. Chattering may also indicate the cat is feeling a degree of frustration (see Chapter 8).

Body Language – Visual Communication

The body language, or visual communication, of cats was thoroughly explored by the German ethologist Paul Leyhausen. His classic book about wild and domestic cat behaviour has been translated into English and is well worth reading for those interested in detailed descriptions and explanations of cat body language. Leyhausen found that cats can simultaneously show signs of two opposing behavioural tendencies by displaying both defensive and offensive signals at the same time. These signals involve body postures (including the tail), which provide general information about the cat's mood and behavioural tendencies, and facial expressions (including the ears), which provide finely tuned, rapid information about moment-to-moment changes in motivation. Therefore, to correctly interpret your cat's intentions, you must note the body posture and tail movements while directing your main attention to the head and eyes, and especially the ears.

Facial expressions

The famous Austrian ethologist Konrad Lorenz once wrote that 'few animals show their moods by means of facial expressions as markedly as cats do'. In Fig. 4.4, you can see what different facial expressions mean. The most non-aggressive cat face is shown in the top left. The diagram has two axes – a horizontal, offensive, axis and a vertical, defensive, axis. If we go to the right of the chart, we see faces showing a gradually increasing *offensive tendency*, that is increasing motivation to attack if necessary to repel an opponent. What do we see then? The ears are swivelled around until they point backwards. Displaying the backs of the ears is a strong offensive signal that shows that the cat is ready to attack. In lynx and tigers, the back of each ear has a bright white spot surrounded by a dark border, making it easy for an opponent to notice that the ears are back even at night.

The Cat's Language

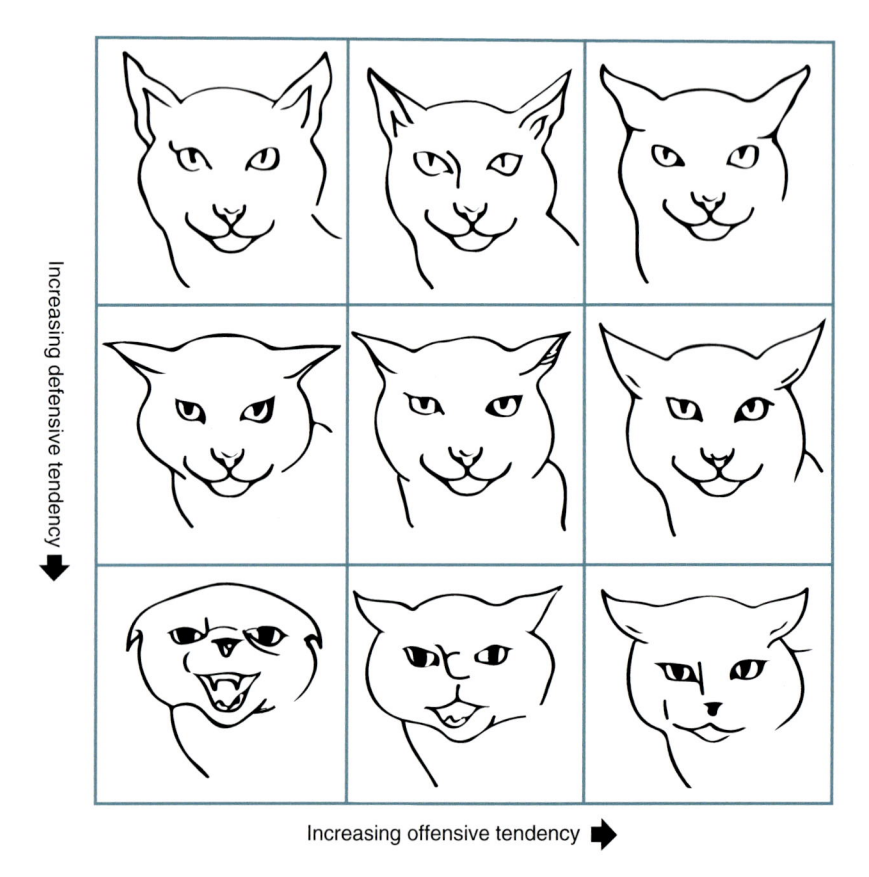

Fig. 4.4. Facial expressions, showing different combinations of increasingly offensive signals (towards the right column) and defensive signals (towards the bottom row). See the text for further explanation. (After Paul Leyhausen, *Verhaltensstudien an Katzen*, Verlag Paul Parey, Berlin, 1956)

Domestic cats almost always have single-coloured ears, but the 'ears back' signal nevertheless means the same: 'There is a great chance that I will attack you if you do not go away right now'.

If we go *down* the chart, we see faces with a gradually increasing *defensive tendency*. Now we can see that the ears are more and more flattened towards the skull. The more the ears are folded down, the stronger is the motivation to defend the body from attack. The cat at the bottom left has flattened its ears so much that they are almost invisible. When cats flatten their ears, their defensive signals cannot be interpreted mistakenly as offensive. This reduces the risk of provoking a dominant cat to attack them unnecessarily. A highly defensive cat will also open its mouth, signalling its readiness to bite if attacked.

Also note the size of the pupils. The most defensive face, shown in the bottom left, has the widest pupils. This is a sign that the sympathetic nervous system has been activated, with excretion of adrenaline from the adrenal glands. This stress response means that the cat is alert, scared and mobilizing energy to defend itself if this becomes necessary. At the same time, we usually see that the hair rises on the back of the neck, called *piloerection*. In a short-haired cat, this makes the cat look bigger, which may help to deter an attack. In contrast, the purely offensive cat at the top right is confident and does not need adrenaline to claim its interests. Be aware, however, that the pupils of all cats will open more widely at night, as this allows them to see better in the dark – this is a reflex unrelated to adrenaline release. The pupils may also widen in other situations, such as when a cat is playing or hunting a bird.

The four drawings in the lower right part of Fig. 4.4 show intermediates between offensive and defensive signals. These cats are partly offensive and partly defensive, and are in doubt, or conflict, about whether to attack or defend themselves. By looking at how turned backwards the ears are, and how flattened down they are, we can see the relative balance between offensive and defensive tendencies. The cat at the bottom right is the most conflicted. In this state, it might do something unpredictable, or perhaps attempt to calm itself by doing something irrelevant to the situation – a displacement activity (see Chapter 8).

Lip licking

A clear indication that a cat is worried or anxious can be seen when it quickly licks its lips two or three times, while closely watching another animal, person or object of concern. This suggests that the cat's mouth has become dry out of fear, as happens also to people when stressed. Normal licking of the mouth, as seen after the cat has eaten, is much calmer and more carefully directed.

Body postures

At a distance, when the face is hard to see, the most conspicuous signals come from body posture. As with the different facial expressions, we can interpret body postures using a diagram with an offensive axis and a defensive axis. The drawings in Fig. 4.5 show cats exhibiting offensive and defensive tendencies to varying degrees. We see a non-aggressive, relatively relaxed body posture at the top left, with increasingly offensive tendencies towards the right column and increasingly defensive tendencies towards the bottom row.

When assessing the cat's intentions, pay attention to the distance between the body and the ground. The more offensive a cat is, the more upright the cat will be. On the other hand, the more defensive the cat, the lower it will crouch. The head, particularly, will be held low. On the bottom left, we see a purely defensive cat. It is close to the ground, with its tail tightly tucked between its legs and flattened ears. The confident cat at the top right shows pure offensive signals, with raised body, straight legs, the tail down and the ears back. Such a cat will display the side of its body to the opponent rather than just the front. This lateral display shows off its big body: 'Look at me! I'm huge and strong. You should go away for your own safety.' Note how this visual communication signal to another cat differs from the body posture of an alert cat engaged in a non-social type of offense, the hunt (Fig. 4.6).

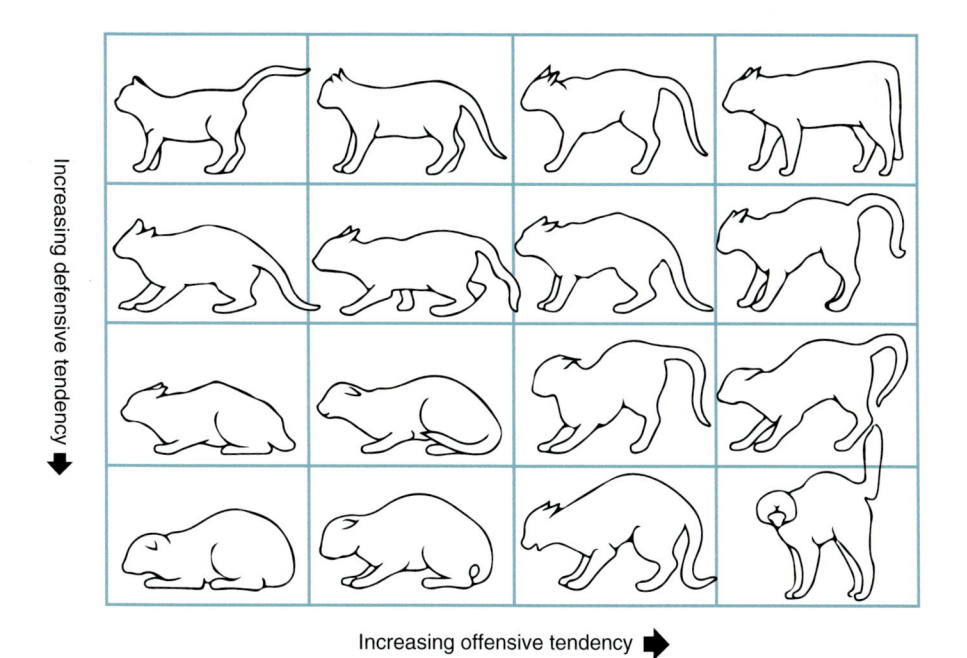

Fig. 4.5. Body positions, showing different combinations of offensive signals (to the right) and defensive signals (downwards). (After Paul Leyhausen, *Verhaltensstudien an Katzen*, Verlag Paul Parey, Berlin, 1956)

The Cat's Language

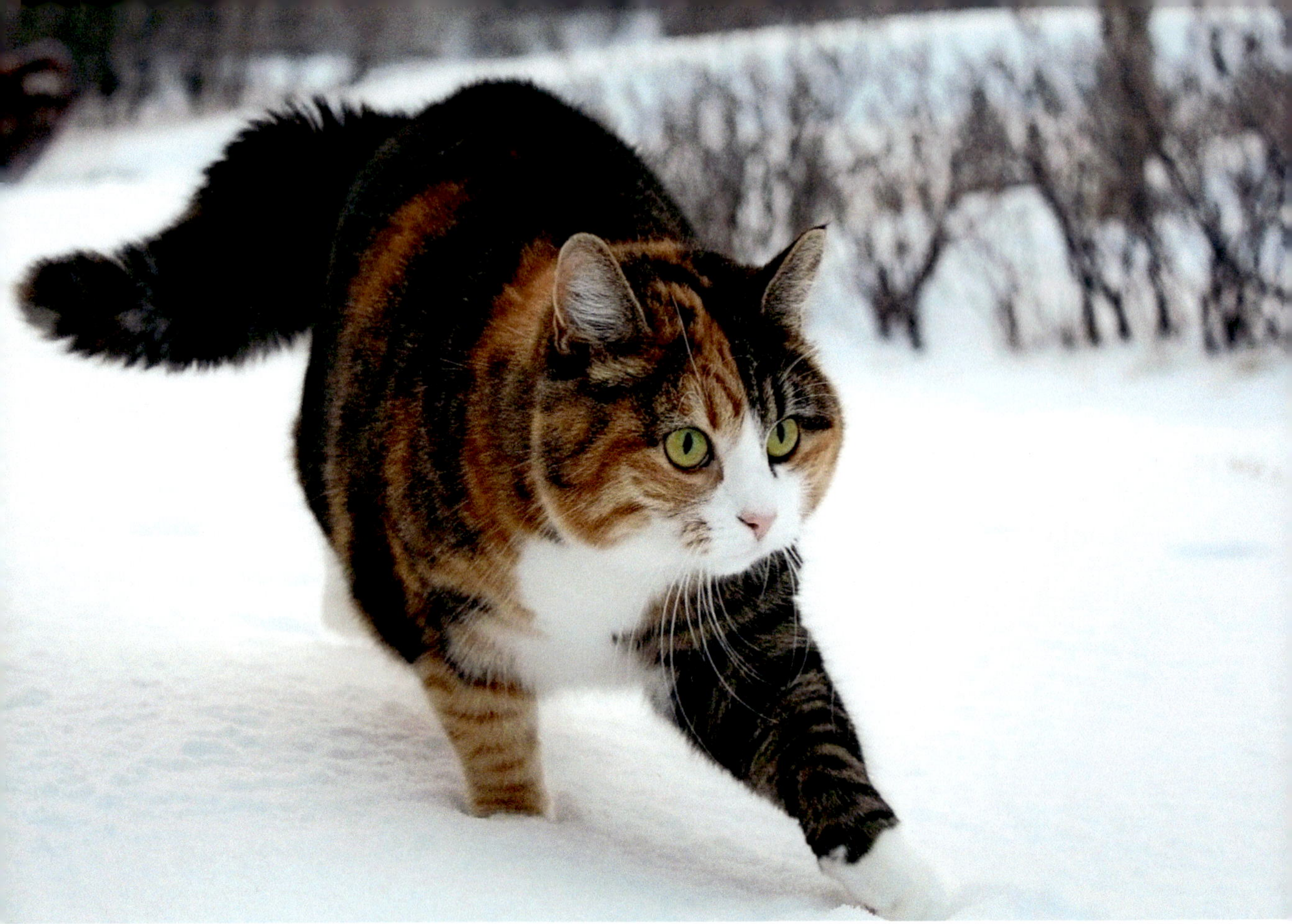

Fig. 4.6. This cat is out hunting, showing an alert posture with ears forward, normal pupil size and a slightly lifted tail. (Photo: Janne Helen Lorentzsen, 2019)

In a social contest, a somewhat arched back and partially raised tail indicates mild conflict between approach and withdrawal. The conflicted cat on the bottom right of Fig. 4.5 has the most arched back, showing that the tendencies to attack and defend are both strong. Leyhausen describes what is happening as a conflict between the front half and the back half of the cat. The cat has a fighting spirit, but the front end of the body closest to the opponent is retracted for safety. The centre of gravity moves backwards, making it easier to escape from the opponent if suddenly needed, bending the spine into an arch (Fig. 4.7). Suppose a mother cat with kittens nearby is facing a scary dog. She would love to chase away the dog but does not dare. Escape is out of the question, as she does not want to desert her offspring, so she stays and makes the best of it. She may also raise her tail, showing that she doesn't want to fight. Below, we explain other social contexts involving a raised tail.

Great boldness is required to launch an attack because it is easy to get wounded in the heat of battle. When two similarly matched cats are in a dispute, each cat carefully evaluates the resolve of the other, watching for tell-tale visual signals from the face, ears, eyes, tail and overall body posture. They are also evaluating the sound signals, especially the yowl, as described earlier. In this battle of nerves, the balance of power is on a knife-edge and a moment's loss of concentration, or an impulsive signal, can cause the other to attack. All movements are very slow to avoid provoking an unnecessary attack. From time to time, the hindquarters of one or both cats may slowly sink down (see Fig. 4.8). This seems to act as a signal of ceasefire, giving the cats a much-needed thinking break. If one cat exposes its teeth, it becomes clear that it is more defensive than the other. Usually, defensive signals are respected, and the more confident cat will not attack. This cat's dominance has been recognized and it can proceed to other important tasks.

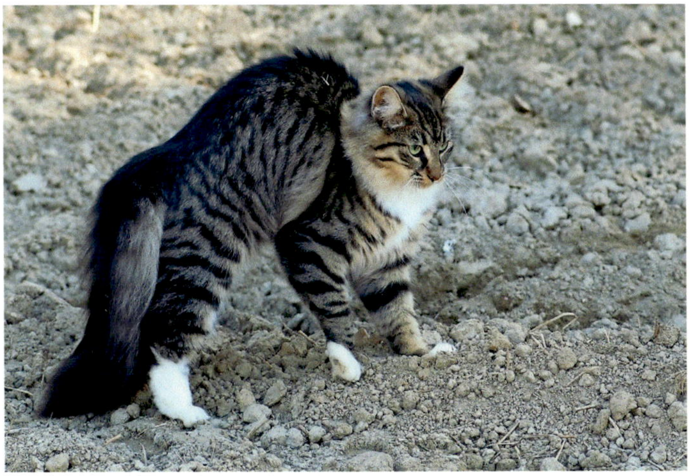

Fig. 4.7. This cat arches its back, displaying conflict between offensive and defence motivations. The ears are erect, showing that the cat is not very frightened at the moment. (Photo: Maria Myrland, 2019)

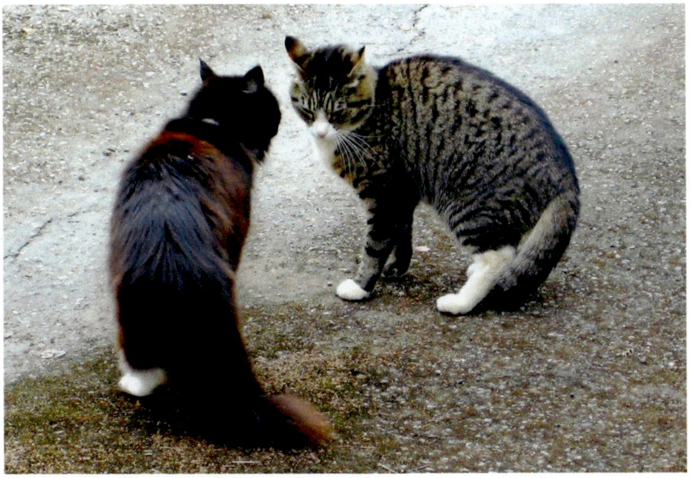

Fig. 4.8. Two equally matched cats in a ceasefire. Both have their ears turned somewhat backwards and lowered hindquarters. (Photo: Bjarne O. Braastad, 2011)

Rearing

Fortunately, the cat uses its body language not only in conflict situations but also when approaching a friend. It may then lift both front paws up off the ground for a couple of seconds, assuming a more vertical posture, and then put them back down again. If greeting a person, the cat may also rest the front paws briefly against the person's legs while rearing.

Lifted paw

You sometimes see that a cat suddenly stops and lifts a forepaw, the paw hanging in a relaxed way. The cat looks like it is concentrating, perhaps attending to a sound or odour that has caught its interest. A dog will do the same. This is referred to as an *intention movement*. The animal shows its intention to move on but pauses to evaluate if this is wise. It is saying 'Hey, what was that?'. It indicates mild conflict over what to do next.

Exposing the belly

If you stroke an unfamiliar cat on its belly, you can quickly get a scratch. The cat aggressively defends

The Cat's Language

its belly using its claws if it does not feel completely safe with those nearby. This is an important survival response that protects the body's most vulnerable region. The abdomen is not covered by bones and an injury here could fatally expose vital organs. The chest has some protection from the ribs, and the head is well protected by the skull, so cats more easily accept strokes there.

However, when a cat has full trust in you, it may roll over on its back and present its belly, like a mother cat presenting her udder for suckling by her kittens. This is an invitation to gently caress the belly. If the cat is unknown to you, be careful not to reach for the belly if it rolls on its back as it is probably doing so just to scratch its back.

Tail signals

Tail up

A 'tail up' signal involves a stiff upward motion that lifts the tail quickly until it is more or less straight up. This is a greeting signal that can be addressed to both cats and people. It is usually accompanied by a slightly curved back and a greeting sound *mrrrt* or *mhrrrn*, that rises in pitch at the end. The cat can use this as a short greeting even if it is just passing by. Then we see the tail go up and down again after a couple of seconds, without any sounds. This is a 'Hi' in passing. The cat has seen us but is not seeking to make close contact at the moment.

The 'tail up' is a signal used by kittens when greeting their mother, and adult cats use the same towards people and other friends. It can be the start of a more elaborate greeting in which the nose is rubbed against the cheek or body of the one being greeted. Kittens do this to their mother when they are hungry. Adult cats direct this greeting to cats of higher social status, signalling their friendly intentions.

Tail over the head

Sometimes you can see a male cat walking with lifted tail, but with the tip of the tail tilting forward towards the head. This is a sign of high self-confidence. It may be a signal to females that it is high-ranking, and a signal to less confident males that they should stay away. At a lower degree of self-confidence, a cat can hold the tail partially lifted. In juveniles, when the tail is tilted forward, it shows that they feel safe in their surroundings and may be playful.

Lashing tail

This is a common tail signal and means something completely different from the dog's tail wagging. It consists of rapid jerks of the tail from side to side and shows that the cat is annoyed. The stronger the lashes, the stronger the irritation. Often, this signal is accompanied by other body signals that indicate irritation, or growling. The cat wants to be at peace and if we do not respect this, the cat may suddenly bite.

Slight tail movements

When resting, if something disturbs a cat, or if it does not feel completely safe, we may see small twitches of the tip of the tail. This is a warning that, while the cat looks relaxed, it is alert and ready to react if necessary. If the cat becomes drowsy or falls asleep, these tail movements will stop. But if the cat is in our lap wanting to sleep and we keep touching it in ways that keep it awake, the tail movements can become stronger, and may even develop into tail lashes. In the end, the cat may suddenly bite our hand, not hard, but as a warning. The cat has had enough and is telling us, 'Stop! Don't you understand that I want to sleep?'. This can be startling if we thought the cat was resting contentedly. From the cat's perspective, the cat asked us to stop when it was twitching its tail and we ignored the signal, so it gave a stronger signal.

Tail rub

Sometimes you can feel that the cat swings its tail against you, perhaps twisting it partly around your leg or cheek. The cat uses its tail to caress you. Occasionally, this friendly signal will be followed by rubbing its cheek against you. In addition to the visual signal, this behaviour can involve scent and touch signalling (see below). The cat usually gives such signals only to close social partners, so we must regard this behaviour as a statement of great trust and desire to maintain a close relationship with us.

Odour Language – Olfactory Communication

Like many mammals, cats use their sharp sense of smell to receive important messages. The odour language, or olfactory communication, involves production of specialized chemical signals, called *pheromones*, which are perceived by other cats and influence their behaviour. Whereas hormones convey chemical messages within the body, pheromones take chemical messages out into the environment where they can be detected by other cats. They can be delivered via urine, faeces, footprints, udder or by rubbing their head and body against objects. When odour molecules are sniffed by other cats, they attach to cells in the nose. From there, the signal is passed along nerves to the olfactory bulbs of the brain for processing. However, unlike us, cats also have a whole other system for processing pheromones, which we describe in the next section.

Urine marking

A cat can urinate in two ways: using the regular squatting posture or standing upright with elevated tail to send small squirts of urine straight backwards. The first method is for eliminating waste products from the body, and cats usually cover this urine. It is the second method that is mainly used for olfactory communication. It is termed *urine marking*, or *spraying*, and we notice it only too well when an intact tomcat has been urine marking. The strong odour comes from glands located by the urinary opening. The secretions from these glands are released into the urine stream during urine marking and in intact males, they have a particularly pungent odour. Urine marks are usually directed towards prominent vertical objects such as trees and walls, making it more likely that other cats will find them. While they can smell them from a distance through their nose, close-up investigation allows cats to use another odour-processing system to learn more about the cats who produced them.

One can see that after carefully sniffing another cat's urine mark, a cat will partially open its mouth, raise its head and lift its upper lip. This is called a *flehmen response*. The movement of lifting the lip causes two tiny ducts to open in the roof of the mouth, allowing the odour cocktail to enter a specialized organ called the *vomeronasal organ*. During flehmen, the cat may also flick its tongue to direct the odour into this organ. The vomeronasal organ contains nerve cells that transmit signals to the accessory olfactory bulbs of the brain. This part of the brain works like a chemical laboratory to process pheromones. Horses and cows have the same mechanism. However, while we may screw up our nose when we smell something unpleasant or breathe in deeply a pleasant smell, we do not have a functional vomeronasal organ.

Both males and females can urine mark and show flehmen, though these behaviours are more commonly seen in males. Tomcats often urine mark when they are courting a female cat in heat. Their urine has a high content of the amino acid felinin, a substance that smells strongly and is believed to signal the male's skill in finding high-quality food. Therefore, the urine marking behaviour is probably sending a message about how successful he is – the tomcat's way to boast to the females and convince them to mate with him. Males also show flehmen when sniffing the urine of females, which contains pheromones telling males when they are in heat. It is *not* common for males to urine mark or perform flehmen as part of a face-to-face confrontation with another male.

Faeces can also be used as a scent mark. Then cats deposit faeces in open places where the odour signal can spread well. When cats want to conceal their presence, they carefully cover both urine and faeces with soil or litter. If none is available, they may scrape the floor for an extended period in an unsuccessful attempt to bury the excreta.

In many animal species, individuals use olfactory communication to mark the boundaries of their territories, but in cats, urine marking acts more like a business card. Cats do not treat scent marks as territorial boundaries. By sniffing the mark and performing flehmen, the cat can identify *who* was there and how long ago the mark was deposited. The scent contains distinctive characteristics of the individual cat. While cats may still be able to detect a scent mark seven days later or even more, Jaap de Boer in Amsterdam showed that fresh urine marks deposited within the last four hours receive the most sniffing and flehmen responses. Because different substances in urine break down at different rates, the chemical composition of a mark changes over time, providing information about how long ago it was deposited.

Pheromones play an important role in the social system of cats. As soon as a cat goes outdoors, it will sniff around to check if other cats have been there. Then it will probably know both who and when, so the cat becomes updated about the cat traffic in its neighbourhood. In Chapter 5, on social behaviour, we shall see how cats use such knowledge in regulating their movements. Some insecure cats may even use urine marking in an attempt to attract an owner who has been away for a longer time than usual, though this is futile as well as being unwelcomed by people.

Scents from skin glands

Cats have many other ways to send olfactory signals besides urine marking. When they scratch on a post, they are depositing pheromones from glands between their toes, called interdigital glands (Fig. 4.9). Rubbing against objects such as poles, trees, chair legs or trousers results in transfer of pheromones from glands in the corner of their mouth, cheeks, mid-forehead and the root of the tail. Sweat glands around the teats of nursing mothers produce a pheromone that appears to have a calming effect on kittens. Synthetic versions of some cat pheromones can be used to calm down cats, which could be helpful when addressing problems with tension and conflict between cats in the household. (Read more about how to solve behaviour problems in Chapter 11.)

The composition of odours produced by the body is influenced by genetics and by diet. Therefore, closely-related cats and cats eating the same type of food have similarities in odours that cause them to seem somewhat familiar to each other even if they have never met before. They may be quicker to accept such cats as friends than other strangers that smell more different. In addition, cats learn to recognize the odours of the other members of their group and distinguish them from strangers. They pay particular attention to the scent marks of unfamiliar cats, especially intact males, presumably attempting to learn as much as possible about them before encountering them face-to-face. When two cats first meet and eventually dare to approach each other, they want to sniff each other, first at the mouth, then the cheek, body and back. Sniffing the hindquarters is often not allowed, as it feels unsafe to have a stranger behind them. The smell of close group members often seems comforting to cats. This may explain why they love lying on clothes that belong to their owner, especially when the owner is out.

There is still much we don't yet know about cats' scent language. As we do not distinguish the differences between their scents in the sophisticated way that they can, it is not easy to investigate this topic. We do not know if the different glands around the head give the same signal, or if rubbing the cheek sends a different signal to rubbing other parts of the body. Cats often deposit scents from several glands in succession, such as when rubbing with their mouth, cheeks, head and tail, and some suggest that they just use the most accessible part of the body for scent marks from skin glands. This would imply that the information is more-or-less the same: 'This is how I smell'. However, the cheek glands alone may include several components, each with a slightly different meaning.

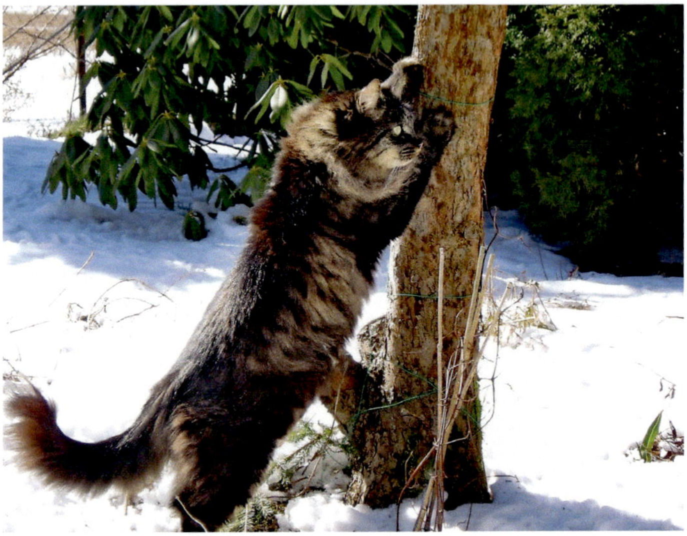

Fig. 4.9. When a cat scratches with its claws, it deposits pheromones from glands between the toes. (Photo: Nina Svendsrud, 2019)

Touch Language – Tactile Communication

When a cat rubs itself against another cat or person, touch language is involved. This is called *tactile communication* by ethologists. Among cats, rubbing is probably a means of ingratiating themselves with other cats. Kittens rub more against adult cats than *vice versa*, and female cats rub more against male cats than *vice versa*. They are saying: 'Be nice! I want to be with you'. When a cat rubs against us and we respond by gently stroking it, we are accepting the invitation. Through this tactile contact, both parties are depositing scent on each other. The mixture of individual scents shared between group members creates a familiar group scent that cats perceive as showing that they belong together.

Another important form of touch comes through *social licking*. In contrast to rubbing, it is usually a more dominant cat that directs licking towards a more subordinate one. Licking signals care. When the mother cat returns from a hunting trip, she informs her kittens of her presence. If the kittens are younger than five days and the ear canals are not yet open, she cannot give them *mhrn* or miaow sounds even if the kittens give distress calls, *miiiy*, because they are cold or hungry. The queen licks the kittens before lying down to nurse them. They associate this licking with milk and comfort as the queen also grooms them while nursing, and they quickly settle down to suckle. Similarly, if a cat hesitates to accept the food we offer, it is more likely to start eating if we gently stroke it. We can avoid interrupting the feeding session by only continuing the stroking for a short while as it eats, before slowly withdrawing our hand. In this way, we use the touch language of cats to achieve our goal.

Communicating with Cats

In the sections above, we have pointed out several cases where we can use our knowledge of cat signals to communicate with cats in their own language. We must consider the message we want to give and ask ourselves how the cat would convey the same message. We can call our cat with a *mhrn* or miaow, increasing the pitch at the end. We can 'smile' with half-closed eyes and accept its presence with gentle stroking. Of course, we cannot have detailed conversations with cats using human words. Nevertheless, cats can learn to understand specific words, such as their name. They can learn how we want them to respond when we give a specific signal as long as we train them appropriately, as we explain in Chapters 10 and 11.

When we encounter an unfamiliar cat with whom we wish to make contact, we should not just go straight up to it and touch it. Many cats will perceive this as a threatening situation and run away. You must first *greet* the cat and announce that you have no aggressive intentions. Sit down to get closer to the cat's height, slowly extend a paw (hand) towards the cat and let the cat sniff it while you talk with a welcoming sound that goes up in pitch at the end (see Fig. 4.10). If the cat shows

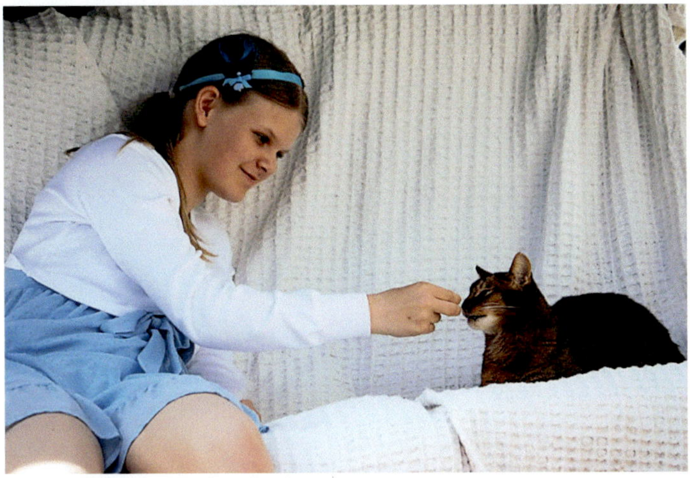

Fig. 4.10. Initiate contact with a cat by letting it sniff your hand. (Photo: Gry Løberg, 2019)

defensive signals, be particularly patient. Let the cat approach you when it feels safe enough to do so. Then you can stroke it gently on the cheek (Fig. 4.11), on the head and eventually on the flank, but avoid its back and hindquarters until it knows you better.

When looking at a cat's eyes, it is not only the size of the pupils that can provide useful information;

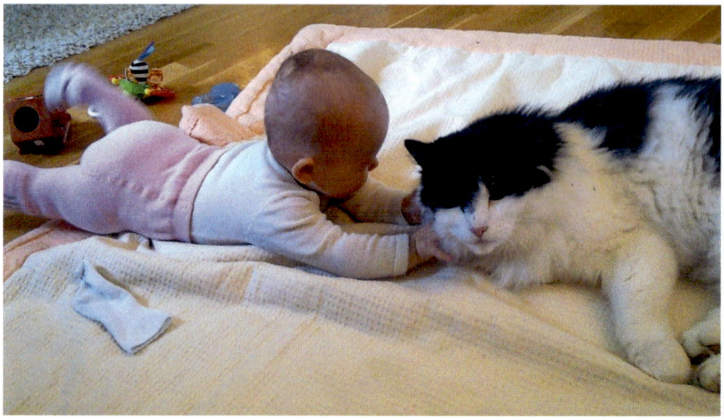

Fig. 4.11. Then you can gently stroke the cat on its cheek. This baby has already understood this. (Photo: Agnethe-Irén Sandem, 2019)

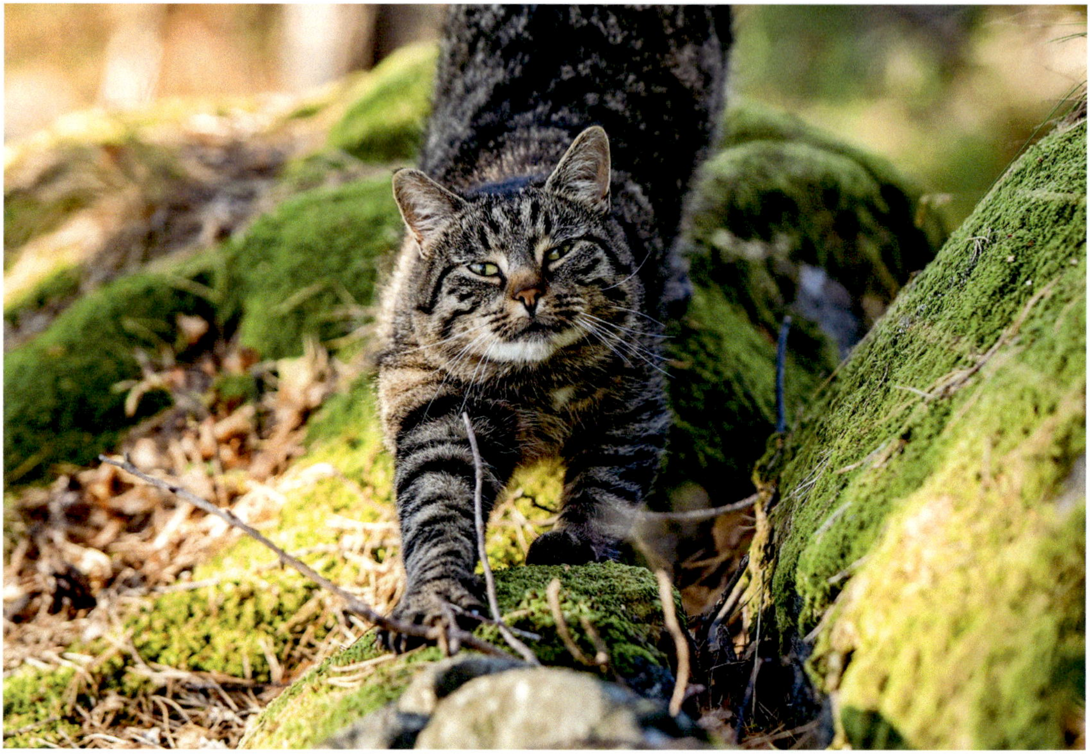

Fig. 4.12. When a cat approaches you with half-closed eyes, you can rest assured that it has good intentions. (Photo: Audun Braastad, 2019)

the position of the eyelids is also important. If a cat stares at you with wide-open eyes, its head slightly lowered and back slightly arched, it is sending you a threat signal. This means 'Do not try something stupid or you'll be in trouble'. Half-closed eyes, on the other hand, send a friendly signal showing that the cat accepts your close presence (Fig. 4.12). Therefore, when you meet an unfamiliar cat, it is important not to stare. First, look slowly away from the cat before turning your gaze back towards its face. While doing this, close your eyes halfway before making eye contact. When you are looking at each other, blink your eyes repeatedly but slowly; keep your eyes shut for a second each time and only half open your eyes between every blink, sometimes moving your gaze away to the side. If the cat responds with the same eye signal, it has calmed down and accepted your presence. Now you can go one step further and offer your hand for sniffing.

The *blink signal* can be used when talking to your own cat as well. It will help strengthen the bond between you. You can use this signal, blinking markedly a few times, if your cat becomes anxious for some reason, for example due to sudden loud sounds or lightning. It will serve as a calming signal and show the cat that you do not detect any danger. This can work well with other animal species, too, such as dogs and cattle.

Bjarne has observed that both his previous cat and the present one seem to react instinctively to a smooth whistle tone of around 440 Hz (an A note in music). As he calmly gives a long whistle at this pitch, the cat stands up and approaches him as if in a trance. It seems to be a calling signal. Perhaps the kitten's *miio* to attract its mother is most effective if it has a fundamental tone around A, possibly with higher octaves. You can try this on your cat. You may need to vary the tone somewhat, as the optimal pitch may vary between cats.

If we provide signals that our cat does not understand, we have not communicated with the cat. All too often, animal owners scold their cat or provide other signals that are not recognized by the cat. The result is a confused or insecure cat. To signal to a cat that a particular behaviour is unacceptable, we must use the principles of proximity in time and space during training. Our reaction must come immediately after the cat's unacceptable behaviour, and the cat must still be in the same place. The cat can then make the connection between its behaviour and our reaction. If the cat has defecated on the carpet in the living room and you come home an hour later and scold the cat as it approaches you to greet you, you will be punishing the cat's approach and not its actions an hour previously. Your cat may interpret your behaviour as social rejection. Is it strange that the cat then gets confused? However, it is better not to punish your cat as this is not a very effective training method and places your social relationship at risk. You will learn more about this in Chapter 10.

Further Reading

Leyhausen, P. (1979) *Cat Behavior: The Predatory and Social Behavior of Domestic and Wild Cats*. Garland STPM Press, New York.

McComb, K., Taylor, A.M., Wilson, C. and Charlton, B.D. (2009) The cry embedded within the purr. *Current Biology* 13, R507–R508. DOI: 10.1016/j.cub.2009.05.033.

Moelk, M. (1944) Vocalizing in the house-cat: a phonetic and functional study. *American Journal of Psychology* 57, 184–205.

Supplementary materials entitled 'What does the miaow mean' and 'The cat's body language' can be accessed at: www.cabi.org/the-cat-behaviour-and-welfare/

5 Social Behaviour of Cats

It is a common belief that the dog is a social animal while the cat is an unsocial, selfish animal that prefers to walk on its own. This is only partially correct and applies best to wild-living cats in areas with a low-density cat population. If cats were unable to live socially, they would not be successful as companion animals. In fact, all animals are selfish to some extent. When they co-operate in a group, it is because the benefits they receive outweigh the costs. This chapter considers how cats can live in a community of cats – outdoors or in the home. The English ethologist David W. Macdonald and co-workers have conducted a particularly nice, long-term study of cats living in social groups in the English countryside. Both this and other research helps us to understand how owned cats respond to others they meet outdoors and how it is possible to have more than one cat in the same household without frequent aggression between them. In Chapter 12, you will learn how cats adapt to a social life with people to the benefit of both parties.

Basics of Social Behaviour

We must first explain three ethological concepts: territory, home range and personal space, to better understand the dynamics of cat social behaviour. These terms apply to animals in general, including cats.

Territory

Some animals establish and live within a territory. A territory is an area used almost exclusively by a particular animal or social group and defended against intruders of the same species. The territory contains all the necessary resources for living, such as food and water, and safe locations for resting and giving birth to offspring. Territories usually don't overlap, and territory holders regularly patrol their territorial boundaries to check that no intruders are trespassing or watch their territory from a lookout (Fig. 5.1). They may also deposit scent marks along the boundaries warning others to stay out. A territory is vigorously defended, and any foreigners who enter the territory are chased away. Territory holders usually succeed in this defence. They have the most to lose and are familiar with the area, which boosts their self-confidence. Confidence declines with increasing distance from their own territory and great boldness is needed to enter the territory of another.

Cats can be territorial, but they do not generally defend the whole area in which they roam or specifically mark territorial boundaries. Instead, they deposit scent marks in places they habitually use, such as urination and defecation sites, sleeping sites and along pathways (see Chapter 4). In areas with a low cat population, free-roaming cats sometimes have non-overlapping living areas, which do not need to be defended as territories. In areas with a higher density of cats, the residents may defend a small territory but share more peripheral hunting grounds with others. At even higher densities, they tolerate the presence of others throughout their living area but may defend specific resources such as a food bowl or nest site. This is called *local resource defence*. Intact, free-roaming tomcats move over larger distances than do females, covering an area that can include the living areas of multiple females. They may defend a small territory during winter but spend too much time away to defend one during the breeding season. Then, they engage in local resource defence, with the resource in this case being females in heat.

Home range

A home range is the total area used by an animal over the course of an entire year, regardless of whether it is a defended area or not. For owned cats that are allowed outdoors, this is not just their owner's home but also includes the whole outdoor

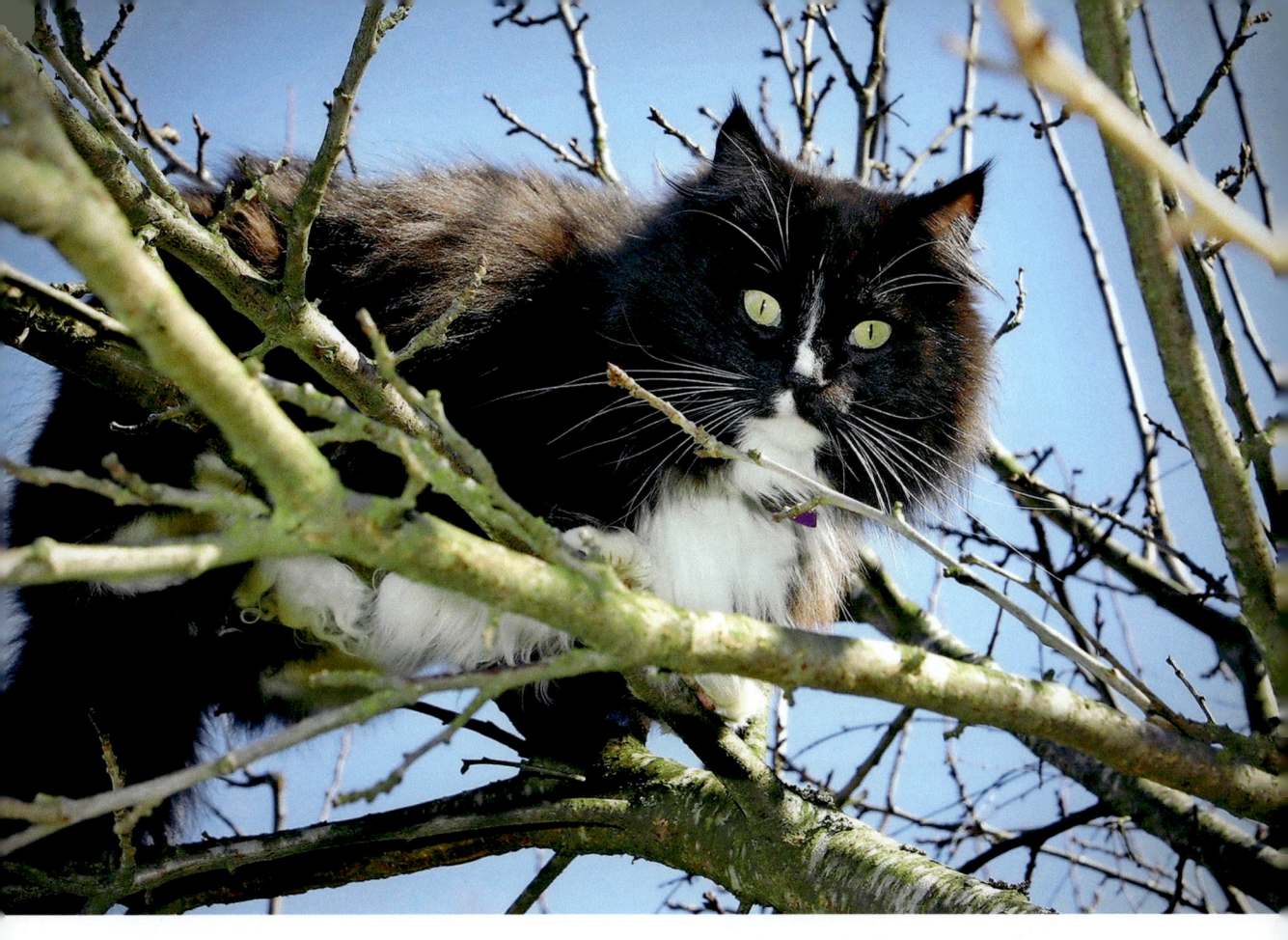

Fig. 5.1. Up in the tree, Rampoline has a good view over her territory. (Photo: Audun Braastad, 2019)

area over which they roam. For cats that share parts of their home range, the home range is larger than their territory. Cats that only show local resource defence have a home range without a territory; that is, they defend resources in their immediate vicinity such as the food they are eating or the place where they are currently resting.

Rather than being a particular shape or size, a cat's home range may be a somewhat fragmented space, including areas that are used only during part of the year. For example, tomcats with outdoor access will use more of their home range during the breeding season than in winter. In contrast, in the first few weeks after giving birth, a mother cat will use less of her home range as she needs to return to the nest regularly and frequently to nurse the kittens. An outdoor cat's home range contains a network of trails leading to good hunting areas and several safe resting spots. Cats do not always go back to a single location to rest. It is more efficient to rest near where they are currently hunting. Even mother cats take naps away from their kittens, especially once the kittens are a few weeks old. An owned cat probably does not imagine that its owner is becoming worried when its return to the house is delayed because it decided to stop for a nap.

The core area of a home range is the area where an animal spends the most time, what we might consider 'home'. This is the area most likely to be defended as a territory. For breeding females, this area is centred on the concealed nest site where they keep their kittens. The core area will usually include concealed resting places, areas with loose soil or litter used for elimination, safe places to sunbathe, lookouts for monitoring the surrounding area and access to some food and water. Cats living in social groups have overlapping home ranges with a common group core area that they may defend from non-group members. For owned cats, the apartment or house and garden is their core area, shared with humans and any other cats in the household.

Social Behaviour of Cats

Personal space

Most animals prefer to maintain a certain minimum distance from other individuals, termed an *inter-individual distance*. This results in a *personal space* around the individual, often oval in shape and largest in front of the head. The personal space is like a mobile mini-territory around the animal. If another enters this personal space, the individual will feel uncomfortable and may retreat or threaten the other, thereby freeing up this buffer zone. In humans, this space is typically about 0.5–1 metre, explaining why many do not feel comfortable close to strangers on a crowded train or bus. In cats, a confident individual is likely to send threatening signals on the close approach of an intruder, causing the intruder to steer clear, whereas an anxious individual would rather move away itself than risk conflict. If kept in a confined area where they are unable to regulate the distance between them, cats may live in a state of heightened social stress.

A personal space does not have fixed dimensions. Its size depends heavily on who is nearby and what they are doing. With social partners and offspring, the inter-individual distance may well be zero when resting without causing any problem. Cats who do not have a particularly close relationship with another cat or a person prefer to stay at least 1–3 metres away. They may attack by leaping upon another cat or your hand if it comes closer than this. When hunting outdoors, a cat will usually keep many metres away from unfamiliar cats, not only avoiding direct attacks but also avoiding threat signals. In a multi-cat house with cats that tolerate each other but who are not best friends, the cats are usually careful to maintain an inter-individual distance of at least one metre.

Do cats prefer a single or a social life?

The biologist and author Desmond Morris once stated: 'A lonely dog is a miserable, unhappy creature. A lonely cat is often just relieved to be left in peace.' This implies that adult cats prefer a solitary life over group living. In fact, for free-living cats, the local ecological conditions are crucial in influencing which option a cat chooses. In areas with a high population density of cats and variability in the distribution of prey – that is, having some areas with an abundance of prey and other areas where prey animals are scarce – cats are likely to be found living with others in a social group. The group can collaborate on maintaining a common group territory and keeping other cats away from their rich hunting areas. David Macdonald showed that such group-living cats tend to be healthier than the solitary cats that are excluded from such areas and forced to live in marginal areas with limited food. On the other hand, if the density of cats is low and they are hunting small prey that are relatively evenly spread out, most cats prefer to live apart from other adult cats. In dense urban environments containing many cats, they hardly have a choice. They must try to adapt to the close proximity of other cats. Flexibility is a keyword for cat social behaviour.

When people feed a cat and provide it with a place to live, the cat may settle down and establish social contact with the people living in the household. If socialized to people as a kitten, it will continue to seek care from people in adulthood. When let outdoors, however, the cat will behave similarly to free-living cats.

Traffic-handling among cats

When a well-fed owned cat uses an outdoor area where cats from neighbouring households are present, their scent marks regulate the 'cat traffic'. These do not prevent others from using the same area but minimize face-to-face encounters. Cats can be quite careful to avoid each other, and they use both sight and smell to check when the coast is clear. Since the scent marks inform them about who was at a certain place and how long ago (see Chapter 4), they can establish a kind of shift schedule for the use of a popular area. If Jasper finds that Oliver typically hunts in a particular area in the early morning, Jasper may hunt there in the evening. If Luna finds that Bella uses a particular resting place in the afternoon, she can use the same place in the morning. In this way, they avoid conflict. This is the cat form of a shared economy.

If two cats should find themselves walking towards each other along the same path, it is normal for one to sit down and wait for the other to pass. There is no reason to attack another that makes no threat. If two more competitive cats meet, maybe at short distance, they do not fight for the right to use the path but instead sit down and threaten each other by staring. Eventually one will give up and carefully take a different direction. Perhaps it is safest to return from whence it came.

Indoors, it is common for group-living cats to respect each other's first right to a particular place. If a cat arrives first at a food bowl and there is no room for additional cats, a latecomer is likely to wait until the first one has finished eating. If a cat has occupied a resting place, another cat will usually not chase it away but, instead, find another place to sleep. This 'courtesy' depends upon the cats perceiving that resources are plentiful and that they can get enough of what they want (see Chapter 11).

Rank order

The social system that these 'traffic rules' reveal has been termed a *relative hierarchy* because an animal's social rank is influenced by time and place. This concept was developed in the early 1950s by the famous cat ethologist Paul Leyhausen. A cat can be said to have a higher relative rank the closer it is to its core area, where it feels more confident and determined to stay. If a cat meets another somewhere else during the time of day when it habitually uses that area, this also adds to its confidence, and it is more likely to prevail in a staring competition.

An *absolute hierarchy*, on the other hand, follows the well-known peck order described in the 1920s by the Norwegian biologist Thorleif Schjelderup-Ebbe, based on his studies of the social behaviour of domestic chickens. An absolute rank order applies regardless of time and place, and determines who has priority of access to resources based on the relative competitive ability of each individual. A hierarchy emerges within a group based on the dominance relationship between each animal and each other animal in the group. One individual dominates another individual, which typically dominates a third, and so on, in what is called a linear rank order. It may also occur that this third individual in fact dominates the first one, and this is an example of a triangular ranking.

To a certain extent, dominance relationships between cats are decided based on body size, which is in turn influenced by age and sex. If body sizes are very different, the difference in competitive ability is obvious and there is no need for a competition to decide who is dominant. Thus, adult males will usually have a higher rank than adult females based on their larger body size. It is the individuals who are close to each other in apparent competitive ability that show the most conflict with each other. Once the ranks have been settled, though, it is rare for them to change.

Leyhausen found that it is particularly in very dense populations of adult cats that an absolute hierarchy can emerge. There may be too many cats for social regulation based solely on relative ranks. More dominant cats regularly exhibit threatening signals that remind others of their priority of access to resources. This can happen in laboratory colonies of cats or when there are many cats in a household. A simple type of absolute rank order can be seen within litters of kittens, where certain kittens have priority of access to the milkiest teats. These

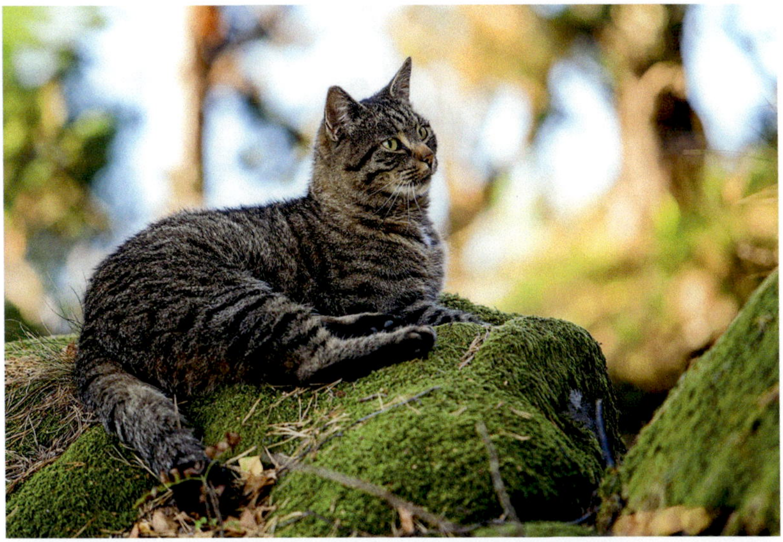

Fig. 5.2. At this time of the day, this is my resting place. (Photo: Audun Braastad, 2019)

kittens were perhaps the biggest and boldest at birth, and with access to the best teats they grow faster. This is also termed a *teat order*.

Since female and male cats mostly live separately in nature, we shall describe their social behaviour separately.

The Female Cat's Social Behaviour

Adult females can have a home range varying in size from a quarter of an acre to about 500 acres (2 km^2). Food availability plays the main role in determining the size of the area needed by an adult female cat. When nursing kittens, this is especially important. As the kittens grow bigger and demand more milk, she will need to find two or three times as much food as usual. It is common that the female's home range overlaps with others, even though she is not living in a group. This is particularly true in an area rich in small prey scattered in unpredictable locations where it is not practical to defend the whole area from intrusions by others.

A female cat living singly can be quite territorial; that is, defending her territory against other cats of both sexes. But when she is in heat, she may tolerate males nearby. She is most aggressive towards other cats when she has kittens. This is partly due to the need to defend her kittens and partly to the need for a larger hunting area when nursing her increasingly demanding growing kittens.

Cats living in groups

The density of cats living outdoors can range from less than 300 m^2 to over 1 km^2 per cat. This variation results in differences in social organization. The prerequisite for cats to be able to form a social group is a concentrated food source. This is often associated with human activity – people feeding free-roaming cats, cats exploiting landfill or rubbish bins, and cats on farms where they find an abundance of small rodents or steal food intended for the farm animals. Mink farms are popular with cats, as the nutritional needs of mink and cats are very similar.

An accumulation of cats in one area does not always constitute a social group. Instead, it is possible to talk about a colony of cats that stays in the same place for the same reason, but without real co-operation. In such cases, this is considered an *aggregation* of single cats rather than a social group. Such cats frequently snarl if they get too close to one another while dining on scavenged food.

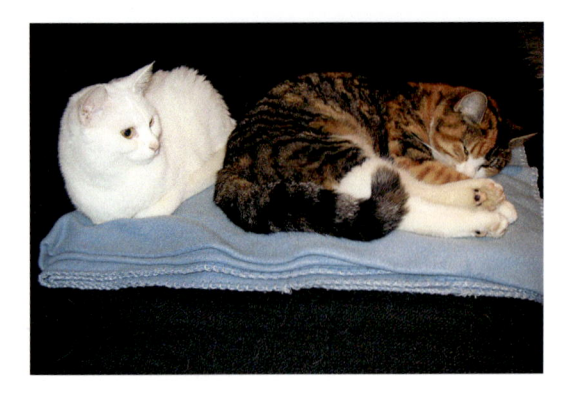

Fig. 5.3. Isis and Moshe, two female cats living together without social conflict. (Photo: Janne Helen Lorentzsen, 2019)

The most basic social unit in cats is a female cat with her offspring. This is termed a *core group*. It does not include the father of the kittens, who may be far away and the father of offspring in several such core groups. Larger social groups of cats usually consist of several female cats with their offspring, that is several core groups. The adult female group members are called *central females*. Such groups can include juvenile daughters and sons of the adult females in the group. In addition, a few adult tomcats may be associated with the group. These have contact with the adult females especially when mating during the breeding season, but otherwise stay on their own. Usually, these males are not closely related to the adult females, as adult males emigrate away from the area where they were born, a mechanism that reduces the likelihood of inbreeding. There are rarely more than ten individuals in a social group, but groups of more than 50 cats may occur if there is a large enough, predictable food supply, as reported by Macdonald and colleagues in England. In other regions, colonies with several dozen free-living cats are found in cities with large populations of homeless cats.

The central females of a social group may attack intruders of both sexes. Apart from this central group and their young offspring, other females and males live alone. These are called *peripheral cats* when living on the periphery of a social group, usually under harsher living conditions. Peripheral cats may, nevertheless, hunt for prey within the core area used by cats in the social group, so this is not a watertight territory where intruders are completely shut out. The social dynamics can vary widely between such groups, related to the group size, ecological factors and personality characteristics of the individuals within the group. Small colonies of cats in the countryside can consist of two or three core groups, where the cats have more contact with those within their own core group than with cats from other core groups.

Collaboration on kitten care

Females living in a social group can be very friendly towards one another. In naturally forming groups, they have usually remained in the group from birth, and rarely move over to another group. Since they hunt alone, their home range sizes can differ, but the group has a common core area where they give birth to kittens and where their main food sources can be found. Here they can have a common nest and help each other with the care of the kittens. They tend to have synchronized heat cycles and give birth around the same time, and their kittens may have the same father or fathers. David Macdonald has observed that a female cat can help another female by biting the umbilical cord of a newborn kitten. It is not unusual for them to nurse each other's kittens. This is called *communal nursing*. Sometimes a female brings prey to another nursing cat. Nevertheless, the females regularly stay closer to their own kittens than to those of the other cats. It appears that they recognize and preferentially care for their own offspring.

Female cats living in social groups can produce larger litter sizes than solitary females. In Macdonald's study of a large colony of farm cats, females that co-operated in kitten care and joined forces to defend food resources had lower offspring mortality than those living alone. Communal nursing is a type of *helper system*, or what we could call *aunting behaviour* among humans. The females in cat social groups are usually closely related – mothers, daughters, sisters and half-sisters, and perhaps grandmothers. Therefore, in evolutionary terms, such helping also benefits those who help. Genetically, a female cat is 50% related to her full sister or mother and 25% related to her half-sister. If she helps her full sister to produce two more weaned offspring than she would have been able raise by herself, the helper will have contributed as many of her own genes to the next generation as if she had weaned one kitten herself. This phenomenon is termed *kin selection* and is thought to play an important role in the evolution of social behaviour.

The Male Cat's Social Behaviour

The home ranges of intact male cats are, on average, 3.5 times larger than those of females. In extreme cases they can reach up to 2000 acres, or 8 km^2. More commonly, a male's rural home range area is 2–3 km^2. The males obviously do not need such a large area to catch food. The reason for roaming over such a large area is the tomcat's urge to seek out females in heat. Therefore, a tomcat's home range often overlaps with the core areas of several females. At the same time, this means that they also overlap with the home ranges of other males. Outside the mating season, however, the overlap can be small. High-ranking tomcats usually have larger home ranges than males with lower ranks, probably because they can roam more freely without being threatened by other males. In more densely populated areas, both females and males have smaller home ranges. These cats usually receive food from humans, and uncastrated males can have good access to fertile females nearby. However, when many female cats are spayed or kept indoors, it becomes harder for tomcats to find females accessible for mating.

When male cats quarrel

Kittens are usually tolerated by adult males. When young males reach around 10–12 months of age, older males can invite them to battle using special call sounds. Initially, the fights are trivial and usually playful. Only in the second year of life does male rivalry become more serious. Then the young tomcat must show his competitive ability. After sniffing each other, both males show aggressive signals, where the body posture, ear position and sounds inform the other one how bold he is currently feeling. Sometimes it seems that the competition is all about making the largest yowling noise. If two males are quite evenly matched and neither exhibits pronounced defensive signals, there may eventually be a fight. This is a last resort, however. The cats can easily incur bad bite injuries, and they try to win the contest using offensive threat signals. Therefore, we should put up with the loud sounds of competing tomcats that wake us from our nightly slumber during early spring.

When one of the males finally accepts the dominance of the other, he will show his defensive attitude by crouching down, hissing and maybe lifting his paw if the opponent gets too close. Cats do not show submission like dogs, exposing their vulnerable neck or belly. As noted in Chapter 4, a defensive cat informs his opponent that he will defend himself if attacked. Usually, the dominant male will accept such signals and end the dispute. At subsequent meetings, the conflicts will become shorter. Both now, and later, the dominant male will urine mark, and scratch and rub against tree trunks and other prominent objects. These actions send visual signals of dominance, and the scent marks provide a reminder.

Among lions, a small coalition of adult males lives together with the lionesses and their offspring continuously until, after a few years, they are chased away by a new coalition of younger, stronger male lions. The main difference in free-living cats is that males generally live alone rather than within the female group. Unlike lions, they do not need to co-operate during hunting because their prey is much smaller and can be caught by a single individual. We shall say more about this in Chapter 6. They also do not need to co-operate to gain access to females. Not surprisingly, then, tomcats do not appear to form co-operative alliances. In dense populations, adult males are rarely friendly towards one another. However, where they live more spaced out, adult males that have clarified their dominance relationships can coexist peacefully and share overlapping home ranges. The most dominant males are rarely tyrants, although bullying may occasionally occur depending on the individual personalities involved.

What is the function of conflicts between males?

The most aggressive tomcat rarely has priority of access to important resources such as food and mating of females. Males can be surprisingly tolerant of one another. A cat that eats is rarely disturbed by a more dominant cat. The last one waits his turn, at least so long as there is enough food for all. In the same way, the 'first come, first served' rule may apply to popular resting places as well as to the opportunity to mate with a female cat. The latter is more likely in larger than smaller cat colonies. In larger colonies it is too difficult for one dominant male to chase away all other males. The queuing system means several males can mate with the same female, and she can give birth to a litter where the kittens have different fathers. Since all these males can be fathers, this probably reduces the risk of infanticide of young kittens by males, unlike in lions.

In small colonies, it is not unusual for one tomcat to be the father of almost all kittens born. In this case, a dominant tomcat manages to threaten other males to stay at a good distance from female cats in heat. However, the female cat herself decides whether she wants to mate with a particular male or not. She will not necessarily accept the most dominant male cat. As with some other mammals, and birds, if you had excellent reproductive success during the last season, why take the risk of substituting your partner? 'Never change a winning team' can be a good rule for animals, too. Bjarne has even known a wonderful and huge male cat that was rather lazy and not very interested in courting females. Instead, the females were queuing up to solicit his attention.

Perhaps the most important reason why male cats fight is related to the struggle for access to a habitat rich in food resources. A young male cat who is clearly lower-ranking than his neighbours will often emigrate from the area and settle in a less favourable area, with less food and few females. Here he can live in relative peace until he becomes older and stronger, and more likely to succeed in competition with other males. This may be the reason why some two- to three-year-old males suddenly disappear from home (see Chapter 7). Even though they have had a good relationship with their owners, competition from other males encountered in the neighbourhood may have led them to seek a new living area. At this age, it is natural for male cats to leave the social group of their mother. Biologically, this is an important mechanism for preventing inbreeding.

The male cat can be a good father

It is a common belief that male cats may be dangerous to small kittens. Occasionally, a tomcat may kill kittens he comes across. Perhaps he considers them as regular prey. In lions, males can kill cubs that are not their own offspring, leading the lionesses to come into heat more quickly. The males can then mate with these lionesses and father offspring themselves. It is possible that such a reproduction strategy may also be found in some domestic cats, but it appears to be rare.

In Norway, there are many stories about male cats who gave care to kittens. In Trondheim, a large male cat carried, in his mouth, a kitten that had

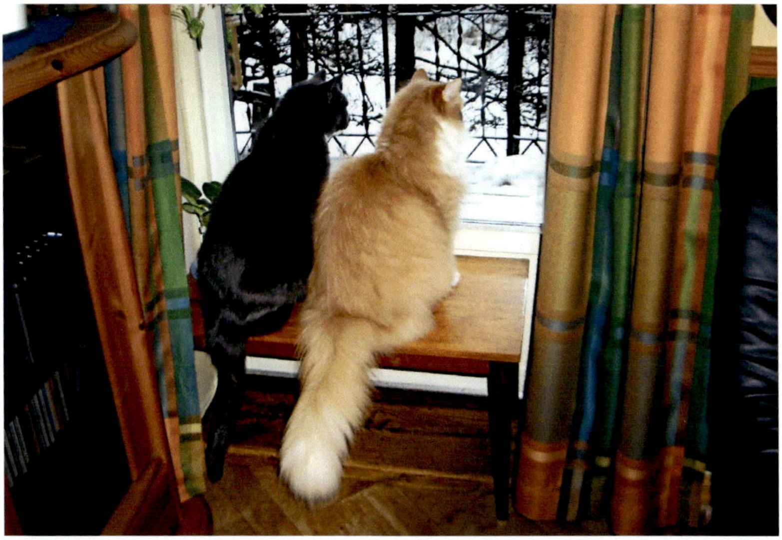

Fig. 5.4. Two male cats can get along well together as long as they are not competing for female cats in heat. (Photo: Leif Aslaksen, 2019)

been hit by a car. Unfortunately, the kitten had to be euthanized, but the male did what he could. In another case in Trondheim, a homeless female cat was shot. Her young kittens, who were born outdoors, were fed by a tomcat. He collected food and brought it to the kittens. At Nes, in Hedmark county, on the farm where Bjarne was born, a female died some weeks after giving birth to kittens in the barn. The resident tomcat, who might have been their father, carried the kittens, one by one, from the barn into the kitchen of the farmhouse. He knew that food was available there. Another story from Trondheim is about a cat family where the cat mother and her offspring were killed. It turned out that one of the kittens had escaped and was hiding outdoors. The tomcat took food in his mouth and ran outdoors, where he was thought to be giving it to the kitten. Eventually the kitten became so sick and cold that she entered the house. Here she was cared for and cleaned by the tomcat. It was thought that the tomcat was probably the kitten's father. Much later, when the kitten had her own kittens in a completely different home, far away, one of the kittens looked very similar to this male, suggesting that he was the kitten's grandfather.

In the 1980s, in the research cattery of the University of Trondheim, Bjarne saw that some male cats were particularly adept at taking care of kittens. After the kittens were weaned and separated from their mothers, they were placed in a separate room. Here an old male was used as a 'kindergarten teacher'. He carefully licked the kittens, and it was obvious that they appreciated his presence.

Such stories indicate that there are relicts of paternal instinct in domestic cats. This is another sign of their descent from the African wildcat, *Felis lybica* (see Chapter 1). In this species, the male and female sometimes live together in monogamy. In such cases, the female is probably dependent on the male helping her to provide enough food to raise kittens in the barren semi-deserts where they live.

Castrated male cats

A high rate of neutering is practised in many countries. For example, in Norway, about 85% of owned male cats are castrated, or sometimes chemically sterilized, especially those living in densely populated areas. These males do not have the same motivation to compete with others as seen in intact males. Rather, they may live in social groups with females and other castrated males and, like females, co-operate to chase away intruders from the group's core area. When a castrated male seems to be bolder within its territory than elsewhere, this he a sign that he has more to defend in that area.

Social Behaviour of Cats

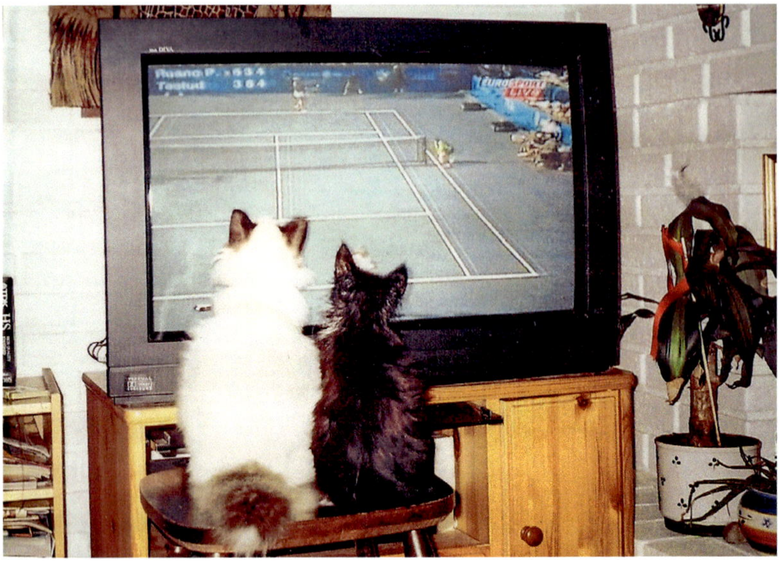

Fig. 5.5. Two cats with a common interest. (Photo: Bjarne O. Braastad, 2003)

Multiple Cats in the Same Residence

Many people are unsure whether it is possible to have two cats in an apartment, especially if they have one cat already and now would like an additional cat. Will they become comrades or feud for evermore? There are large individual differences in social behaviour among cats. This has a lot to do with the personalities of the different cats, and whether they will be compatible can be unpredictable. A cat may accept one newcomer but be aggressive towards another. Often, it is more successful to keep a female and a male together rather than two females, unless the females are closely related (e.g. sisters or mother and daughter) or the newcomer is a kitten. In an American study of 60 homes with two neutered indoor cats, two male cats were closer to each other, on average, than two females or one female and one male. Aggression between the cats was most frequent during the first two years and became less frequent the longer the cats lived together. Another study indicated that, in half of the cases, the newcomer was accepted before one month has passed. In England, the ethologist John Bradshaw showed that two adult cats from the same litter spent more time together than two cats from different litters did. Littermates more often ate together and groomed each other's fur. If you wish to have two cats, it is therefore a good idea to obtain two from the same litter.

People with four cats in their household often believe that they have one social group consisting of four cats. They might instead have four cats that would rather live alone. In such cases, the cats must establish a kind of balance of power, staying by themselves and finding ways to avoid provoking the other cats. However, many people have multiple cats living together in harmony. Like in nature, the most important means for achieving this is that the cats do not have to compete for resources. There must be enough food for everyone, with a separate food bowl and litter tray for each cat, and possibly extra ones. There must be plenty of resting places. Finally, yet importantly, each cat must get the same amount of friendly contact and petting by people in the household.

It is difficult to predict the outcome when introducing a new cat. The easiest advice is just to try. If you are unsure how it will be received by your existing cat, ask for a two- to four-week trial period from the seller with the option to return the cat if the introduction is unsuccessful. A person who is selling or giving away a cat should take an interest in ensuring that it will thrive in its new home.

When the new cat arrives it is normal that the two cats will initially want to stay apart. The existing cat has something to defend and is likely to

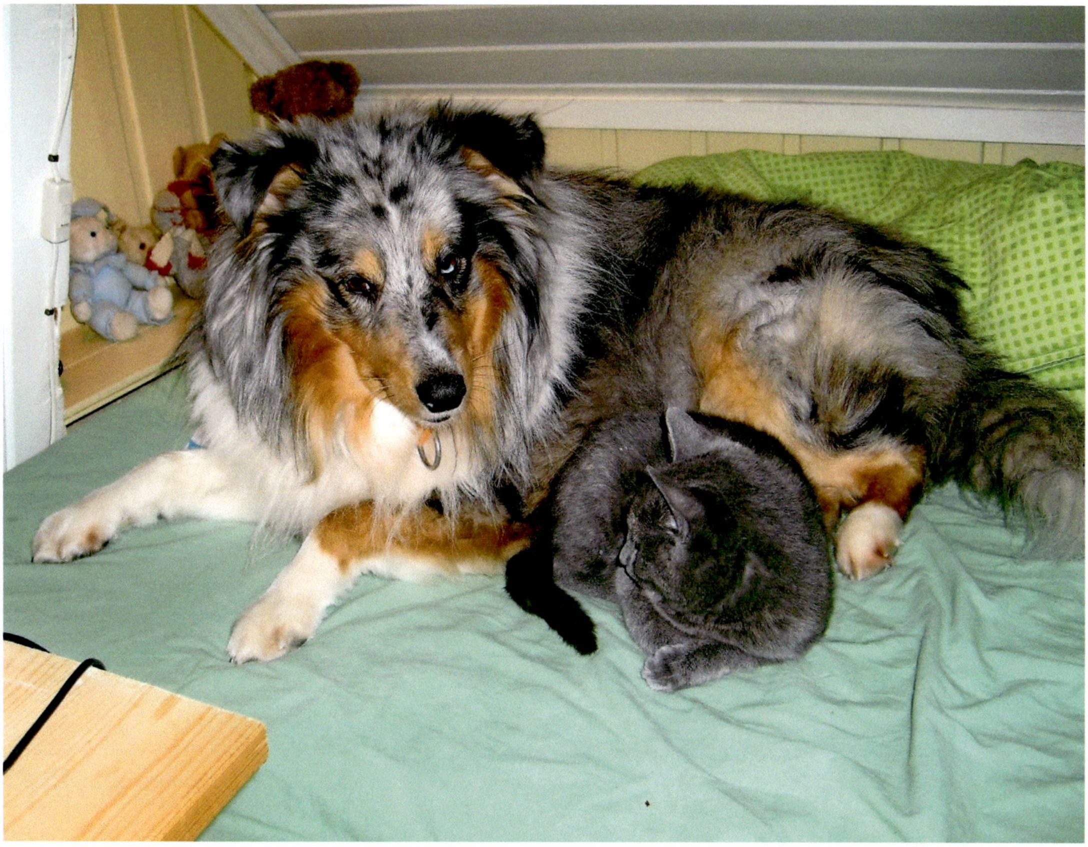

Fig. 5.6. A dog and a cat, like Amigo and Molly, may get along well together. (Photo: Kjersti Teig, 2019)

hiss at the intruder if it comes too close. The newcomer feels insecure in the unfamiliar environment. It is best to keep the newcomer in a separate room (such as the bathroom) for the first few days. Once it is relaxed in that room, eating well and willing to play with you, you can open the door. By then, the existing cat has also got more used to the smell and sound of the new one. Leave the new cat's food bowl and litterbox in the original room (the bathroom in this example) for another week or more until both cats are comfortable being together in the same room. Do not expect them to become friends in the first two weeks, even if some cats become friendly more quickly. Make sure that there are separate places for them to retreat to. Do not force them to come closer together than they are comfortable with. Playing with each cat using a toy dangling from a wand may be helpful in placing both in a playful mood and encouraging them to come closer to each other. Eventually, the cats should accept each other, but it takes time, so be patient. They may never do so completely. In that case, the best you can hope for is that they will respect each other without frequent threats or fights, or one always feeling it must run away if the other is around. If they share space through mutual avoidance, this is often acceptable to the cat owner.

A Cat and Dog Together

Many people find it easy to have both cats and dogs (Fig. 5.6). The Israeli ethologists Feuerstein and Terkel examined this systematically in 2007, with behavioural observations on dogs and cats kept together in 170 homes, and questionnaire responses from the owners. They concluded that both animal species were equally inclined to enter into a friendly relationship. This is easiest to achieve if you get the cat before the dog, so that the cat has the psychological advantage of established residence before the arrival of the, probably larger, dog. It is advantageous if the cat is younger than six months and the dog is younger than one year when they meet for the first time. The researchers found that dogs and cats living together largely understood each other. The younger they are when they first meet, the easier they will learn to understand each other's body language and avoid misunderstandings. Further advice on introducing cats and dogs is given in Chapter 2.

Further Reading

Feuerstein, N. and Terkel, J. (2008) Interrelationships of dogs (*Canis familiaris*) and cats (*Felis catus* L.) living under the same roof. *Applied Animal Behaviour Science* 113, 150–165.

Levine, E., Perry, P., Scarlett, J. and Houpt, K.A. (2005) Intercat aggression in households following the introduction of a new cat. *Applied Animal Behaviour Science* 90, 325–336.

Leyhausen, P. (1979) *Cat Behavior: The Predatory and Social Behavior of Domestic and Wild Cats*. Garland STPM Press, New York.

Macdonald, D.W, Yamaguchi, N. and Kerby, G. (2000) Group-living in the domestic cat: its sociobiology and epidemiology. In: Turner, D.C. and Bateson, P. (eds) *The Domestic Cat: The Biology of Its Behaviour*, 2nd edn. Cambridge University Press, Cambridge, pp. 95–118.

Supplementary materials entitled 'Social behaviour of female cats' and 'Social behaviour of male cats' can be accessed at: www.cabi.org/the-cat-behaviour-and-welfare/

Video

The cat comrades Kaos and Mio playfighting

video.cabi.org/BCHIU

6 The Cat as a Predator

The cat is a carnivore, a predator and, at the same time, the most common companion animal in western Europe and North America. Depending on the ecological conditions, the cat can be a threat to the local fauna and perhaps, most obviously, to birds. However, the threat to vulnerable species of mice, amphibians or reptiles is often overlooked. The conditions differ enormously between places where domestic cats are found, so we cannot generalize from a single study to cats in general. Research on this topic is still scarce or lacking in many countries.

Since the hunting ability of the cat was an important reason for its domestication (see Chapter 1), it is a paradox that it is this ability that can cause problems today. Many owners appreciate that cats catch mice and rats near their home whereas bird catching is less welcomed. The cat's popularity as a companion animal is often related to its independent nature. It can be let outdoors if the conditions permit and is less demanding than a dog. Yet the cat also satisfies our desire for social and physical contact. Research reveals that having a companion animal such as a cat is associated with positive effects on people's physical and mental health and quality of life (see Chapter 13). It can be argued that this is important from a public health perspective. Therefore, authorities should not put unnecessary restrictions on the keeping of cats. However, the interests of cat owners may conflict with the consideration of birds and other wildlife, just as there are often conflicts between conservation interests and development interests. In such cases, we should endeavour to find solutions that can take into consideration both the cats and their prey species.

Predatory Behaviour

The cat's predatory behaviour has been thoroughly analysed by Paul Leyhausen, including comparisons with other cat species. An overview is available from Fitzgerald and Turner (2000). Cats usually hunt in relatively fixed areas. They move away from home, often up to about 1 km, though the variation is great. The cat is mainly a nocturnal hunter, but domestic cats also hunt during the daytime.

In a hunting area, the cat may patrol slowly through the area, watching for opportunities, or lie in ambush, patiently waiting for signs that a prey animal is nearby. When such signs are detected, it will trot towards the prey in the cover of vegetation, and then slowly stalk closer with its head completely immobile and eyes fixed rigidly on the prey. When close enough for an attack and still undetected by the prey, the cat runs or jumps with lightning speed and seizes the prey in its mouth. If a bird flies up, the cat can leap up and catch the bird in mid-air. The cat will not necessarily kill the prey immediately. It may release the animal and then catch it again, often repeatedly – this includes birds that it has injured so they cannot fly away. Cats are highly motivated to catch prey, and this motivation must subside before delivery of the kill bite. Prey-catching behaviour allows cats to hone their prey-catching skills, which are maintained through practice throughout life. Such practice begins at around five weeks of age, when mother cats (and some males) first start bringing live prey home to the kittens. This early exposure to different types of prey animals allows the kittens to learn about the characteristics of the prey species in the area. Such experience influences their choice of prey in the future.

Cats are especially adapted to hunting small rodents. The most important prey are different species of mice and voles, young rats, passerine birds and young rabbits. At night, cats also catch a surprising number of moths and other night-flying insects. In one study on free-roaming cats fitted with a collar carrying a GPS tracker and video camera, it was found that nocturnal insects were

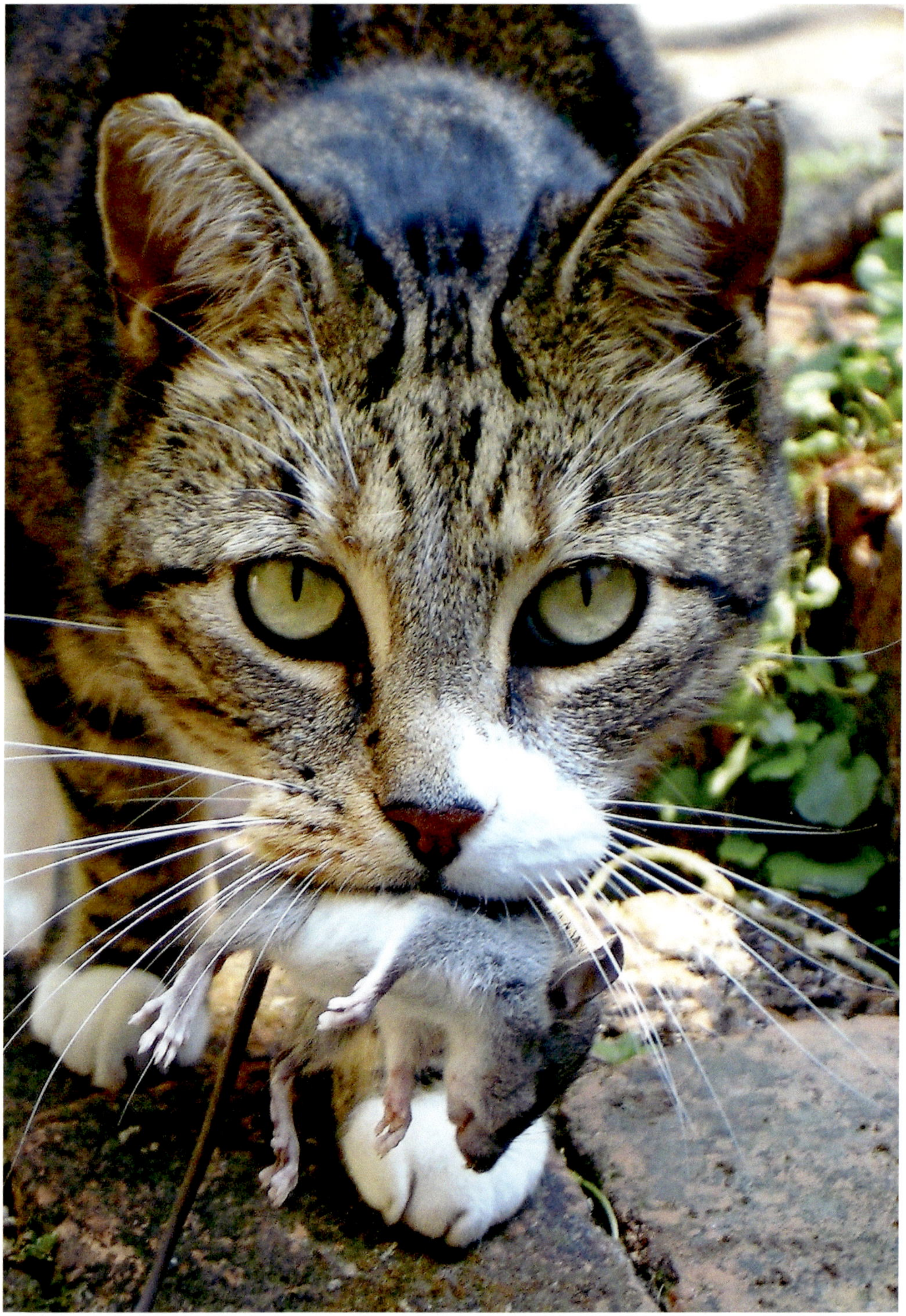

Fig. 6.1. Small rodents are the most typical prey of cats. (Photo: Lxowle, Creative Commons Attribution-Share Alike License, CC BY-SA 3.0, https://commons.wikimedia.org/w/index.php?search=lxowle&title=Special:MediaSearch&go=Go&type=image)

particularly favoured prey. Less commonly, cats prey on larger rats and rabbits, hares, squirrels, ducks, pheasants, quail, fish, frogs, spiders, lizards and small snakes. There are many stories about cats that entice snakes to stretch out and bite, after which they jump unbelievably quickly to one side and then pounce onto the neck of the snake and bite. In a study at a bird sanctuary in western Norway, it was observed that cats preyed on multiple wading bird species. An English study described more than 70 prey species taken by cats, including 20 species of mammals and 44 species of birds.

According to Eriksen's 2014 survey of Norwegian cat owners, approximately 82% of non-pedigree house cats and 27% of pedigree cats were allowed to roam freely outdoors (see Chapter 12). The effectiveness of prey catching varies greatly between these free-roaming cats. Multiple studies show that the distribution of prey caught per cat is extremely skewed; some cats take many prey, while most take relatively few. This is influenced by how cats are kept. Cats that are more often out at night take more prey than other cats, in particular more mice. Also, on average, cats living in rural areas take around twice as many prey as do urban or suburban cats. Rural cats tend to take proportionately more mammals and reptiles than birds whereas urban/suburban cats may catch a relatively higher proportion of birds, depending on the location.

It is estimated that, on average, cats need to make two to four attacks per successful catch of small rodents and birds and five attacks per rabbit caught. Younger adults take the most prey while cats tend to become less effective hunters after five years of age, particularly when it comes to catching birds. Pedigree cats are often poor hunters, although some have excellent hunting skills. These include Bengal cats and the forest cat breeds (Maine coon, Norwegian forest cat, Siberian cat). Siamese cats are shown to have weaker stereoscopic vision compared to non-pedigree cats and this may be a handicap when it comes to prey catching.

Effects on the Fauna

There is great variation in results about cat predation across studies. Mean values from several European studies suggest that domestic cats take around 60% mammals (mainly small rodents), 21% birds, 2% reptiles, 1% amphibians and 11% insects. In the USA, an estimated population of 94 million owned domestic cats (in 2017) is calculated to cause the death of at least 1.3 billion birds and 6.3 billion mammals annually. In Canada, a cat population of about 10 million (in 2013) is believed to cause between 100 million and 350 million bird deaths annually. In a scientific report to the Norwegian government in 2022, cat predation levels were estimated based on several studies in northern Europe and South Africa. From radio-tracking, video cameras attached to cats or analysing scat (faeces) and gut samples, it was estimated that, on average, only 20% of captured prey are brought home. Based on cat owner reports, this worked out to roughly ten prey per year. Hence, cats with outdoor access may take around 50 prey per year on average, although this will vary considerably between cats.

Such estimates must be viewed with caution, as there are differences in the methods used to collect the information across studies. Care must also be taken when extrapolating results from one region to another due to the unique ecology of different regions. One must take into account the population density of the cats in relation to the population density of each prey species, bearing in mind that this differs greatly between rural, suburban and urban habitats. To understand the impact of cats on local fauna, studies are needed not only on cat predation but also on other causes of mortality and reproductive failure in the different available prey species. Such causes can include diseases, climate change, loss of habitat due to the construction of new roads and buildings, non-wildlife friendly gardens, and predation by species other than domestic cats. Estimates of the overall number of birds taken by cats each year often represent only a small proportion of the total number of birds hatched or dying each year. Nevertheless, even low numbers become significant when cats prey on endangered species.

Cats do not take only the unwanted rats and house mice that infest our buildings and food supplies. They also catch other species of small rodents that may be vulnerable species in certain areas. Cat owners easily underestimate this impact, especially if not paying close attention to the specific types of rodents that our cats deposit on the doorstep. The extent to which cats are catching vulnerable species of small mammals and reptiles is often uncertain and should be investigated further.

In addition to predation by owned cats, we must also take into account the predation by populations of stray and feral cats. The sizes of these populations are often unclear, especially in natural areas. Many stray cats live in inner cities, where rodents may be more important prey than birds. Such cats typically scavenge on food leftovers in garbage, beg for food from passers-by or are fed by animal welfare organizations and other volunteers. Without analysing the contents of their faeces, it is hard to estimate the proportion of food they obtain from catching live prey.

Can cats eradicate prey species?

Neither Fitzgerald and Turner nor other researchers have reported cases where cats have completely eradicated populations of birds or other fauna on the mainland, but this can happen to local populations on islands, especially where there have been no predatory mammals before cats were introduced. This applies, for example, to the Galapagos and Ascension Islands, as well as islands near Florida, Honduras, Bahamas, Mexico, Fiji and New Zealand. On such islands, it is usually native reptiles, birds and small mammals that are at risk. In some cases, it is poorly documented whether it is cats or other environmental factors that have played the main role in damaging the local fauna.

In Australia and New Zealand, authorities are particularly concerned about hunting by imported carnivores, and studies show that cats (and rats) are a larger threat to the native bird species than to imported bird species. Unlike the native species, the imported species evolved in places with ground predators. These species, such as the house sparrow,

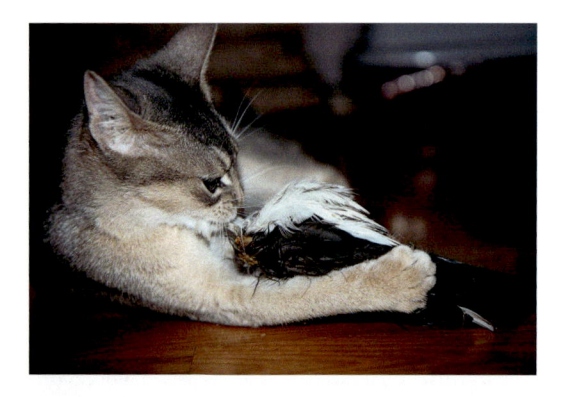

Fig. 6.2. Milli enjoys a bird, in this case a toy bird. (Photo: Heide Kvaløy, 2019)

blackbird and song thrush are termed exotic or invasive species, and they have effective *anti-predator behaviour* that helps them to avoid predation by cats. In contrast, the native bird species are either unable to fly or fail to fly away due to lack of fear of animals that approach them from the ground (including people). They may also be adapted to nesting on the ground or in burrows instead of in trees. In Australia, feral cats are now considered a serious pest and are estimated to substantially threaten the survival of at least 142 native species on the mainland as well as on offshore islands. In 2015, a governmental plan was developed to address this problem.

In the scientific report to the Norwegian government, it was estimated that cats, both owned and feral combined, annually take 4.6% of the bird population in areas with cats. In Sweden, ethologist Olof Liberg conducted a study on predation by owned and feral cats in Skåne, an area of cattle pastures and moors, and to a lesser degree forest land. He estimated that cats were consuming approximately 3.6% of the annual production (i.e. the new generation) of the predominant prey species, which were wild rabbits and small rodents, and, to a lesser extent, hares and birds. On average, the feral cats were killing four times more prey than the owned cats.

Owned cats live and hunt close to where people live. Naturally, cats most readily come across the most abundant prey species around human settlements, such as common species of small rodents and passerine birds. In western Europe, these include the Eurasian tree sparrow, yellowhammer, great tit and blue tit. In a study in two Swiss mountain villages, cats were found to reduce the productivity of the black redstart (*Phoenicurus ochruros*) by 12%, mainly because young birds were caught. So long as the vast majority of bird species live far away from human settlements, cats will hardly pose a major threat. Endangered bird species usually include some birds of prey and seabirds that live in areas with few or no cats. However, for endangered or vulnerable passerine birds, predation by cats may add to the many other factors that are reducing their population numbers.

In places where cats have existed for over 1000 years, the local fauna has likely adapted to some extent to their presence. We can assume that when birds choose to nest near residential areas, they are likely to reproduce more successfully there than if they nest elsewhere. Many birds benefit from food provided by people, but this must be balanced against the opportunities for nesting safely and the number of predators that take eggs and baby birds. Some species of birds appear to avoid nesting in areas with many cats. In urban areas of England, it has been found that the denser the cat population, the lower the diversity of bird species overall. This particularly affects species that nest in hedges such as wrens and hedge sparrows in the UK, as their nestling young are easily taken by cats.

Cats prey on other enemies of birds

By hunting rats, particularly young rats, cats reduce the number of these predators. This is perhaps especially beneficial for ground-nesting bird species. Using mathematical models, scientists have shown that a reduction in the cat population does not necessarily always give the best outcome for conservation of bird populations. On the contrary, it may be more beneficial to preserve a predator like the cat that is high in the ecological hierarchy. Cats are so-called *super predators,* taking rats and, occasionally, other small mammals like squirrels that pose a threat to eggs and young birds. If you reduce the cat population, you will need to increase your efforts against rat populations.

Measures to reduce predation by cats

Although cats are not always a serious threat to populations of birds and other native fauna, several measures can reduce the risk of predation by cats. Keeping cats indoors at night, especially during the nesting season and early summer, can reduce predation on mammalian prey. Some studies report no effect of attaching a bell to the collar, while others report a 34–53 % reduction in prey catches. This variation may be influenced by the size of the bell, as small bells probably have a negligible effect. Cats can move so stealthily that the prey does not hear the bell before it is too late. Ultrasound devices probably should not be used on cats, as cats have acute hearing of ultrasound and these devices could be a source of stress.

Most birds are diurnal and use their colour vision to detect predators. If a cat wears a colourful collar cover or bib, such as a Birdsbesafe®, this provides a visual sign of the cat's presence (Fig. 6.4). Swiss researchers reported a 37% reduction in the number of birds brought home when using a coloured collar cover. The numbers of mammalian prey brought home were reduced by 54–62%, but only if the cat was also equipped with a bell. Most of the cat owners that participated in the Swiss study stated that they would like to continue using the coloured collar cover after the study. Several different types of such equipment are on the market.

Another method of reducing bird predation is to attach a CatBib® to the cat's collar. This device hangs in front of the chest and flaps upward when the cat pounces towards the prey. An Australian study found that their use was effective in reducing predation on birds, mammals, reptiles and amphibians.

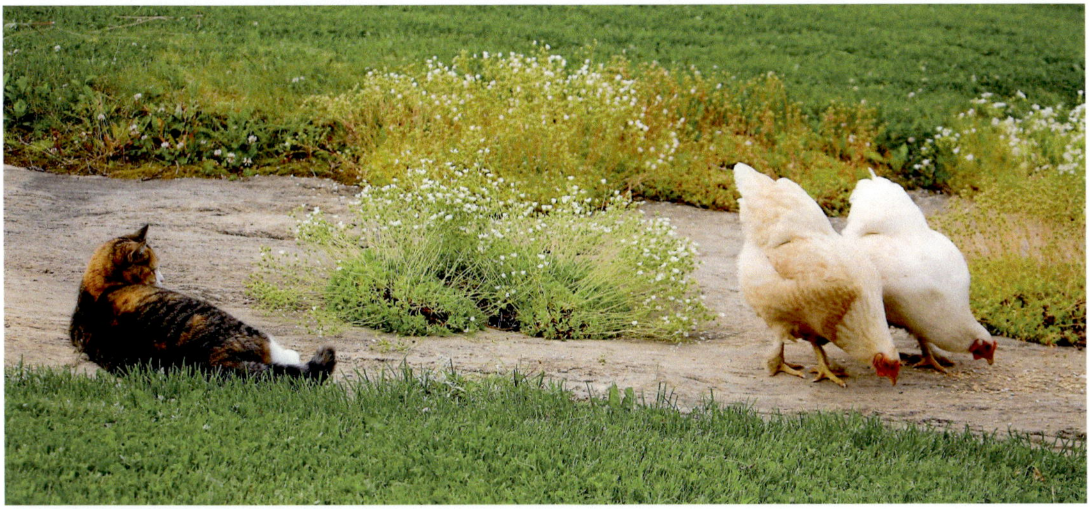

Fig. 6.3. Moshe leaves the garden hens in peace. (Photo: Janne Helen Lorentzsen, 2019)

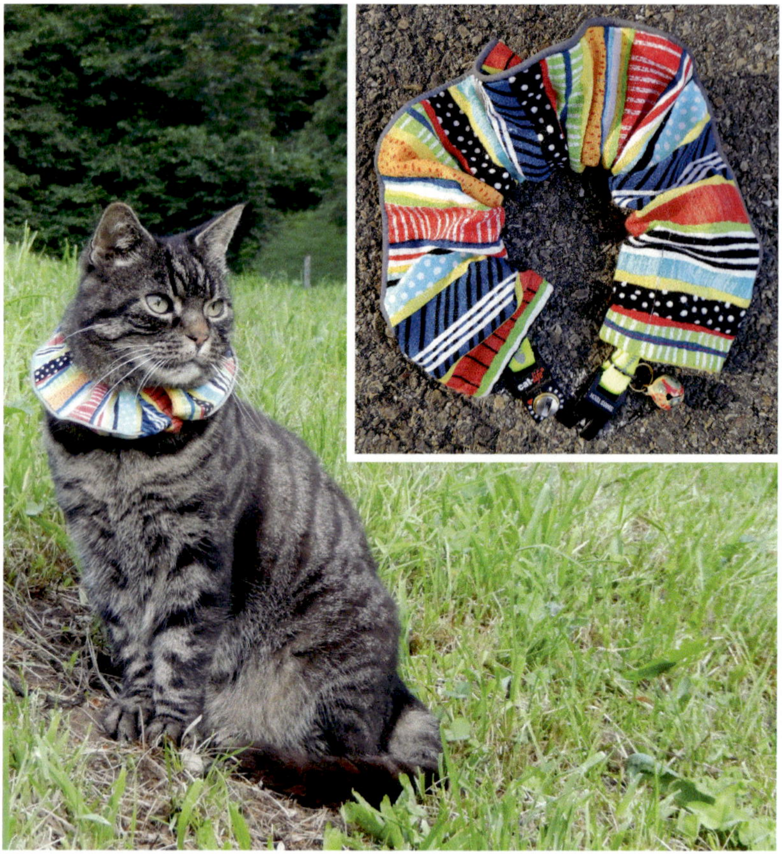

Fig. 6.4. A cat wearing a colourful collar cover to warn birds, the Birdsbesafe®. (Photo: copyright Kathi Märki/swild.ch and Madeleine Geiger/swild.ch, 2022)

Furthermore, Martina Cecchetti and colleagues at the University of Exeter, UK, found that when owners spent five to ten minutes per day in object play with their cat, the cats brought home 35% fewer mice and other small mammals, although this method did not reduce bird predation.

Cat owners must be responsible and not let their cats roam freely if they live near a bird sanctuary or any area where they could prey on vulnerable wildlife species, including city suburbs which are increasingly recognized as important potential havens for wildlife and biodiversity. Since Liberg's investigation indicated that feral cats took more prey than owned cats, there can be benefits to controlling populations of feral and stray cats. Chapter 9 addresses the issue of unowned cats, including in cities where their density can be high.

What should the cat eat?

Since the cat is a carnivore, it must get food suitable for carnivores. Cat food produced by reputable animal nutrition companies contains the nutritional elements that cats need. These companies also produce food formulated for kittens, senior cats, indoor cats and cats with specific health needs. Be sure to provide food that contains the essential amino acid *taurine*, as cats, unlike dogs, cannot produce this protein building-block in their body. You may occasionally give your cat fresh meat and fish. It is not possible to turn cats into vegetarians, even if you are a vegetarian yourself. Cats have a very low ability to utilize carbohydrates and have no tastebuds for sweetness. This indicates that sweet things do not belong in their diet. Furthermore, in the University

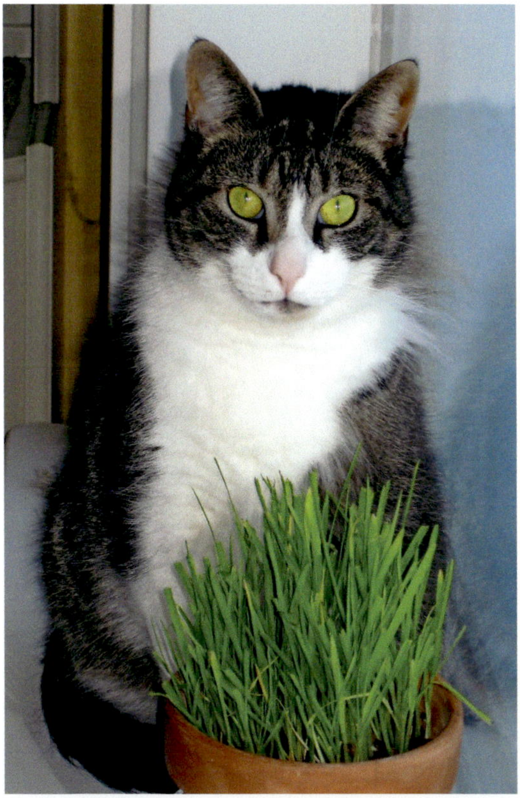

Fig. 6.5. Offer grass to your cat during winter to prevent constipation. (Photo: Kari Kristiansen, 2019)

of Exeter study, feeding a diet high in meat protein was found to reduce the number of mammalian and bird prey brought home by about a third compared to feeding cat food containing carbohydrates, indicating that a meat diet is more nutritionally satisfying.

Occasionally, cats will eat grass. This serves as fibre that can help to prevent constipation and may help the gut cope with hair balls. It may also be an evolved adaptation for reducing intestinal worms. In winter, if the ground is covered in snow, cats appreciate it if you provide them with a small grass garden indoors. This grass can be grown in a plant pot or plant tray. At the same time, be careful to avoid keeping indoor plants that are poisonous for cats.

Further Reading

Australian Government, Department of the Environment (2015) Background document for the threat abatement plan for predation by feral cats. Available at: www.environment.gov.au/system/files/resources/78f3dea5-c278-4273-8923-fa0de27aacfb/files/tap-predation-feral-cats-2015-background.pdf (accessed 9 April 2022).

Cecchetti, M., Crowley, S.L., Goodwin, C.E.D. and McDonald, R.A. (2021) Provision of high meat content food and object play reduce predation of wild animals by domestic cats *Felis catus*. *Current Biology* 31, 1107–1111.e5. DOI: 10.1016/j.cub.2020.12.044.

Fitzgerald, B.M. and Turner, D.C. (2000) Hunting behaviour of domestic cats and their impact on prey populations. In: Turner, D.C. and Bateson, P. (eds) *The Domestic Cat: The Biology of Its Behaviour*, 2nd edn. Cambridge University Press, Cambridge, pp. 151–175.

Geiger, M., Kistler, C., Mattmann, P., Jenni, L., Hegglin, D. *et al.* (2022) Colorful collar-covers and bells reduce wildlife predation by domestic cats in a continental European setting. *Frontiers in Ecology and Evolution*, 10: 850442. DOI: 10.3389/fevo.2022.850442.

Leyhausen, P. (1979) *Cat Behavior: The Predatory and Social Behaviour of Domestic and Wild Cats*. Garland STPM Press, New York.

Norwegian Scientific Committee for Food and Environment (2022) Assessment of the risk of negative impact on biodiversity and animal welfare from keeping domestic cats (*Felis catus*) in Norway. Scientific Opinion of the Panel on Alien Organisms and Trade in Endangered Species of the Norwegian Scientific Committee for Food and Environment. VKM Report 2022. Available at: https://vkm.no/english (draft accessed 1 October 2022, to be published late in 2022 or early 2023).

Royal Society for the Protection of Birds (n.d.) Birds of conservation concern 5. Available at: https://www.rspb.org.uk/globalassets/downloads/bocc5/bocc5-report.pdf (accessed 19 May 2022). A full report is available at: https://britishbirds.co.uk/sites/default/files/BB_Dec21-BoCC5-IUCN2.pdf (accessed 19 May 2022).

Supplementary materials entitled 'The cat as a predator' can be accessed at: www.cabi.org/the-cat-behaviour-and-welfare/

7 The Cat's Ability to Navigate

There are many stories about cats that have found their way home after being given away or sold, disappearing from a summer cabin or getting lost in other ways. What does the cat do when it has gone astray? Does the cat have a good navigational ability, and how does it work? This chapter considers these questions and offers advice on what you can do to find a lost cat.

Tales of Cat Wanderings

All over the world there are stories about long journeys taken by domestic cats. Finding their way home is called *homing*. Homing usually occurs over a few kilometres but can occasionally cover hundreds of kilometres. A journey may take from a few days to a couple of years.

Sam disappeared during a caravan tour in Wales, more than 400 km from its home in East London. Local newspaper ads and messages to local police stations brought no response. Two years later, when Margaret Adams, the cat's owner, went outside to fetch in the laundry from the washing-line, she saw a tired cat sitting on the fence. Margaret noticed that the cat had the same white spot on the stomach and the same short, thick legs as the cat she had lost. She called 'Sam', and the cat responded immediately. The family was in no doubt that it was their long-lost cat that had managed to find his way home.

In Norway, Petter Tiedemann related that in April 1940, during World War II, his family was evacuated from their home to a cabin 7 km away. There was no road to the cabin so they travelled there on skis, carrying their two-year-old cat in a dark box with a few air holes. The ski tracks were soon obliterated by fresh snow. On the third day, the cat suddenly disappeared, and they thought a fox must have caught it. Five days later, Petter had to go home to pick up something. To his great surprise, the cat met him on the doorstep, scruffy and desperate for affection.

A most impressive feat by a Norwegian cat was achieved by the three-year-old tomcat Hampus. In the summer of 1976, its family, who lived near Oslo, went to visit relatives living north-east of Trondheim, bringing Hampus with them. At the end of their holiday, it was decided that the relatives would keep Hampus. During the first month, it appeared that Hampus had settled well into its new home, but in early September he suddenly disappeared. One day in early May, the following year, the family back home was awakened by a cat standing outside the door, miaowing. The mother opened the door and to her astonishment she saw a big black male cat that absolutely wanted to enter. The astonishment became great pleasure when she realized that it was Hampus who had returned home. He must have walked nearly 600 km in eight months – from autumn through to spring! No-one in the family was in any doubt that it really was Hampus. Hampus had a characteristic way of answering when one of the family members called its name. After he had eaten, he jumped straight up into his favourite chair. The cat had clear marks of having been on a long journey. He had sore and torn paws. Hampus was a great mouse hunter, so the family thought he was able to catch food for himself and perhaps manage to scrounge some food from people living along the way. When a national newspaper, *VG*, wrote about this story in 1977, the family was contacted by a lady from Lillehammer district. She explained that in late autumn, a big black cat had arrived and stayed with her until spring before disappearing. The description fitted Hampus. While we cannot be sure it was the same cat, it makes sense that Hampus stayed with this kind lady rather than travelling under harsh winter conditions.

Many years ago, with help from a radio programme and *VG*, Bjarne gathered stories of long cat journeys in Norway. Of nine cases where the gender was stated, there were seven male cats. None was less than a year old and most were over

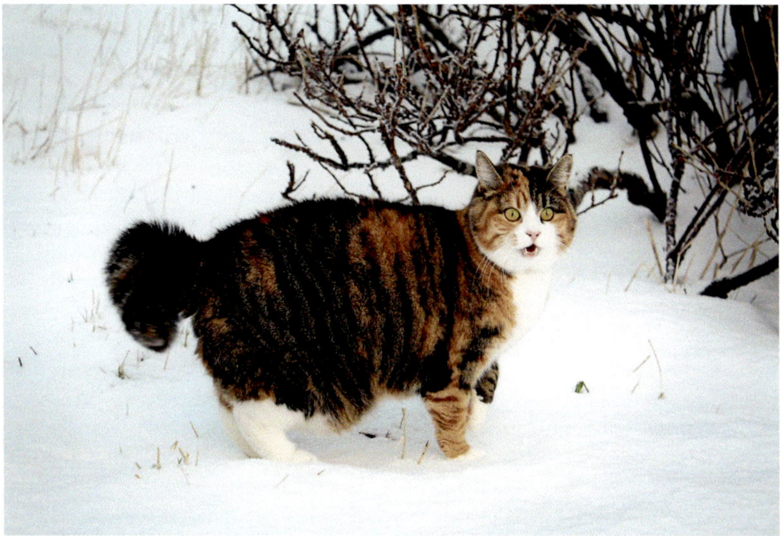

Fig. 7.1. Which way should I choose now? (Photo: Janne Helen Lorentzsen, 2019)

two years old, suggesting that these cats had previous experience of roaming. The speed of travel ranged from 0.6 to 9 km per day. The fastest cat travelled an average of 9 km a day for 22 days. It must have been walking for a large part of the day, with success in finding food to fuel its journey.

How credible are such stories of homing over long distances? It is hard to be 100% certain about these stories without being able to check the cats' identities, something that is easier today with ID chips. However, a common feature of such stories is that the cat – in addition to looking exactly like the lost cat – behaves in a similar way, seems to recognize the family, the house and its usual resting places, and has very sore paws. A cat will not get sore and torn paws without having wandered a very long distance.

Research on the Cat's Orientation Ability

Joseph Rhine and Sara Feather at Duke University in the USA collected hundreds of accounts of animals that had made long journeys to get home. They then imposed strict conditions to investigate them further: there was a reliable first-hand source, the animal had unique characteristics such as scars or specific colour markings, there were eyewitness reports from independent people, and the animal was still alive. After winnowing out cases that met these criteria, the researchers were left with 22 well-confirmed stories about long cat journeys. They pointed to parapsychological explanations but, as we shall see below, there are quite normal explanations for the remarkable navigation skills of cats.

In 1921, Professor Francis Herrick, of Cleveland, Ohio, performed a series of trials where he drove male or female cats 1.5–7 km in different directions from his home and released them. In all cases, the cats managed to return home within one to four days. Herrick was sure that the cats could neither hear, see nor smell anything from their home where they were released. All cats seemed to take a direct way home rather than retracing the route used to transport them. In one case, the cat was even anaesthetized so that it slept during the outward journey.

At the University of Kiel, in Germany, Precht and Lindenlaub (1954) used another research method. They wanted to investigate if cats knew which direction to take when walking home from an unfamiliar place. They transported 42 cats, one at a time, in a closed box that prevented them from seeing where they were heading. During the outward journey, detours were taken to various places in different directions and at different distances from home. The box was opened in the middle of a covered circular maze with six exits, at 60^0-angles apart. By chance, one-sixth of the cats would be expected to come out of each exit. But half of the cats, 21 out of 42, came out from the exit pointing in the correct direction of home. This is a statistically significant result showing that it is unlikely that the cats chose the exit just by chance.

The Cat's Behaviour in Unfamiliar Terrain

Bjarne was inspired by the research conducted by Precht and Lindenlaub when choosing the topic for his Master's thesis research in 1979/80. He decided to investigate more closely how cats behave when in unfamiliar terrain and what cues they might use to navigate home. He borrowed 14 cats from benevolent cat owners around eastern Norway and drove each one by car some kilometres from its home along a route with big detours. In most cases, the cat was placed inside a closed box during the drive so that it could not see the road. Each cat was released in a forest at a site where the wind was blowing in the direction of home. It was therefore impossible for the cats to see or smell something that could direct them home.

Before the car ride, each cat had a small radio transmitter (weight 50 grams) mounted to its collar. The cat quickly got used to this, in a matter of minutes. The carrying basket was opened from at least 30 metres away using a rope attached to the lid, while Bjarne was hiding behind a bush. As the cat travelled, Bjarne repeatedly took its bearings using a radio receiver and plotted the cat's location on a map. He was careful to keep a few hundred metres away from the cat. It soon turned out that many of the cats settled down in the area where they were released. Only four tried to find their way home by walking away from the release site, but all those that tried succeeded in making it home. None of the cats got lost, and none went far in a completely wrong direction.

Every cat that went home did so during the first day. To investigate whether a cat that did not go home immediately would try to go home later, Bjarne followed the cat for several days and carefully observed what it was doing. The cat rested in dense thickets, and occasionally in a barn if one was available. One of the cats was out for a whole month without showing signs of wanting to go home. This tomcat was more interested in the female cats nearby.

The cats in this study were used to getting all the food they needed from humans. During the trials, which lasted from May to September, it seemed that they were doing well on their own. They were active for about 12 hours a day, mostly in the late evening and early morning. None used a disproportionately large part of the time for hunting, and when they hunted, they were often located along a stream where there were likely to be small rodents to prey upon. It was therefore hardly vital for the cats to go home. Had it been winter, the situation might have been different.

The cat owners were naturally miffed when their cat seemed to lack the motivation to return home. However, several of these cats probably made no attempt because they were stressed when released in the forest. Instead, they hid, making it difficult to find them. Nevertheless, as soon as they were brought home, all the cats quickly settled down. The cats now showed signs of well-being and a desire to be with their owners – purring and rubbing their heads and body against the legs of their owners. So even if a cat stays away from home for some time, this does not mean that it feels uncomfortable at home; the cat may simply have different needs at different times. It is also possible that many of the cats in this study did not try to walk home because they did not know in which direction to go. If their orientation skills were weak, what factors limited this ability?

Bjarne's results suggested that the distance from home to the place of release was a critical factor. None of the cats went home from distances over 2 km as the crow flies. This limit may have been related to the way the cats were transported. A few of them were given the opportunity to look out of the car window during the drive, but none of these cats followed the road home. Some of the cats that

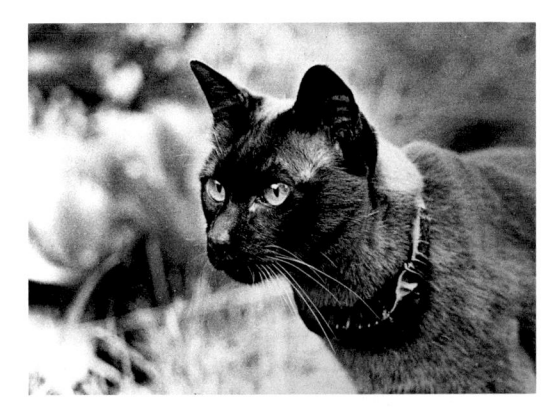

Fig. 7.2. Lady Femina, with a radio transmitter, informing the researcher where she was. (Photo: Rolf M. Aagaard, Aftenposten A-foto, 1979)

went home took detours, probably so they could travel in the most protected terrain, which would reduce their risk of being caught by a predator. Each of the four homing cats travelled at approximately 0.5 km per hour. Since a cat normally rests for at least 12 hours a day, this would mean that cats on longer journeys would cover 5–6 km daily if travelling at the same speed.

How Can the Cat Navigate in Unfamiliar Terrain?

Many animals are well known for having good homing ability. The best known are pigeons and migratory birds. Also, whales, salmon and insects – perhaps most animals – have impressive *orientation* skills. Biologists often distinguish between orientation and *navigational* ability. An animal's orientation ability is the ability to find its way over known areas and then follow the same path back home, otherwise known as *tracking*. This may be part of how cats initially learn about the immediate environs around their core territory. For an animal to be said to have navigational ability, also termed *scouting*, it must know where it is in relation to home so that it can take a direct route home even from an unknown area without needing to retrace its steps.

Which orientation methods could the cats in Bjarne's study have used? Those that went home could not have used their sense of smell, or visual input from home, when they started homing. Two cats went home in completely cloudy weather, so they could not see either the sun or the stars during their journey, though we know that these are used in navigation by some species such as certain migratory birds (e.g. starlings). The fact that Bjarne took many detours made it difficult to retrace the route, and this could have been part of the reason why few of the cats got home. If you drive an adult cat straight to a new home, it may be easier for the cat to use tracking to return in the direction from which it came.

Scent map or sound map?

Jay Rosenblatt, at Rutgers University in Newark, New Jersey, found that kittens, even during the three first weeks of life, can orient themselves towards a core area around their nest. Both the queen and her kittens deposit pheromones in this area. When the kittens notice the familiar scents, they feel more comfortable and relax. As the kittens grow, they expand the size of this area and scent mark in the additional space. It is therefore likely that cats use *olfactory orientation* along with visual landmarks to find their way within their home range and could potentially use these methods over longer distances as well.

Cats have a very good sense of hearing. It is not unthinkable that they can perceive and locate particular sounds from factories, waterfalls or roads several kilometres away. The German ethologist Paul Leyhausen put forward the idea that cats may have a kind of *acoustic map*, a type of mental map of their memory, by which they can orient.

However, scent maps, visual maps and acoustic maps cannot explain cases of navigation over long distances when transported in a manner that prevents tracking. Perhaps cats can use some additional navigation methods that are found in other species with excellent navigation skills. Besides using the sun and stars, which require clear weather, we shall point to two possible explanations – a magnetic sense, and continual registration of the direction in which the animal is moving.

Magnetic sense

Some animals, such as pigeons, dolphins, turtles and honeybees, have a *magnetic sense* based on an internal magnetic compass. When you change the magnetic field, such animals will take off in a direction that is wrong, but which corresponds to the size of the change in the magnetic field. One theory is that they know where they are relative to the Earth's magnetic field by using information from cells in their body containing tiny crystals of the

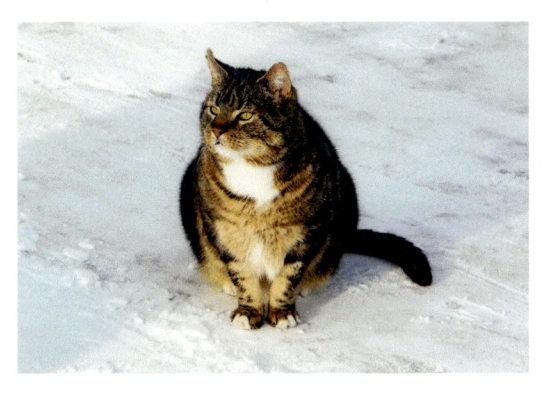

Fig. 7.3. Isn't there a familiar smell in that direction? (Photo: Ragnhild Mykleby, 2019)

The Cat's Ability to Navigate

iron compound magnetite (Fe_3O_4). Most animals, including cats, have cells containing magnetite. Another possibility is that the Earth's magnetic field induces an electromagnetic field in the semi-circular canals of the inner ear. Some animals, such as dogs, have a compound in their eyes that is activated by the magnetic field, but this is lacking in cats.

Even people may have a magnetic sense, although we are not consciously aware of it. Experiments by Reginald Robin Baker and colleagues at the University of Manchester, UK, showed that blindfolded students who were transported by bus with intricate detours up to 65 km from the university were able to point out the direction to the starting point quite accurately. Without the blindfold, their answers were more often wrong. Visual impressions may have interfered with their magnetic sense. In a subsequent study, 16–17-year-olds were tested with a helmet on their head in addition to the blindfold. In half of the helmets, a magnetic rod altered the magnetic field by 90 degrees, while the other half had a rod without this effect. Those who wore the helmets with the magnetic rod typically pointed out the direction with an error of 90 degrees. These results were later disputed by other scientists, so the issue of human magnetic sense remains uncertain. Further research will no doubt shed light on this matter.

Directional summation

Considering that the semi-circular canals of the inner ear provide a three-dimensional coordinate system that measures head movement, a theory proposed in the 1960s was that animals can know where they are in relation to home, based on their head movements. According to the principle of *vector addition*, the direction and distance from home can be described by the double integral of all head accelerations over the duration of a journey. Spacecraft can navigate based on this principle though it is unclear if animals use this method.

The brain's Global Positioning System (GPS)

There is evidence that animals can use sensory information about their location to form a brain map of their location in space. This evidence comes from the work of researchers May-Britt and Edvard Moser at the Norwegian University of Science and Technology. In 2014, they received the Nobel Prize for describing the GPS of the rat's brain. The hippocampus in the limbic system of the brain stores information about the body's geographical positions in special *place cells*. Nerve cells that integrate signals from the inner ear's semi-circular canals are found in the medial entorhinal cortex, which is closely connected to the hippocampus. Here, the so-called *grid cells*, which are organized in a nerve grid, store information about the direction in which the animal moves and how far in this direction it has moved. Other nerve cells store information about how fast the animal moves. Close by, in the lateral entorhinal cortex, there are neurons that are specific to objects. This makes it possible for the brain to associate objects with locations. In the same brain region, there is also an analysis of time in a newly discovered *time sense*. This part of the brain can therefore compare information about objects, place and time.

The Nobel laureates have put forward a theory that this spatial mapping ability forms the basis for the more general role of the hippocampus in memory formation. They suggest that spatial memory came first, and then there was further evolution that extended brain function to the other memory functions found in many animals today, such as social memory. The evolutionary importance of spatial memory is probably why we can easily remember what happened the last time we were in a certain place if we go back to the same place again. Both time and place are important in learning, and objects are often the focus of learning. Bear this in mind when reading Chapter 10 about training your cat.

Studies on homing pigeons show that they do not rely only on a single sense for navigation but can use different senses according to which are providing the best information at the time. The same is probably also true for cats. When travelling home from an unfamiliar location, a cat may head off in approximately the right direction using magnetic sense – and perhaps also have an idea of how far away it is, based on vector additions in the brain. As it gets closer to home, it may begin to detect certain familiar features of the terrain, sounds and scents that allow it to home in on the correct place.

How Can You Find a Lost Cat?

Unfortunately, many people experience the distress that occurs if their cat escapes or disappears, either from home or from a place unfamiliar to the cat. The owners search desperately, but the cat is nowhere to be found. Few are as lucky as a couple from Oslo who owned a Tonkanese, a rare pedigree cat. The cat could not be found when they were about to return home from a holiday at a cabin almost 100 kilometres from home. They had to go home for work, but the next weekend they drove back again to search further. To their astonishment and great joy, they saw their cat through the car window, wandering along the roadside in the direction of Oslo. It had already travelled many kilometres from the cabin. They just had to open the car door and pick it up.

If a cat disappears voluntarily from a home where it knows the surroundings well, it may be roaming far away, especially if it is a tomcat. Such wanderings are quite normal, and the cat will most likely find its way home by itself – when it is ready to return home. As seen in Chapter 5, adult tomcats can travel far in their search for females in heat. Also, those around two to three years of age are occasionally expelled from the area by more competitive males living in the vicinity, so they may not return home until they are older, if then.

Other types of disappearance can have a lucky outcome. These are the cases where a newly arrived cat leaves its new home and finds its way back to the old home. This is more likely if the cat is an adult. Likewise, a cat that does not feel a strong connection to its owners may walk home if, for example, the owners take it with them on a holiday. A cat can also get lost during a trip without any intention to return home. In such cases, many people have been able to find the cat using the following tips.

If the cat is young and inexperienced, it is important to start searching for it immediately. If the cat is an adult, used to roaming in nature, and the distance to home is less than about 2 km in a straight line, the cat will probably return home by itself. Over larger distances, there is a risk that the cat will settle in the new area rather than return home.

When a cat first gets lost, it is likely to be close by. Most of the cats in Bjarne's study stayed near the place where they were released for several days. The cat will likely spend a couple of hours getting acquainted with the immediate surroundings, usually within a few hundred metres. After a rest break, it will gradually increase the area over which it moves. It will now be looking for hunting grounds, safe sleeping places and lookouts. Hunting often takes place along a stream where small rodents can be found, and the cat will prefer to sleep in a barn or thick scrub if available nearby. In many cases, people have found cats within a couple of hundred metres from where they first disappeared, up to one to two weeks after they disappeared.

Owners are often surprised at how quickly their cat becomes timid in unfamiliar terrain. Cats will usually avoid walking across open areas such as

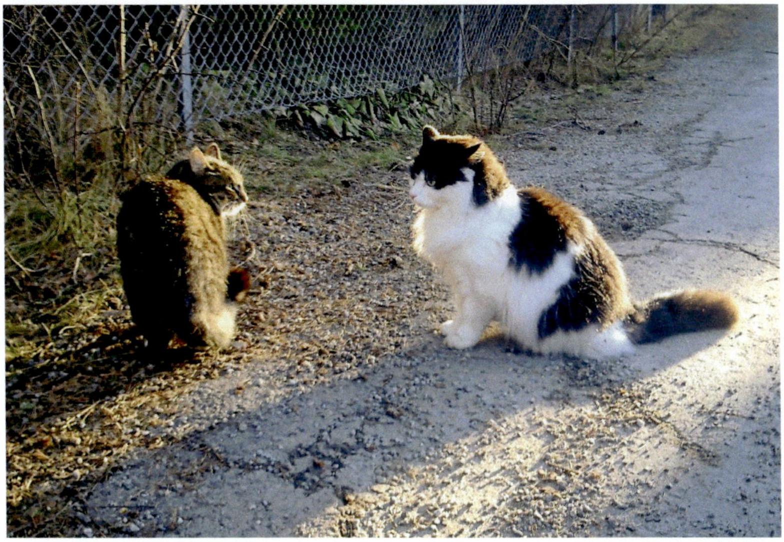

Fig. 7.4. Male cats aged two to three years can be expelled from the area by a dominant male. (Photo: Agnethe-Irén Sandem, 2019)

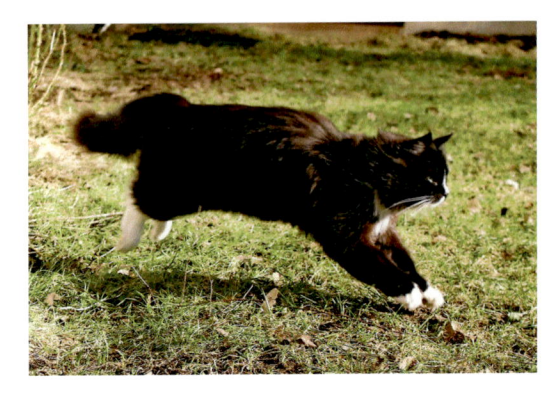

Fig. 7.5. The cat can run away if you try to catch it, so be patient. (Photo: Audun Braastad, 2019)

fields and pastures. These are spaces where they are exposed to being caught by birds of prey or other predators. Instead, they will usually keep themselves well hidden in thick grass or hedges. In a forest, they will hide in dense ground cover. In an unfamiliar place, a cat will not necessarily come to you even if it hears you calling. It is important to be aware of this. The more nervous and reserved the cat is normally, the more difficult it will be to lure it from its hideaway. It does not dare come out even if it wants to. If you cannot lure the cat to come to you, put out strong-smelling food like fish at regular intervals in places where the cat is likely to be, such as barns, dense undergrowth and along streams. If you can figure out where the cat is, you can eventually try to get it to come out and eat from your hand. Placing out a litter tray with the familiar odour of the lost cat or other cats in the household may also help to attract it. If it has become very timid, you must be extremely patient and avoid sudden movements. This is particularly important if it is an unfamiliar person, rather than the owner, who finds the cat.

In Bjarne's study, he used a specially made cat trap to recover cats. It had a trapdoor that dropped down and closed the exit when the cat stepped on a food tray inside the trap. However, such a trap must be used with care and requires frequent supervision, several times a day. Be prepared for the fact that other animals may get trapped instead. The trap must be adjusted correctly so that it works at the cat's first attempt. If the cat manages to escape, it will never try again. If you intend to use such a trap in nature, check whether you need permission from the wildlife authorities. Hunting regulations often restrict the use of traps.

If your cat has already left the area in which it disappeared, it will probably be more difficult to find, especially if it has a shy personality. A tracking dog might be useful if it can be presented with materials doused in the cat's scent so that it knows what to search for. If you find no sign anywhere nearby, try searching in the homeward direction, or towards the cat's birthplace/previous home if it is a cat that you have recently acquired. Even though none of the cats in Bjarne's study went far in a totally wrong direction, one should not expect them to travel home along a straight course. They will usually travel along the edge of woods or hedges even if this requires a detour. Remember, they will generally avoid open areas. Consider that the cat may start walking in a direction ± 45 degrees from the correct direction. Cats feel safer at night and there is a greater chance that you will see the cat if you search in early dawn or at dusk rather than during the daytime. In a quiet residential area, try searching at night – you may even find your cat walking down the middle of a street.

While the cat travels, it will probably move at a speed of about 0.5 km per hour, measured in a straight line across the cat's more meandering route. This includes time for eating and taking short rest breaks. A cat will never run in unfamiliar terrain, unless suddenly frightened by something. If the cat is travelling more than a few kilometres to reach home, it will need longer rest breaks during its journey.

Advertise a lost cat

If you lost the cat in a residential area or the cat is likely to pass through residential areas, then you can put up posters with a photo of the cat on posts and on noticeboards in shops, even in schools and community centres. You can also place a notice with a photo of your cat in local newspapers, on local community media, on Facebook and on web pages dedicated to lost and found pets. Here you may also find more tips on what you can do to find your cat. Furthermore, you can check with the police and veterinary offices in the area in case they have received messages about cats that have been found. When you have found your cat, remember to take down all the posters and online posts.

Ensure that your cat is ID-tagged

All cats should be ID-marked, even if they are indoor cats. There is always the possibility that, one day, they might get out accidentally. Although not usually mandated by legislation (which it should be), it is in the interests of cats that their owners can be contacted if a member of the public finds them. This can be done by attaching a tag with your phone number to a quick-release collar. Never use a collar that won't come off if it gets caught on something, as this could strangle the cat. However, given that a quick-release collar can come off, it is important to back up this method with a more permanent mark. In some places, a number may be tattooed in the cat's ear, but nowadays it is more common to use a microchip that a vet injects under the skin on the back of the neck. In some countries, such as the UK, the microchipping of dogs and cats is a legal requirement of ownership.

If it is not a legal requirement or common practice to have cats microchipped, you may also decide to have a letter M tattooed in one ear to show that the cat is microchipped. In regions where microchips are commonly used, vets, animal rescue centres and, sometimes, the police have equipment for scanning the microchip. Identification can be complicated by the availability of incompatible microchip systems requiring different scanners. If you are moving to a different region or country, check which microchip system is commonly used at your destination and get your cat chipped with that system in addition to the microchip it already has.

All found cats should be scanned, as they may be chipped but not tattooed. Even if the cat seems to be very timid or wild, it may have owners who miss it.

Taking Your Cat on Holiday

Despite all the stories about cats that disappear, do not fear that they get lost so easily. When considering the many millions of cats in the world, the stories about long journeys taken by cats are still rare. When you are going on holiday, you should not leave the cat alone to fend for itself. You have several options – good neighbours who will care for your cat in your absence, a boarding cattery, or

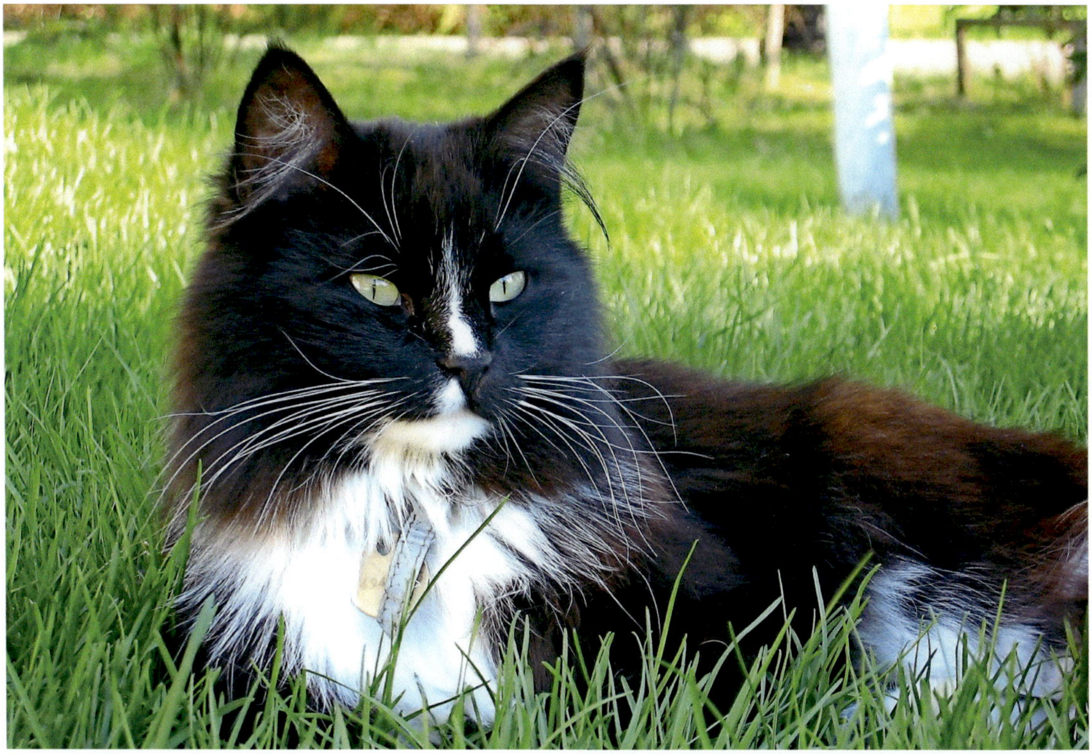

Fig. 7.6. Rampoline has a medallion on her collar with a phone number and is also labelled with a microchip. (Photo: Bjarne O. Braastad, 2004)

a professional cat-care person who will come to your home. If your cat has a good relationship with you and is used to being fed by you, you can also consider bringing your cat with you, especially if you are going to a single, suitable place that it can get used to, such as a summer cabin that you drive to regularly. You should familiarize your cat with car trips from an early age, starting with short tours and then gradually increasing in length. You should also train your kitten to walk on a leash (see Chapter 10).

Once at the holiday location, allow your cat time to get well acquainted with the indoor accommodation (at least a day or two). Then you can take the cat on short trips around the outside of the accommodation on a leash, and, once comfortable with this, and if a safe place to do so, let the cat go outside without a leash but under your supervision. It needs to take small trips to inspect the surroundings and learn where to return to find you. This is important so the cat can feel safe there. When the cat is taking frequent trips back to the accommodation to receive food and attention from you, this is a sign that it feels comfortable there.

Nowadays, it is possible to fit your cat's collar with a GPS device allowing satellite tracking of its location. You can practise tracking your cat at home before using it on a trip. However, this is a back-up system only and does not replace the above steps.

For most cats, it is advisable to keep them on a leash if travelling from place to place, unless you are prepared to be significantly delayed by a frightened hiding cat. Note also that cats prefer to be at home following their familiar routines, and some cats experience motion sickness, so they may not appreciate the opportunity to join you on a road trip. Moreover, bear in mind that there are always risks for a cat when outdoors and the risk is magnified in an unfamiliar area because the cat does not have a strong knowledge of where to find you, where dangerous traffic and predators may be lurking, and where to hide in safety. If travelling to other regions, be aware of local regulations, possible disease risks, and risk of cat theft. Although there are remarkable stories of lost cats finding their way home over long distances, the odds are, sadly, rather low. Nevertheless, there are a few famous cats that have travelled widely with their owner on a bicycle, a motorbike, a boat or on skis.

Further Reading

Herrick, F.H. (1922) Homing powers of the cat. *The Scientific Monthly* 14, 525–539.

Moser, E.I., Moser, M.-B. and McNaughton, B.L. (2017) Spatial representation in the hippocampal formation: a history. *Nature Neuroscience* 20(11), 1448–1464. DOI: 10.1038/nn.4653.

Precht, H. and Lindenlaub, E. (1954) Über das Heimfindevermögen von Säugetieren. I: Versuche an Katzen. *Zeitschrift für Tierpsychologie* 11, 485–494. [In German]

Supplementary materials entitled 'Orientation and navigation in cats' can be accessed at: www.cabi.org/the-cat-behaviour-and-welfare/

8 Motivation, Behavioural Needs and Emotions

The previous chapters introduced the ethology of the cat. We learnt about its natural behaviour and how this is influenced by domestication and our deliberate, selective breeding for different shapes and colours. We have also learnt about how an individual's development and personality is influenced by both genetics and environment. In this chapter, and the chapter on learning, some important and fundamental mechanisms that control behaviour are described. What makes the cat perform a particular behaviour at any given moment is examined, namely its motivation and behavioural needs. When the cat has different options, how does it know which behaviour to choose? We shall see that the cat's emotions, combined with its knowledge of the world, guide it to act in a way that makes it feel safer and happier.

Motivation and Behavioural Needs

Motivation has to do with what the cat wants to achieve in any given situation, while behavioural needs consist of the various behaviours the cat needs to perform to fulfil this motivation. Fig. 8.1 shows how different factors can influence what the animal does at any moment. It shows that stress results from the animal not being able to meet its behavioural needs and thus not satisfy its motivation to achieve its goals. Short, acute stress is part of life. For example, if I am feeling chilly, my motivation is to get warm, and my behavioural need is to put on some warmer clothing. I shall feel stressed until I can fulfil this need. If an animal, or human, frequently feels acutely stressed, or feels continuously (chronically) stressed, then their welfare is likely to be compromised and behaviour problems can develop (see Chapter 11).

All behaviours have a *genetic* basis, although the extent to which a behaviour is genetically influenced varies. Experience that the animal obtains throughout life, especially during development from pre-birth to full social adulthood, affects both when and how it will use a certain individual behaviour pattern. Some examples were described in Chapter 3. The behaviour patterns usually used by the individual cat may be termed its *behavioural phenotype*, or personality. For example, some cats show more exploratory behaviour around a new object in the room, and we may describe them as being confident/bold, compared to another more cautious/nervous individual.

The behaviour displayed is affected by internal stimuli such as hunger or being hot or cold. Another set of internal stimuli are hormones. Obvious ones that affect behaviour are those that initiate sexual maturity and consequent changes in behaviour from those of a kitten to those of an adolescent cat, such as a tomcat starting to spray mark. The release of reproductive hormones is triggered by the lengthening daylight of spring. It is these that result in a queen becoming quite flirtatious.

At any moment, the cat is also affected by external stimuli, which may be something or someone in the environment. This could be a noise, a smell, a touch, or something the cat sees like a bird outside the window, or a highly competitive neighbourhood cat, or the gentle stroke of its owners. Such external stimuli can also cause the release of hormones, such as adrenaline or cortisol that prepare the cat for action, or oxytocin that helps it relax (Chapter 13).

Together, both internal and external stimuli contribute to the cat's motivation. The motivation is the driver for the behaviour that will enable the cat to reach its goal, its *behavioural need*.

Behavioural needs can be defined more precisely as behaviours that are necessary to maintain:

- normal physiological and physical condition, such as eating, body care, keeping warm, resting and sleeping (Fig. 8.2); and/or

Motivation – Needs – Behaviour – Consequences

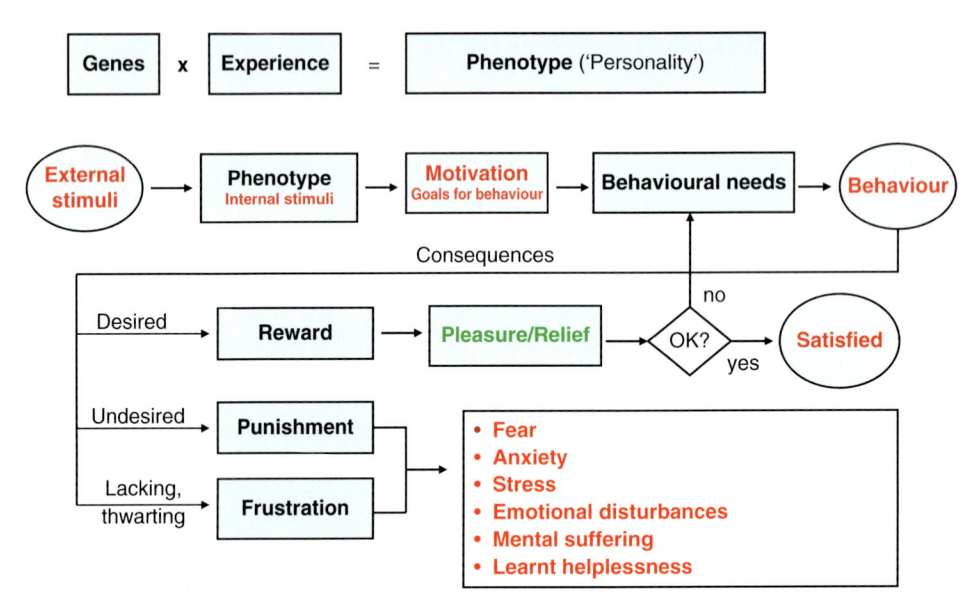

Fig. 8.1. Basic concepts describing how animals choose a behaviour.

- a normal psychological state, both emotionally and cognitively. This includes, but is not limited to, avoiding unpleasant or scary stimuli and experiencing pleasure through both social and intellectual behaviours, such as playing, solving puzzles and exploring.

Since behaviour is influenced by learning and experience, individuals will vary in the strength of their different behavioural needs. Just as in T.S. Eliot's range of feline characters, some cats will be more social, playful, confident or predatory than others. Therefore, it is important to know the personality and preferences of each individual cat to ensure that they have the best possible welfare.

It is not uncommon for two competing motivations to occur at the same time and then the cat will have to decide what to do. Just as when we are in a similar predicament, the cat will choose to satisfy the motivation that is strongest and produces the least objectionable outcome. Let us imagine a hungry cat, Missy, who is motivated to eat, but Tommy appears on the scene and sits down near the food bowl. Tommy is bigger and more confident than Missy. Now Missy is also motivated to make Tommy go away. After all, he may eat the food that she wants to eat. Missy cannot approach the food and chase Tommy away at the same time, so she must choose. It has been a long time since Missy ate and her hunger overrules her anxiety around Tommy. He must leave first. This gives Missy a behavioural need, namely, to find a way to get Tommy to leave. This need stimulates the behaviour that Missy chooses to perform.

Missy chooses to show her annoyance and puts her ears back and yowls, whilst keeping a watchful eye on Tommy. She waits to see his response, the consequence of her behaviour. An important principle of how both we and cats learn is that a performed behaviour pattern has a *consequence*. This may be the desired consequence, an undesired consequence, or thwarting of the desired consequence. In our example, we can imagine each of these three scenarios:

- **Desired consequence:** Tommy shows some signs of retreating. This works as a reward for Missy, who therefore continues with her signals (more of the successful behaviour). When Tommy is far enough away, Missy moves to the food bowl and eats well. This gives *satisfaction* – both pleasure from eating nice food and relief from feeling hungry. In a similar situation in the future, Missy is likely to choose the same solution, as she has now learnt that this behaviour lets her reach her goal of moving Tommy away from things she wants to access.

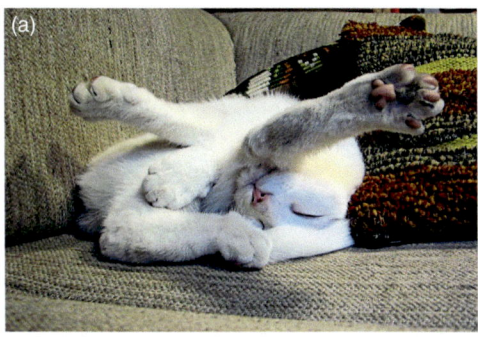

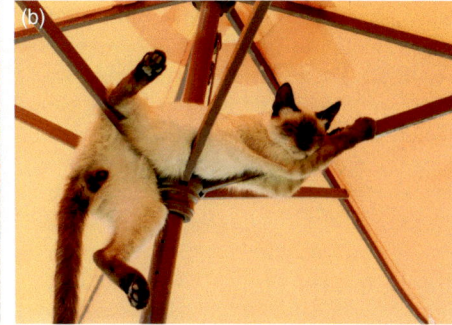

Fig. 8.2. Resting is an important behavioural need in cats, associated with the emotion of relief/pleasure. (a) Cats decide for themselves how and where they want to rest (Photo: Ann Kristin Solvang, 2019); (b) cat sleeping in a seemingly precarious place, but it likely feels safe as it is high off the ground. (Photo: iStock 509829621)

- **Undesirable consequence:** Tommy responds by putting his ears further back than Missy and stares at her as he slowly moves towards her. This acts as a positive punishment for the choice Missy made, and she must decide on another strategy, perhaps making a curve and approaching the food bowl from another side to avoid him. If she finds Tommy's response particularly threatening, she may retreat and come back later when he is no longer around. In this case, the aggressive nature of Tommy's response has strengthened her motivation to avoid conflict and stay safe, overriding her original motivation to eat.
- **Thwarting of the desired consequence:** Tommy does not care about Missy's signals. He simply ignores them and remains sitting calmly near the food bowl. This makes Missy frustrated. She tries some alternative behaviours, but Tommy does not budge an inch. His actions mean she is denied access to the food, a negative punishment. She may leave and take out her frustration elsewhere. Alternatively, she may stay, become increasingly frustrated and show increasingly aggressive behaviour towards Tommy. In that case, what happens next will depend on Tommy's response.

Sometimes an animal is in a situation of strong conflicting emotions, as in Missy's predicament, or if it cannot decide whether to chase away an intruder or retreat itself. In this case, it likely will choose a third, irrelevant behaviour, such as to sit down and groom its fur. This is a *displacement activity*. This behaviour choice provides an opportunity for the animal to 'halt proceedings' and consider its options.

In the first scenario of the Missy and Tommy encounter, the consequence led to pleasure and a good welfare state. The consequences in the latter two scenarios led to emotions of anxiety and frustration, respectively. These unpleasant feelings may last only for a little while and cause short-term (acute) stress – this is not of concern. However, if an animal is frequently exposed to, or cannot get away from, situations that cause anxiety or frustration, then it may suffer despair and chronic, long-term stress. As with humans, this is harmful, both physically and psychologically, as we shall see in Chapters 9 and 11. Thus, it is important to be able to read your cat's behaviour and identify which emotions it is feeling, and to consider how frequently it is experiencing any unpleasant emotions and how quickly they are replaced with pleasant ones. We also need to understand how emotions control behaviour and influence how and what an animal learns.

How the Cat's Emotions Control Behaviour

Clearly, the consequences of behaviour lead to emotional reactions. These, in turn, help the cat decide what to do next, as the Missy and Tommy story illustrates. Emotions are how we feel and, technically, are known as *affective states*, and these terms are used interchangeably in this book. Emotions are crucial to our interactions with the physical and social environment. Both pleasant and unpleasant emotions act as behaviour advisors, enabling the animal to choose a behaviour that is beneficial and adaptive, that is one that helps it to avoid unpleasant feelings. Of course, unpleasant emotions are essential to life and maintaining the individual's welfare. For instance, without feeling fear you will be too foolhardy, and without feeling pain you will not take care and can easily suffer even more damage. Emotions also regulate our social interactions, as with Missy and Tommy. They are the foundations of the relationships and attachments individuals form with each other, be that between friends and partners, or parents and offspring, or individuals who are less than amicable.

The Canadian researcher Michel Cabanac described the concept of feelings (emotions) as being 'intense mental events aroused by exposure of the subject to situations more or less related to motivation, either positive or negative, but all resulting in behaviour oriented to, or away from, the stimulus. Emotions are felt internally and affect our external behaviour'. Researchers in various scientific fields, like Marc Bekoff, have provided evidence that numerous and diverse animals have rich and deep emotional lives. Thanks to the work of the neuroscientist Jaak Panksepp and others, we have learned much about the interconnections between emotions, different areas of the brain and how these are linked in determining how the brain generates behaviour. Such research is a hot topic these days, with much remaining to be discovered.

Emotions vary in both type and nuance, that is the strength with which they can be felt. For example, one may be mildly or greatly amused, mildly irritated or greatly frustrated. No doubt future research will identify more emotions in animals, and even more in humans, but here is a list of 19 that many species experience, including cats and humans. We have tried to put these 19 on a scale from the most unpleasant to the most pleasant: panic, despair, pain, anxiety, fear, sadness, anger, frustration, loneliness, boredom, satisfaction, pleasure, joy, hope or positive expectation, love for a partner, parental love, sexual lust, pleasant surprise, and relief (feeling safe). The order can certainly be discussed, and it may vary between individuals and at different times in an individual's life. Of course, emotions can occur together and influence each other. For example, we may be lonely, sad and anxious; or bored and frustrated.

In the following chapters on welfare and learning, we shall be focusing on only six emotions. Three are aversive (unpleasant/negative) emotions, namely anxiety, fear, frustration – though in this chapter we shall also consider startle/shock. The other three are appetitive (pleasant/positive) emotions, namely anticipation (also called hope or positive expectation), relief and pleasure/joy. We shall now look at all of these in a bit more depth and how they relate to each other (Fig. 8.3).

Aversive (unpleasant) emotions: frustration, startle, fear and anxiety

Frustration

Frustration is an important emotion in the context of animal welfare. This occurs when an individual expects a reward but does not get it, or when the animal has a high motivation to perform a behaviour but is prevented from doing so. It may be prevented because of a lack of opportunity (a lack of triggering stimuli); for example, a lack of toys to

Anticipation (hope) ⟶ predicts ⟶ Pleasure (Joy) / Relief

Anxiety ⟶ predicts ⟶ Fear / Frustration

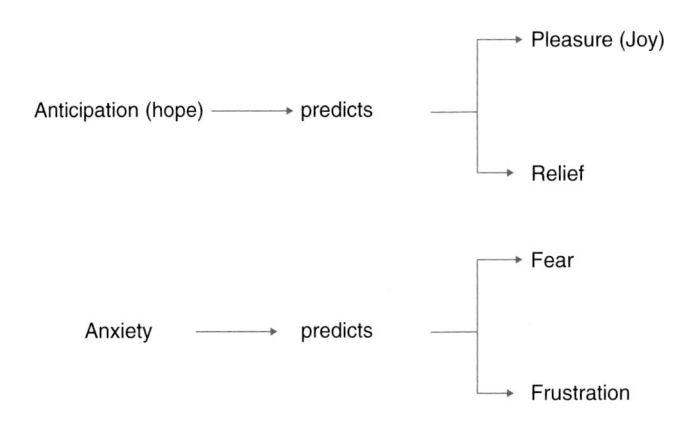

Fig. 8.3. The relationship between the six emotions.

play with. Alternatively, there may be social or physical barriers, as with Tommy's presence frustrating Missy in her desire to eat, or the window stopping the cat from getting to the birds feeding outside, causing it to swish its tail and chatter its teeth in mild frustration (Fig. 8.4). The cause of frustration can lead to different behavioural outcomes.

When the frustration is caused by competing motivations, the animal may then show a displacement activity that is unrelated to either motivation. In contrast, when frustrated because of lack of opportunity, and the animal is unable to find the right stimuli to fulfil its behavioural need, it will likely become restless. Restlessness is when the animal switches between different behaviours, not settling on any one activity. We can find ourselves in just that state.

A little bit of frustration can be a good thing and spur us on to try harder and test new behaviours, as with the authors testing several different possible sentences. We shall see in Chapter 10 that this burst of behaviour is part of how we learn. However, when an animal is exposed to strong and prolonged frustrating or anxiety-inducing circumstances, then both restless and displacement behaviours can develop into pathological forms known as *behavioural stereotypies*. These are short behaviours or movements that do not seem to have any purpose – they are not directed towards any obvious reward. They are repeated in the same way, over and over, often for minutes or even hours at a time and it is difficult to distract the animal. The animal has developed a behavioural disturbance. We shall look at these in more detail in Chapter 11. When true stereotypies develop, they are always indicative of important social, cognitive and/or physical deficiencies or conflicts in the animal's environment.

These abnormal, repetitive behaviours show pronounced individual variation. For example, one cat may pace, another over-groom, making itself bald and sore in places, and another may suck on a blanket (Fig. 8.5). It is thought that behavioural stereotypy may be a way of attempting to cope with stress. These behaviours are often seen in animals that are kept in barren or boring environments (boring from the animal's perspective), or in social environments that they find chronically stressful. Whilst one may show active repetitive behaviour, another in the same situation may show passive 'stereotypies', namely sleeping excessively and not responding to much – symptoms redolent of depression. Though both are showing that they are stressed and suffering, it is thought that these passively depressed animals may be in an even poorer welfare state than those actively trying to cope. Hence, we can see the importance of providing our cats with an interesting environment, compatible (human/cat) company, and cognitive enrichment throughout the whole of their lives.

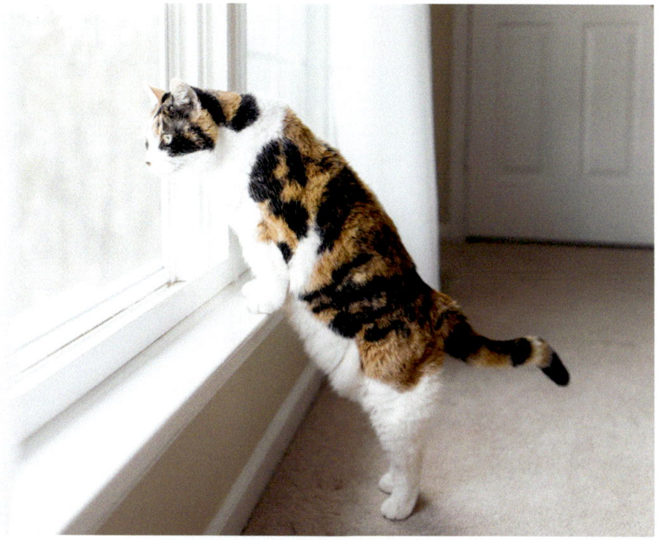

Fig. 8.4. Cat watching birds feeding outside – entertaining, if a little frustrating. (Photo: iStock 960931130)

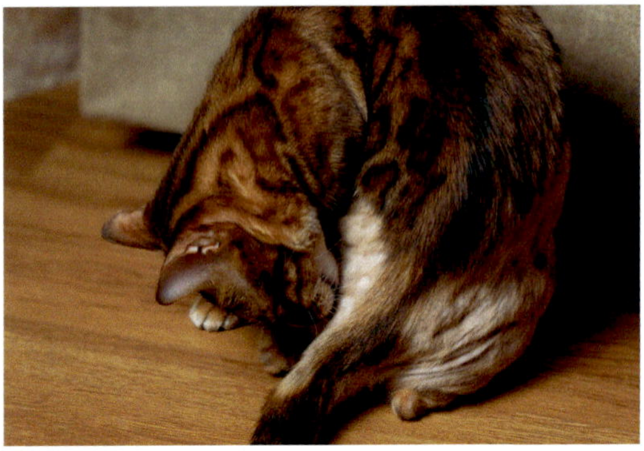

Fig. 8.5. An adult cat overgrooming (note bald flank). (Photo: iStock 1364305846)

Startle (shock)

The startle reaction is caused by a sudden event that takes us unawares. You may have been sleeping, resting or engaging in a pleasurable activity, and suddenly your attention is drawn to a noise, a touch, a flash of light or a scent. We 'jump' – which is the startle reflex. It is a rapid response preparing our body for the next action, which might be to run or fight, and is associated with the unpleasant feeling (emotion) that we call shock or startle – a burst of fear. Think about how you have felt when you have been startled – very unpleasant. The startle response is unconscious, a reflex to help keep the animal alive. It does not think about what to do, it just does it. It is the reason why we should leave sleeping dogs, and cats, alone. Their immediate response is likely to be defensive aggression. After all, it is better to respond as if the stimulus is a threat rather than find out when it is too late.

Only after this initial response has occurred will the brain have had time to process the information and ascertain whether the stimulus was a threat or not. If not, then the animal will recover its homeostasis quickly and go back to snoozing or whatever it was doing. However, if it *was* a threat, then the emotion experienced will be fear, and further action will be taken that helps the animal feel safe again. As we shall see in the next chapter, fear is less easy to recover from and the experience that caused it is never forgotten.

Fear

Fear is a natural reaction to what is perceived as dangerous or scary. An outdoor cat should be fearful of large, moving objects, such as cars, and it is quite normal for a cat to show fear if attacked by a large, aggressive cat. When frightened, an animal has three natural ways to respond. It can freeze – that is, go very still, almost motionless. This is an attempt to appear invisible and not be noticed by the scary thing. This is what cats initially do when they see a dog being walked along the street towards them. If that does not work, then they can flee, and run away to somewhere safe such as under a parked car, up a tree or back through the cat flap. The final option is to fight – that is to show defensive aggression using claws and teeth (Fig. 8.6). This is the behaviour of last resort, as the cat may itself be injured, and is only shown when the cat considers it has no means of escape.

In threatening social situations, some particularly social species, including ourselves and dogs, have a fourth possible tactic – appeasement. They use a range of behaviours to try to reduce the threat from the other animal, to appease it. Some are natural behaviours, as with our 'appeasing smile' and looking down, or the dog who looks away and lowers its head (often mistakenly interpreted as the dog 'knowing it is guilty'). Dogs also show behaviours that they have learnt can dispel threats from people, such as play-bowing to start a game or putting on a 'silly, cute face'. Children are quite adept at using similar behaviours, to divert an adult from telling them off. As we have seen in Chapters 4 and 5, the cat's social structure is looser than that of dogs and humans, and appeasement is not as important a part of their social language.

Anxiety

Anxiety is essential for survival. As Jeffrey Gray (1987) says: 'Anxiety is elicited by threats of punishment or failure and by novelty, and which causes the animal to stop, look and listen, and prepare for vigorous action'. The biological purpose of anxiety is to put all senses in a high state of alertness, enabling the animal to assess the situation. This is important, especially when there is something, or someone, new in the environment. It enables the animal to decide if the new thing is safe or scary. If deemed scary, then fear will kick in and the animal will freeze, flee or fight. If the assessment is that it is safe, then the animal may choose to ignore it, or approach for closer inspection.

To survive another day, animals must learn what stimuli predict threats. Anxiety is the emotion that

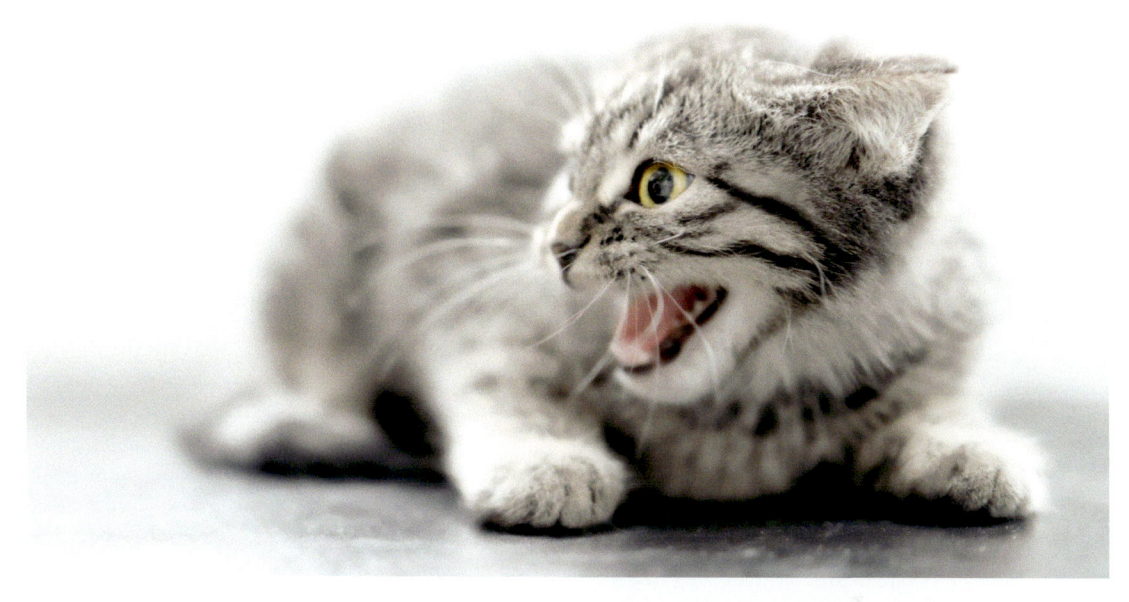

Fig. 8.6. A frightened cat, resorting to defensive aggression. (Photo: Trudi Atkinson, 2018)

is quickly associated with such stimuli – so quickly that the association can be learnt after just one experience. When these or any very similar stimuli are encountered in the future, the animal will become anxious, and its behaviour will prepare it for the possibility of threat and danger. Such preparation may be to hide when these stimuli occur (Fig. 8.7). For example, a cat may find unfamiliar people frightening, perhaps due to too little socialization. It has learnt that the doorbell means a person is arriving, and this leads to a feeling of anxiety. So, as soon as the doorbell rings, the cat hides and assesses if the visitor is a known, safe person or a potentially scary, unknown person, in which case, staying hidden until the person leaves is a sensible strategy from the cat's perspective.

In appropriate amounts, anxiety is an essential part of a long and balanced life. However, sometimes the initial experience was very frightening, or the animal has repeatedly been exposed to the same anxiety-provoking stimuli. This can lead to conditioned (learnt) fears called phobias. Phobias are deeply ingrained fears and resistant to being

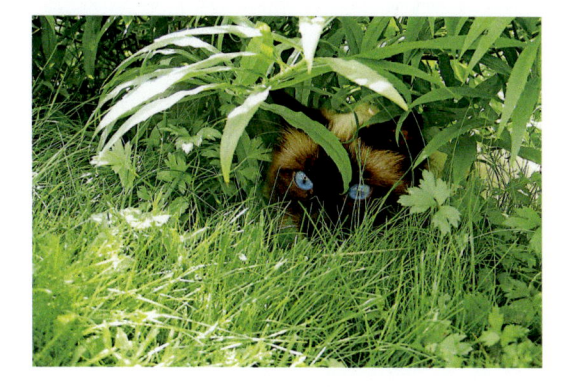

Fig. 8.7. An insecure, anxious cat feels safer when it keeps hidden. (Photo: Audun Braastad, 2019)

changed (Chapters 10 and 11). The phobia may have developed from the original fear- or frustration-provoking stimulus (or any like it), or occur when the animal has associated a random stimulus that was present in a situation where the strong fear or strong frustration experience happened. In this

Motivation, Behavioural Needs and Emotions

case, it has learnt to respond to this random stimulus through *classical conditioning* (see Chapter 10). For example, the cat may have been chased into a corner of the garden by some annoying (but, to the cat, very scary) children. This only needs to happen once for the cat to associate that place with the fear it experienced and to not approach that part of the garden in the future. It will become more anxious the nearer it is taken to that area.

So as with frustration, a little bit of anxiety is a good thing, especially in novel situations. However, if the cat cannot get away from or resolve anxiety-provoking situations, then it will suffer chronic anxiety and stress, which can lead to a variety of problem behaviours (see Chapter 11).

Appetitive (pleasant) emotions: relief, hope, joy and surprise

Relief

Relief is an extremely powerful emotion because it is *the* emotion associated with safety. We, and other animals, feel relief when we know we have avoided or escaped a potential or actual scary or frustrating situation. As we have seen with Missy and Tommy, it is essential to feel safe before one can start to get on with the pleasurable, joyful things in life such as eating. Relief is the emotion you feel when you come home and settle into your own bed, your safe, warm and comfortable resting place where you can sleep peacefully, maybe with your cat alongside.

Hope (anticipation)

Hope is triggered by the anticipation of a pleasant event. As with anxiety, this anticipation is the result of classical learning. Hope is elicited when the animal has learnt that a stimulus predicts that a good thing will occur. This may be something like food or seeing a friend that leads to feelings of pleasure. Hope is also elicited by events that predict safety and feelings of relief, such as the sight of home after a difficult day at work; or, for your cat, the sight of the cat flap when running away from a scary dog, or bully cat, in the street.

When the cat gets signals indicating that something pleasurable may happen, it will exhibit anticipatory, expectant, hopeful behaviour. Imagine that our cat really likes freshly cooked fish. The cat has learnt from experience that it always gets some fish when we cook fish for dinner. When we start preparing the dinner, which signals that something good will occur, the cat shows its expectation with optimistic and pleading miaow sounds, as it walks around our legs and strokes us with its tail, or it may sit and watch us intently.

Giving our animals signals that elicit pleasant expectations is among the best ways we can put them in an appetitive emotional state, a good mood. This contributes to enhancing their welfare. When animals look forward to something, we should not always give them what they want immediately. Within limits, the longer we wait, the longer the expectation phase will last. This is like children looking forward to their birthday, even if it is still three weeks away, or when you have bought a lottery ticket on Monday and you wait in anticipation for Saturday, hoping that, this time, you will win the main prize. In such a state of positive expectation, the brain secretes a lot of *dopamine*, which makes you enlivened. Obviously, if the delay is too long then hope turns to frustration and potentially even despair (hopelessness). So keep your cat waiting for the fish for just a while, such as by letting it cool before putting it into the food bowl, but not for so long that the cat gives up and leaves the room.

Joy (pleasure), hope and surprise

The feelings of joy, hope and surprise have a unique connection with each other. Joy, also known as pleasure, is a complex emotion that acts as a strong motivation for behaviour. To experience pleasure every day is essential for our cat's mental health. Play is joyful, and when the cat can access something strongly desirable it shows joy (Fig. 8.8). As we have seen, hope is triggered by signals that something good will occur and that joy will be experienced.

Surprise, a pleasant surprise, is one of the most enjoyable emotions we can have, even though it only lasts a short time. Unexpectedly and suddenly, we get a strong reward that we did not expect. Not only does it elicit strong feelings of pleasure, but it is also likely to be remembered. That is why you should occasionally give your loved one flowers or chocolates on a day that is not their birthday or Valentine's Day. The delight will be much greater.

Likewise, we can use surprise to really reinforce behaviour we want and increase the bond our cats have with us. Every now and then, give your cat a treat when it is not expecting it, when it is not nagging you, but is simply sitting on the chair or resting in its bed. Your cat will really appreciate you, and possibly reduce its nagging behaviour as well!

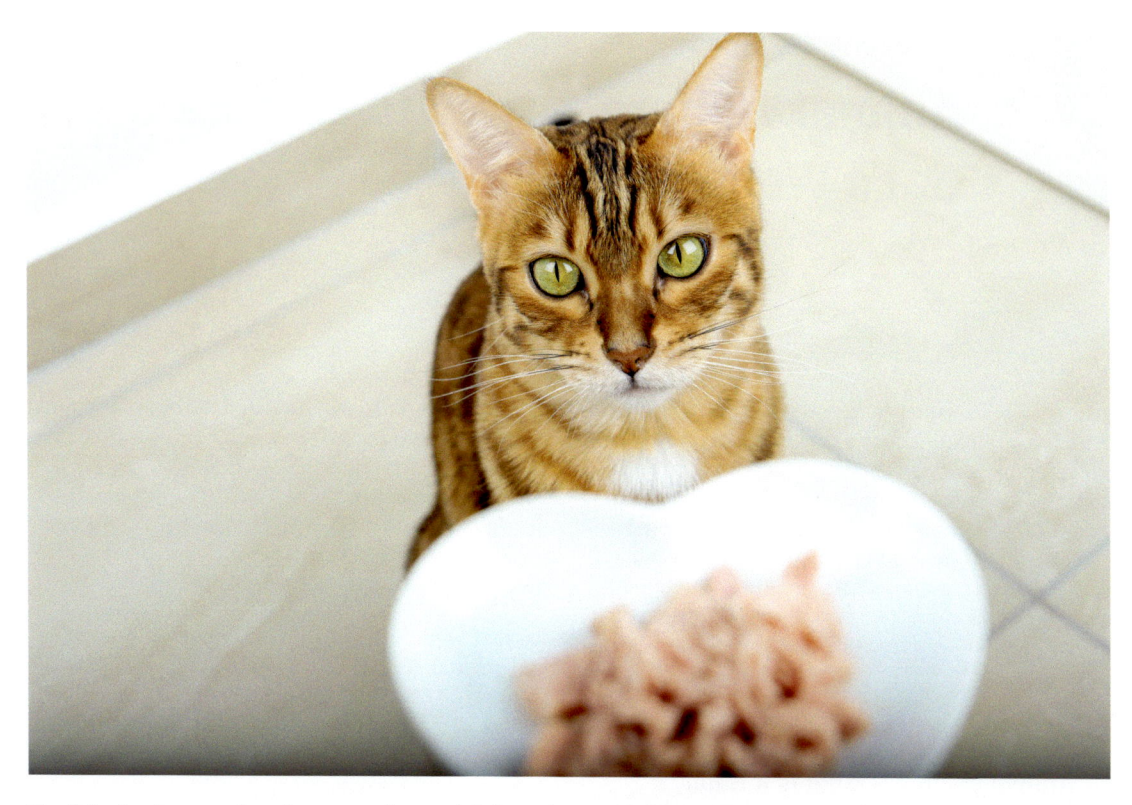

Fig. 8.8. A cat expressing pleasure as its special dinner is served. (Photo: iStock 1359551361)

Further Reading

Atkinson, T. (2018) *Practical Feline Behaviour: Understanding Cat Behaviour and Improving Welfare*. CAB International, Wallingford, UK, p. 249.

Bekoff, M. (2010) *The Emotional Lives of Animals: A Leading Scientist Explores Animal Joy, Sorrow, and Empathy – and Why They Matter*. New World Library, Novato, California.

Cabanac, M. (2002) What is emotion? *Behavioural Processes* 60, 69–83.

Gray, J.A. (1987) *The Psychology of Fear and Stress*. Cambridge University Press, Cambridge.

Panksepp, J. (2004) *Affective Neuroscience: The Foundations of Human and Animal Emotions*. Oxford University Press, Oxford.

9 Animal Welfare – How to Ensure the Cat's Welfare

If we are to benefit from keeping cats, the cats must also enjoy our company. We must safeguard their welfare. This chapter explains further what we mean when talking about animal welfare, how we can recognize a cat's state of welfare, and various welfare problems that cats can experience. It includes discussion about stray cats and hereditary diseases of cats, and gives practical recommendations for ensuring the welfare of cats in the home, in shelters and in boarding and breeding catteries. We hope this information helps cat owners and carers to provide the things that make a big difference to cats' quality of life.

Animal Welfare – What Is it Really?

Animal welfare is about the quality of life of the individual animal. The focus is on the animal itself, rather than what we do (animal care) or ought to do (ethics). Of course, we expect that how we care for animals, and the guidelines we put in place to protect them, will make a difference to animal welfare, but these are separate from animal welfare itself. A cat's welfare belongs to the cat. What we decide to do about it is another thing. Therefore, to understand a cat's welfare, we need to learn as much as possible about cats in general, and the individual cat specifically, and then use empathy to put ourselves in that cat's 'shoes' – to think like the cat. We should avoid jumping to conclusions based on what we humans would prefer.

That a cat has good welfare means much more than just being physically healthy. According to modern understanding, animal welfare encompasses three main dimensions, as outlined in Fig. 9.1. To get a good overview of an animal's welfare situation, we must consider all three dimensions:

1. *natural life* – the extent to which the animal is able to perform a broad repertoire of behaviour typical of the species, with freedom of choice and ability to adapt to the environmental conditions in which it is living;
2. *biological function* – how well the body functions to keep the animal alive, healthy and (in breeding animals) able to reproduce successfully; and
3. *subjective experience* – how the animal itself mentally experiences or perceives its situation or quality of life, which depends on the balance between positive and negative emotions.

Animal welfare has to do with both the physical and mental health of the individual, and how it copes with the challenges and opportunities presented by the environment where it lives. It has been defined by the research group on Ethology and Animal Housing at the Norwegian University of Life Sciences as follows, adapted from Donald M. Broom: 'Animal welfare is the individual animal's subjective experience of its mental and physical state as regards its attempts to master its environment.'

Some scientists hesitate to include 'subjective' experience in the definition, as this can be hard to assess. We cannot directly read the minds of others, whether cats or humans. However, even if we don't know exactly what they are thinking or feeling, this should not stop us from striving to understand how they are experiencing the world; otherwise, we would never get beyond describing them as objects, like cars that can behave in different ways and use sensors to detect nearby obstacles, but not feel what it is to be alive. Here we explain the different concepts used in the animal welfare definition.

Mental states include emotional and cognitive (thinking) states that help the animal to decide what to do next (see Chapter 8). For example, feeling tired often leads to taking a nap; feeling happy may lead to friendly social interaction; feeling frightened can lead to fleeing, hiding or defensive aggression, depending on the situation, and feeling frustrated may lead to aggression or depression.

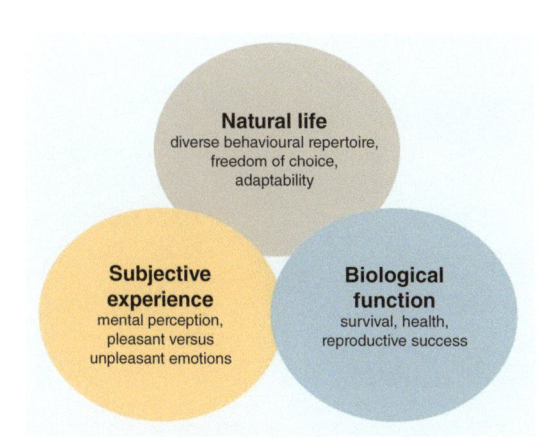

Fig. 9.1. Animal welfare has three dimensions that contribute to overall animal welfare.

Mental states are affected by both current stimuli the animal receives from inside and outside the body, and memory of previous experience with similar stimuli. What the animal does at any moment will depend on the animal's mental evaluation of safety and the relative priority of different possible actions. Mental states imply *sentience* – the ability to consciously experience feelings and thoughts. If cats were not sentient, we would not be concerned about their welfare but only about their usefulness and dangerousness, like cars.

Physical states include physical and physiological conditions that affect mental processes. They include things like skin condition, stage of pregnancy and stress hormone levels.

Environment includes the social, physical and biological environment. The *social* environment mainly comprises members of an animal's own species, but for cats we may include familiar people and other animals with whom the cat interacts. The *physical* environment includes the weather conditions, the terrain and housing conditions. The *biological* environment includes pathogens, parasites, predators, prey and unfamiliar people.

An animal is influenced by multiple aspects of its environment, some positive and some negative. Its overall welfare level will be characterized by the balance between positive and negative experiences. Therefore, its welfare can vary along a scale from very bad on the left to very good on the right. Bad welfare implies that the animal is experiencing predominantly unpleasant (negative) emotions at the time, whereas good welfare implies that the animal is experiencing predominantly pleasant (positive) emotions. At the central point on the scale, the animal is not experiencing any particularly noticeable negative or positive emotions at that moment.

It is not realistic to be able to remove all the problems or frustrations that a cat may experience. Perhaps the cat has a low competitive capacity and is harassed outdoors by the neighbour's cat. What can we do? One possibility would be to go outdoors together with the cat and play with it there. This will give the cat more positive experiences and move its welfare further to the right on the scale. This can be measured by assessing *welfare indicators* for mental and physical states.

The welfare level must be assessed for the individual cat. Although most individuals in a cat colony may have good welfare, we should pay particular attention to individuals that have a poor ability to cope with the social, physical or biological environment. These could be cats with a low social rank or a high degree of fearfulness or anxiety, and, of course, cats that are sick or injured.

Indicators of Animal Welfare

Since the welfare level of an animal is a sum of positive and negative factors, we distinguish between positive and negative welfare indicators. To get an indication of mental states, we use behavioural (ethological) indicators, while to assess physical states, we can measure various aspects of health and physiology. Cat owners can easily evaluate basic aspects of behaviour and health status while more detailed measures and tests are used by vets and researchers. There are various cat welfare assessment protocols that can be used to get an overall measure of cat welfare (see articles by McCune and by Kessler and Turner in the Further Reading section). Here we give some general guidelines on what to look for.

Negative welfare indicators

Behavioural indicators of poor welfare are deviations in relation to what is normal behaviour for the individual that indicate stress, pain, fear, anxiety, panic, aggression, apathy or more specific behavioural disorders (discussed in Chapter 11). Poor cat welfare may also result in incomplete grooming, reduced activity, changes in eating and drinking behaviour, social problems, lack of play and grimacing in pain. The University of Montreal has developed a Feline Grimace Scale© which can help owners recognize when their cat is in pain (felinegrimacescale.com).

Physical indicators of poor welfare include, of course, injuries and symptoms of diseases, but also signs of parasites such as ear mites and ticks, or areas of missing fur which can mean anything from ringworm to over-grooming (see Chapter 11). If you discover such symptoms, you must take the cat to the vet. To assess physiological stress, blood samples can be taken to measure the level of the main stress hormone, cortisol.

Positive welfare indicators

There are several behavioural indicators of good animal welfare. Exploratory behaviour is a sign that the animal is doing well and at present has no other important tasks. A cat with good welfare has normal levels of activity, body care, social contact with humans and other animals, and such a cat will often initiate social contact.

Behaviour patterns that indicate that the cat has a *positive expectation*, looking forward to something, are strong positive indicators. We may stimulate maximum welfare by putting the cat in a state of anticipation, like we feel when looking forward to an upcoming holiday. We can achieve this by providing a signal that is associated with receiving a reward – for example, showing the food dish, but waiting a little while before giving it to the cat. Repeated instances of positive expectation may act as 'stress therapy' for both cats and people.

Other signs of satisfaction and joy in cats include resting in a relaxed manner, purring, keeping the eyes half-shut, rolling, walking with the tail straight up, ears pricked forward, and playing. Play does not occur when cats are stressed, and when your cat is playing, other and more basic needs are covered. Play can help the animal gain experience in coping with the unexpected, which can contribute to improved stress-coping ability. You can read more about kitten play in Chapter 2.

Physical indicators of good welfare include a well-groomed appearance, clear eyes and good body condition (neither too heavy nor too thin). Physiological indicators are linked to activation of the reward system in the brain, such as the neurotransmitters (signal substances in the neural system) dopamine, oxytocin and opioids, but these require special analyses that are normally only made in connection with research projects.

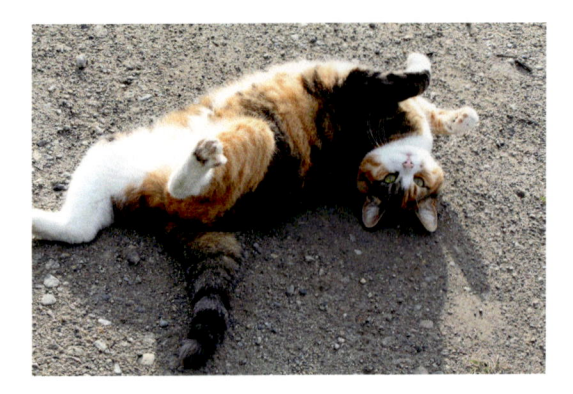

Fig. 9.2. A cat rolling on the ground near familiar people feels safe and has good welfare. (Photo: Janne Helen Lorentzsen, 2019)

Ethical Obligation to Ensure Animal Welfare

Now that we have explained the concept of animal welfare, we move on to the question of how we should care for cats to *ensure* their welfare. When keeping domestic animals, including cats, there is an ethical obligation to protect them from harm. In some countries, an animal welfare law sets out societal expectations regarding animal welfare. Cat owners must be knowledgeable about the general laws relating to animal welfare in their country as well as any specific legal requirements for cat-keeping in their area. The Norwegian Animal Welfare Act provides some general basic ethical principles that we think provide relevant guidance to those keeping cats, no matter where they live (see Box 9.1).

Homeless Cats – What Can We Do about Them?

Problems and obligations

Although the majority of cat owners are responsible animal keepers, in many places there are large numbers of homeless cats. This can have many causes. Some have strayed from home. In particular, male cats around two years of age may voluntarily emigrate if they are uncomfortable in the social environment of the cats in their neighbourhood, even though they have owners (see Chapter 5 on social behaviour). Others are abandoned by irresponsible owners. They may drop unwanted kittens or adult cats in the woods or countryside, or leave them behind when moving or going home from a holiday

Box 9.1. Comments on selected parts of the Norwegian Animal Welfare Act of 2009 of relevance to cat owners.

§ 1. Scope
The intention of this act is to promote good animal welfare and respect for animals.

Comment: Promoting good animal welfare is more than safeguarding against poor animal welfare. One must provide an environment that promotes positive aspects of welfare. The requirement about respect for animals concerns an expectation that animal owners have a positive attitude towards the animals they keep, recognize the animals' distinctive characteristics and show empathy if the animals suffer.

§ 3. General requirement regarding the treatment of animals
Animals have an intrinsic value regardless of the usable value they may have for people. Animals should be treated well and protected from the risk of unnecessary stress and strains.

Comment: Intrinsic value addresses the understanding that animals are sentient beings with lives that matter to them. They are not simply objects here to please us. Having intrinsic value requires that they are given due respect.

§ 4. Duty to help
Anyone who comes across an animal that is obviously sick, injured, or helpless shall as far as possible help the animal. If the animal is kept by people or is a large wild mammal, and it is not possible to provide adequate help, the owner or police must be notified immediately. If it is obvious that the animal will not survive or recover, the person who discovers the animal may kill it at once. However, animals kept by people or large wild mammals shall not be killed if it is possible to alert the owner, a veterinarian, or police within a reasonable period of time.

Comment: The duty to help includes stray and homeless cats who are ill, injured or helpless.

§ 5. Duty to alert
Anyone who has reason to believe that an animal is exposed to abuse or serious neglect regarding the environmental conditions, supervision, or care, shall as soon as possible notify the animal welfare authority or the police.

Comment: We are obliged to alert the relevant authorities if we discover that our neighbour or other people abuse their cat or show serious deficiencies in its care. We must also alert authorities if a homeless cat is obviously sick or injured. The reader is advised to find out who the relevant authorities are in their country.

§ 6. Competence and responsibility
The animal keeper shall ensure that animals are taken care of by appropriately competent personnel. Others should have the necessary skills for the activity they perform. Parents and carers with parental responsibility shall not allow children under the age of 16 to have independent responsibility for animals. The animal keeper shall not transfer animals to people if there is reason to believe that they cannot or will not treat the animal properly.

Comment: Cat owners must have sufficient competence to keep cats, including knowledge of their behavioural and other needs and other matters of importance for ensuring adequate welfare. This knowledge can, for example, be acquired by reading this book. You can give a cat to your child, but you cannot transfer the main responsibility for the cat before the child is 16 years old. If you sell or give away kittens, you should check the knowledge and attitudes of the new owners. If you suspect that the cat will not get proper care from the new owners, you must not give away or sell the cat to them.

§ 12. Euthanasia
The euthanasia of animals and handling in connection with euthanasia must be done with due consideration of animal welfare. Anyone who uses anaesthetic or equipment for euthanasia shall ensure that it is suitable for the purpose and well maintained. Animals owned or otherwise kept in human custody must be rendered unconscious before killing begins and remain unconscious until death occurs. Emergency killing must, as far as possible, be done in accordance with these points.

Continued

> **Box 9.1.** Continued.
>
> *Comment:* A cat should always be euthanized by a veterinarian unless it is an emergency, and the animal must be killed quickly. Even in an emergency, the animal should be made unconscious, so it does not suffer from being killed. Shooting is not recommended because cats are small and there is a risk of causing wounds that do not kill instantly.
>
> ### § 23. Animals' living environment
> The animal keeper shall ensure that animals are kept in an environment that provides good welfare based on species-specific and individual needs. The environment shall give the animals the opportunity to carry out stimulating activities, movement, rest, and other natural behaviour. The animals' living environment shall promote good health and contribute to safety and well-being.
>
> *Comment:* To avoid frustrations and stress, the owner must know the cat's behavioural and environmental needs. This book provides you with this knowledge. Keep in mind that needs may show individual variation. An active breed, like a Bengal cat may have different needs than a less-active Persian cat.
>
> ### § 25. Breeding
> Breeding should promote characteristics that make animals robust with good functioning and good health. No breeding shall be carried out, including using genetic engineering methods, that:
>
> a. Changes the genotype to adversely affect the physical or mental functions of animals, or that maintains such adverse genes,
> b. Reduces the animal's ability to exhibit normal behaviour, or
> c. Evokes common ethical concerns.
>
> *Comment:* Cats with diseases or disabilities that may have a genetic origin should not be used as breeding animals. Nor should cats be bred if that breeding would lead to negative mental functions, such as increased fearfulness or aggression or reduced cognitive abilities. Pedigree cat clubs must adjust breed standards for body form or details of the anatomy that have become too extreme and judges at cat shows must not show preference for such extreme characteristics.
>
> ### § 27. Trading of animals and professional care of animals belonging to others
> A person who sells or transfers animals to others shall give the person who receives the animal the necessary information about conditions of importance for the animal's welfare.
>
> *Comment:* This puts great responsibility on people selling or giving cats to others, whether pedigree or not. One should provide necessary information to new owners, both about cat care in general and about the characteristics of the individual cat that are important for its care, nutrition and health. People who buy or otherwise acquire a cat should really receive a cat manual from the cat breeder. Note that this applies whether you pay for the cat or get it for nothing.

at the cabin. It is incomprehensible that people can abandon cats that they have previously taken care of, but unfortunately this is not so rare, even though being an obvious violation of ethics and, in many countries, of the law. The cats are then homeless unless they are adopted by other people.

Many kittens are born to homeless cats. If they grow up with little or no contact with people, they may be referred to as wild cats, but real wildcats belong to a different species from the domestic cat (see Chapter 1). Instead, these kittens and their homeless parents are properly called *feral* cats, and they are usually very shy of people. If they have not been socialized as kittens (see Chapter 2), these feral cats are rarely adopted as they will never be as friendly as a well-socialized cat. Another concern is that, if living in regions with true wildcats, feral cats may interbreed with the native wildcats. Crossbreeding can make the offspring less able to survive in the natural habitat to which the wildcats are uniquely adapted. Furthermore, wildcat species are often vulnerable to extinction due to habitat loss, and the presence of feral domestic cats and hybrids competing for territories makes their

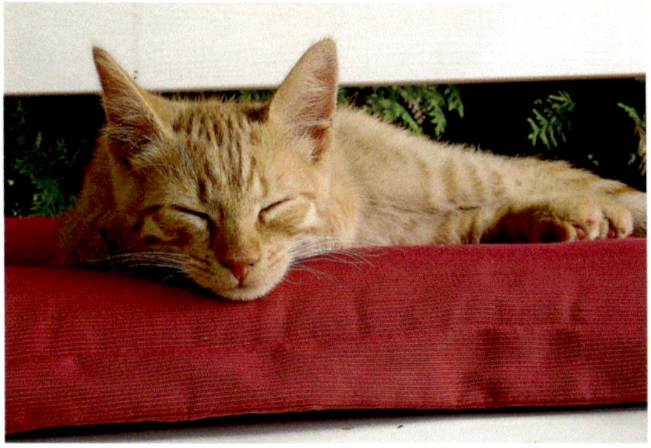

Fig. 9.3. In this environment, I enjoy myself. (Photo: Silje Kittilsen, 2019)

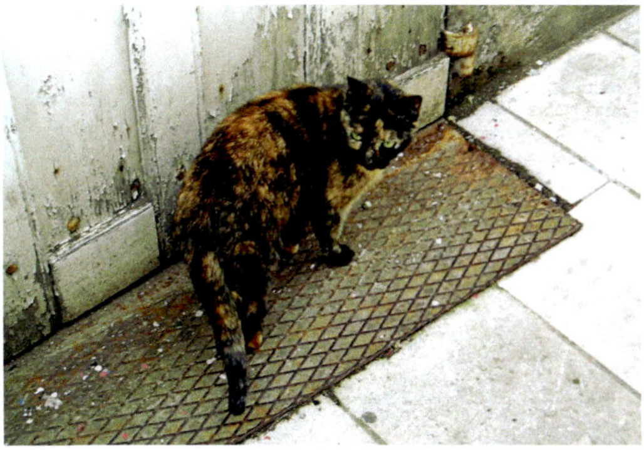

Fig. 9.4. A homeless cat that needs help. (Photo: Anita A. Pedersen, 2019)

conservation far more complicated and tenuous. Feral cats are 'in-between cats', neither valued as wildlife nor suited to living with people.

Homeless cats often struggle to get enough food. Many of the cats are sick and suffer from contagious diseases such as cat flu (feline herpesvirus 1), feline immunodeficiency virus, feline distemper (feline panleukopenia virus, also referred to as cat plague), and feline leukaemia virus. They are likely to have intestinal worms, ear mites, lice, fleas and dental problems, and, in some regions, there is a risk that they have rabies. If they do manage to survive and find food, they can have offspring three to four times a year and contribute to large populations of feral cats. In many places, animal welfare societies and cat organizations take in homeless cats or provide some care *in situ*, but the need for help usually exceeds their capacity.

Earlier, it was common for municipalities to capture and kill such cats to reduce their populations. There are two reasons why society and the public must deal with this in another way:

- The status of the cat in society has increased significantly in recent years. The cat is the most common companion animal in much of the world. Knowledge of the positive significance of the cat for human psychological and physical health gives the cat an important role in community medicine. The cat's increased status and social significance give both cat owners and the public increased responsibility for ensuring the welfare of cats.
- The community has an ethical responsibility for homeless cats. Do people have the duty to care for the welfare of unowned animals of domesticated species? Of course, here we are thinking of cats, though the ethical issues are the same for all domestic animals. We believe the answer is an unconditional YES, because people have created the problem:
  ○ people have abandoned them;
  ○ they have escaped or wandered away from people;
  ○ they are lost and unable to find their owner; or
  ○ they are descendants of such animals.

All homeless cats originate from cats that have had owners, either in the same generation or in previous generations. This means that domestic cats cannot be regarded as wildlife but should have a special position in relation to hunting legislation. Apart from on certain islands or other localities, cats are rarely considered pests to wildlife or people. This makes killing a cat just because it has no owner at present legally unfounded in many countries though there is the recognition that stray and feral cats can become a problem. Hence, there is an ethical and sometimes legal obligation for owners and societies to (i) consider the requirement for permanent ID labelling of cats with numbers maintained in a register; and (ii) encourage the neutering of cats to prevent unplanned breeding.

Current measures

Experience from major cities in the UK, the USA and Italy shows that killing campaigns only have a short-term effect. When cats are killed, their vacant territories are quickly occupied by immigrating cats (for example, peripheral cats who would otherwise have low breeding success; see

Chapter 5), so the killing actions need to be repeated frequently. Different alternative solutions, and their effectiveness, are discussed by Margaret R. Slater in her book *The Welfare of Cats* (see Further Reading).

Trapping and neutering (TNR/TTVARR)

There are several ways to take action that involve castration or spaying of cats. A common method is termed the TNR method – Trap, Neuter, Return. Cats are trapped in live traps, neutered (castrated or spayed) and returned to the spot where they were trapped. Where rabies occurs, the method includes vaccination and is termed TNVR – Trap, Neuter, Vaccinate, Return.

A more elaborate version of TNR may be called TTVARR. This stands for Trap, Test, Vaccinate, Alter, Rehome or Release, which means that allegedly stray cats are *trapped* in live traps and *tested* for an ID marking and for their health condition. Seriously ill unowned cats are euthanized. Healthy cats are vaccinated and altered (i.e. castrated or spayed). They are ID-tagged and rehomed to new owners if they are sufficiently friendly towards people. Cats that have had owners and later have become homeless can get used to a life with people again. If the cats are too shy, they are released again at the place where they were trapped. Cats that are not completely wild by nature but which require more socialization before they can be adopted by new owners can be temporarily placed in a cat shelter run by an animal welfare organization until they are fit for adoption. This method is also called TNR for simplicity. By this method, the number of cats released is noticeably lower than the number captured. Castrated male cats may be more territorial than uncastrated ones, helping to prevent the immigration of new cats. This method ensures a certain population of cats, so unwanted prey species are kept under control. The TTVARR method can produce a longer-lasting reduction in cat numbers than killing actions, though it must also be repeated now and then as existing members of the population die and are replaced by immigrating cats.

Many countries are now using these methods. Several organizations, such as International Cat Care (iCatCare) provide information on cat-friendly methods of controlling stray and feral cats, and how such cats can be housed at cat shelters (see *The Feral Cat Manual*, edited by Claire Bessant, under Further Reading). To be effective, one must trap and neuter at least half of the feral cats in the area and involve an animal welfare organization that can monitor the released cats and, potentially, establish feeding stations. They can establish co-operation with the municipality on implementation and funding, especially to cover veterinary expenses. It is important to combine the TTVARR or TNR method with a strong campaign urging cat owners to ID-mark and neuter their cats to prevent the population of homeless cats from rising again.

ID-tagging

Permanent ID-tagging has obvious benefits to cat owners and cats, whether done by tattooing a number in the ear or placing a microchip under the skin. This greatly increases the chance that lost cats will be reunited with their owners. We recommend that this be mandatory in regions with many cats. Homeless cats can quickly become shy towards humans including their owners, so it is important that they are caught at an early stage and returned to the owners without delay (see Chapter 7). Until most cats are microchipped, they should also be visibly marked with an M (for 'marked' or 'microchipped') tattoo in one ear so people who come across a homeless cat will realize that it is microchipped. In addition, it is a good idea to give the cat a quick-release collar showing the owner's phone number.

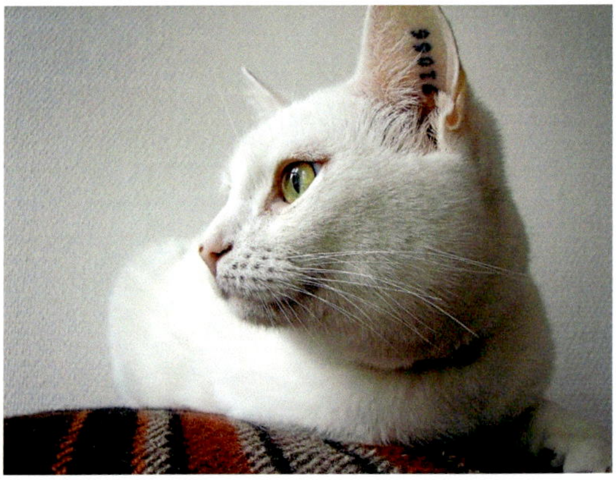

Fig. 9.5. This cat is ear-marked according to an ID scheme. (Photo: Ann Kristin Solvang, 2019)

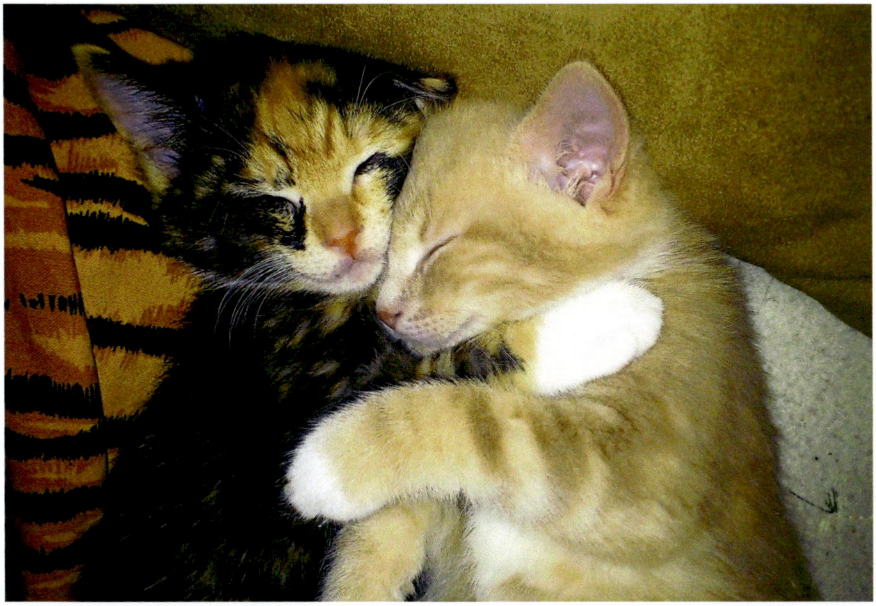

Fig. 9.6. If all cats were neutered, we would not have been born. (Photo: Linda Iren Jensen, 2019)

Propagation control

According to surveys conducted in 1997–98, approximately 82% of Norwegian male cats were castrated, while 25% of females were spayed and 53% received birth control pills. In another study of 1209 cats conducted in 2014, 95% of non-pedigree cats and 60% of pedigree cats were reported to be neutered, suggestive of increased interest in propagation control over the intervening years. The surveys were conducted among cat owners in cat clubs or, in 2014, among Facebook groups for cat owners. Both these groups may be more aware of their responsibilities than the average cat owner. Therefore, the real numbers were probably lower amongst the whole Norwegian cat population. Nevertheless, there is clear potential for conducting attitude-changing work to increase the percentage of neutered cats. Neutering goes a long way towards reducing the number of unwanted cats.

However, if propagation control measures approach 100%, there may be two unfortunate consequences because a small proportion of the cat population will then be responsible for all reproduction: (i) if the unneutered cats have irresponsible owners, those owners may also fall short in other aspects of cat care including failing to socialize the kittens, resulting in an increasing proportion of cats with behavioural problems; (ii) if these few cats have genetically related deficiencies, physical or behavioural, the consequence will be an increasing incidence of such defects. Similarly, if a temporary ban on cat breeding is imposed, one can predict that some people will circumvent the rules and produce kittens, and the genetics of those kittens will quickly dominate the cat population.

Early neutering

Neutering of cats has many advantages, both for female and male cats. They may more easily function in a group, and neutered females tend to have lower levels of the stress hormone cortisol. Vets often recommend early neutering of cats, at 10–12 weeks of age, to avoid unwanted pregnancy. Removing the sex glands avoids sexual maturation, but the cats may retain a more juvenile character and can more easily develop obesity. Neutered adult cats therefore need fewer calories and should be given food that is 30% less energy-rich than that given to intact cats, or be provided with smaller meals.

Based on studies of anatomy and physiology, there appears to be no health reason to discourage even earlier neutering at 7–8 weeks of age. Surveys in the USA indicate that early neutering does not create more behaviour problems for owners than in other cats. However, it is unclear how early neutering affects the social behaviour, confidence and competitive ability of adult cats, especially when outdoors or kept in a social colony. Before we have more knowledge in this field, it may be best to wait until kittens are 4–6 months of age, depending on rate of maturity of the individual.

Limiting the number of cats per household

Occasionally, certain people will take in more cats than they have the capacity to care for properly. Although well meaning, they are often unaware that the welfare of their cats (and themselves) is poor. This is a psychological disorder called *animal hoarding*. Handling of such cases by the authorities requires individual decisions in each case, usually involving removal of the cats and referral of the person for medical assessment and treatment. This should not lead to harsh all-encompassing regulations on the maximum number of cats allowed in a household. In hoarding cases, one cannot establish a rule about how many cats are too many. For some people, three cats would be too many to cope with, whereas ten breeding cats kept by a responsible breeder with appropriate facilities, knowledge and care can be perfectly fine as long as good relations are maintained with the neighbours (see Chapter 12).

Health and Diseases

When you take your cat to a vet once a year to be revaccinated, your vet should also conduct a general health check. However, diseases may occur at any time of the year, and you should be aware of the main symptoms that something is wrong. If you notice any of the symptoms below, you should contact a vet to be on the safe side:

- lack of appetite
- abnormal thirst
- sudden weight loss
- frequent vomiting
- persistent diarrhoea or constipation
- urinates often or with difficulty
- secretions from the nose or eyes
- the third eyelid (the nictitating membrane) covers half the eye or more
- coughing or sneezing
- abnormal breathing or panting

- sudden bad breath or very bad breath
- the cat frequently scratches itself
- unusual aggression, especially when touched
- unstable or peculiar locomotion
- the cat hides, does not play, will not go outdoors (if it usually goes out).

Health Problems in Pedigree Cats

Negative side-effects of breeding on dog health are well known by the public. Unfortunately, side-effects of pedigree cat breeding are less well recognized. Many pedigree cats are more prone to diseases and disabilities than non-pedigree cats. This is related to a strong focus on specific anatomical features and fur colours in breed standards. In the international cat-breeding organization FIFe (Fédération Internationale Féline), there are strict rules aimed at preventing hereditary diseases. However, it is not easy to overcome the problems that have arisen gradually over decades of unfortunate breeding, as well as inbreeding within small populations of the rarer breeds, particularly when the demand for such breeds increases.

Breeding Effects on Anatomy, Health and Behaviour

Here are some examples of hereditary disorders found in various cat breeds:

- *Deafness* mainly occurs in white cats on the side on which they have a blue eye, and on both sides if they have two blue eyes. Not all white, blue-eyed cats are deaf, but most of them are.
- *Fold-ears (osteochondrodysplasia)*, as found in Scottish fold cats, are due to a so-called autosomal dominant gene. Several malformations may be associated with this genetic disorder, such as a short, thick tail and severe abnormalities of the cartilege of bones resulting in subsequent walking problems. This disorder may lead to painful arthritis, although there is individual variation in its severity. The British organization International Cat Care states that it is unethical to continue to breed cats with a genetic mutation that is known to cause a significant painful disease. We fully agree with them.
- *Gangliosidosis* is a disease that was acknowledged some years ago in Korat cats, but it has been around for much longer than this. It is a neural disease caused by a recessive gene. It first appears between one and five months of age as weakness in the hindlegs, but gradually gets worse.

- *Crossed eyes* can occur in all breeds, but it seems to be most associated with certain Siamese selection lines.
- Siamese cats may have an error in the *visual pathways* between the retina and the cerebral cortex, such that the nerve cells end up in the 'wrong place' in the visual brain cortex. This can lead to impaired depth vision (stereoscopic vision), and many owners of Siamese cats find that their cat sometimes makes errors when judging distances to jump.
- *Progressive retinal atrophy (PRA)* is a hereditary eye disease that leads to blindness, primarily a problem in Abyssinians and Somalis, but it can occur in other breeds also.
- A survey shows that if one of the parents has an *umbilical hernia*, 75% of the offspring will get this disorder, while only 3% will have this disorder if it is not present in either of the parents.
- *Polycystic kidney disease (PKD)*: kidney cysts occur due to a dominant gene. The disorder can occur in all breeds, but is only considered to do so to a serious degree among Persian and Exotic cats, with around 40–50% of the cats afflicted in certain selection lines.
- *Amyloidosis*: this involves a metabolic failure. It has caused kidney problems in Abyssinians, while more often causing liver damage in Siamese and some other breeds. The disease occurs in certain family lines and has been reduced by selecting against it.
- Persian cats have a big head with a short muzzle (*brachycephalia*). When extreme, this gives rise to abnormal dental position, narrow upper respiratory tract, difficulty in breathing, inclination to birth difficulties, and several other problems. In a UK study published in 2019, Dan O'Neill and colleagues found that 2099 of the 3235 Persian cats examined had at least one health disorder.

These health problems are unintended outcomes of goal-oriented breeding for colour or shape. They are often caused by mutations and maintained by breeding in small populations. Cats with known health disorders should not be used as breeding animals and usually do not get access to cat shows. Any kittens will not be registered. However, some problems derive from the breed standards themselves, which promote selection of head and body forms that deviate substantially from the natural 'wild' type. Think of show-oriented ideals like the triangular head form of the Siamese and the square head form with flat nose of the Persian. The facial expression of brachycephalic cats such as Persians and Scottish folds is permanently in a grimace, which may make it hard for owners to tell when they are in pain. It is also questionable to breed for abnormally long fur that the cat cannot care for by grooming itself. If you look at pictures of Siamese and Persians taken a few decades ago, you can see that they looked quite different (and more normal) than they do today.

Breeding can also have unintended negative effects on an animal's mental health, for example, resulting in an increased tendency for fearfulness or aggression. Behavioural problems are a frequent cause of euthanasia of dogs and cats. Emotional characteristics have measurable heritabilities, so it is possible to select for cats with lower levels of fearfulness and aggression.

How can we reduce genetic disorders?

Preventing the breeding of cats with genetic disorders is an obligation that pedigree cat clubs and their breeding councils must take seriously. Pedigree cat breeders must find healthy breeding individuals, and for some breeds this means finding cats without extreme anatomical traits so that one can reverse the unfortunate breeding and get more functional and healthy animals.

The international cat organization FIFe states:

- The health and welfare of each individual cat and kitten must be the first priority for any breeder and owner of adult cats or kittens.
- It is necessary to work actively for responsible breeding based on genetic principles, disease prevention and an environment characterized by love and well-being.
- Accurate records must be kept of the health and breeding of cats and kittens.

These are commendable statements, and similar objectives can be found at other international cat organizations as well. In the UK, The Governing Council of the Cat Fancy (GCCF) states that 'Health must be the overriding consideration in any breeding programme. The good (positive) and bad (negative) features of the individual cats should be assessed and weighed against each other before any mating. This includes the risk of passing on genetic faults/anomalies.'

We wish cat-breeding organizations success with this important work. For certain breeds, DNA testing for specific disorders is required before using a cat for breeding. The major breeding organizations – FIFe, GCCF, The International Cat Association (TICA, US-based) and Cat Fanciers' Association (CFA, US-based) – should critically review the different breed standards, not least how these are practised by breeders and judges at cat shows and assess whether any of the standards should be adjusted. The breed standards should include maximum values for the forms that can be allowed with respect to the welfare of the cat. The Council of Europe asked for the same in a resolution on breeding of pet animals in 1995. Andreas Steiger of the University of Bern, Switzerland, has reviewed 16 main types of anatomical disorders in pedigree cats and how to correct them.

It would also help if companies stopped using extremely brachycephalic cats (and dogs) as 'poster pets' for advertising their products. This is an example of what the legendary American ethologist Temple Grandin has called 'when bad becomes normal'. The UK animal charities such as the Blue Cross and the Brachycephalic Working Group (though primarily concerned with dogs) are working to raise awareness on this topic in the hope that this will reduce the public appetite for such pets.

Hybrids cats

A further ethical consideration concerns the creation of so-called *synthetic breeds* based on crossing domestic cats with various species of wild cats. Examples include crosses with the Serval (*Leptailurus serval*) to get the Savannah, the mainland leopard cat (*Prionailurus bengalensis*) to get the Bengal, and the Jungle cat (*Felis chaus*) to get the Chausie. The source and welfare of the wild species should be evaluated. If they are being captured from the wild, this may be impacting species conservation and driving the smuggling of kittens to evade trade regulations. The mating behaviour should be observed to ensure that the male and female are compatible, especially if the breeding animals of the wild species are not well socialized to people and cats, and if they are not used to being confined. Further, the health of offspring should be monitored because such pairings often result in non-viable kittens, especially in the first few generations. While most are aborted before birth (a welfare concern for the queen), it is also a welfare concern if the kittens are born too weak to survive. Because it is difficult to obtain viable crosses, the gene pool may be very limited, leading to unpredictable outcomes across different breeding lines. These ethical and welfare concerns are some of the reasons why FIFe will not approve the Savannah or any later cat breeds formed by crosses with other species. However, some other organizations have approved the Savannah.

It is crucial that people considering buying a hybrid cat have the competence and motivation to keep cats that behave differently to typical domestic cats. These cats are often large, strong and highly active, needing considerable exercise in three dimensions. They can be destructive if confined in an apartment, and powerful, far-ranging predators on local wildlife if allowed to roam outdoors. Unfortunately, people attracted to the beauty and rarity of these cats may get 'more cat than they bargained for', leading to unhappy adult cats that are difficult to rehome.

Requirements for the Cat's Environment and Care

What can we do to satisfy the cat's environmental needs? Cats must have the opportunity for stimulating activities, movement, rest and other natural behaviours, whether the cat is only indoors or is allowed outdoors. As we explained in the section on stress coping (Chapter 8), this requires that the cat is able to predict and control its environment to a reasonable extent. Cats prefer routines and can be stressed by unpredictable events such as unexpected visits by unfamiliar people or cats. Keeping cats indoors does not necessarily inflict poor welfare, as long as the cats are used to it from birth, but it requires more of the owner. This extra input from owners is not always met, perhaps because cats are considered 'easy' pets. This is likely why indoor cats are reported as exhibiting more behavioural problems than cats with outdoor access, although some types of problems are more frequent in the latter group (see Chapter 11).

A range of different cat toys and cat furniture can be bought in pet stores. Check out internet pet shops, and you will be amazed by how much is available on the market. These items can serve as *environmental enrichment* for the cat, with the goal of stimulating natural behaviour and avoiding boredom. Climbing 'trees' and scratching posts are essential cat furniture. 'Trees' exercise the cat and provide elevated resting and lookout spots, especially if placed near a window. Scratching posts are important for claw maintenance and should be located in the rooms the cat uses as living and sleeping areas and anywhere else that the cat is inclined to scratch. Puzzle feeders are made so that the cat must work to obtain food pellets. These should be used to provide a proportion of the cat's daily food, the rest in a bowl. Cats can quickly get bored with working for food, so some should always be available in the bowl, especially if your cat is free-roaming outdoors (Chapter 11) and needs more energy to support outdoor activity. Otherwise, these cats may increase their predation of wildlife.

If you buy a feather teaser toy, an elastic stick with feathers on the end, you're guaranteed fun play with the cat until it is completely worn out. Cat toys do not need to be expensive. You can make such toys yourself. Your cat will enjoy shelves of different heights, open cardboard boxes, table tennis balls, a cloth mouse filled with catmint, a wand that you use to dangle a small toy from, or a simple piece of paper attached to the end of a string. Do not forget that you are also an environmental enrichment for the cat, by talking to it, petting it, playing with it and training it. Some kittens of around 4–6 months will enjoy playing fetch with you, repeatedly returning with their favoured small mouse toy each time you throw it for them.

Catnip

Catnip (*Nepeta cataria*) is a plant to which cats can react either actively or passively. When reacting actively, cats typically investigate the catnip (or object containing it) by sniffing and licking or chewing it. They then rub their face or body against it and roll in it. Less commonly, cats may stretch out, salivate, leap and dash about excitedly, or exhibit aggressive responses. In a passive response, cats seem to be in a trance or hallucinating. Both sexes respond to catnip, regardless of whether they are neutered or not. Kittens show a passive response whereas adults are more likely to show an active response. It is not just domestic cats that respond but also tigers, lynx and other species of cats. Silver vine (*Actinidia polygama*) is a plant found in Japan and China that elicits a similar response.

It turns out that both catnip and silver vine contain insect-repelling compounds called iridoids. A study by Reiko Uenoyama and others showed that these compounds are absorbed into the nose and stimulate the brain to release beta-endorphins. These are *opioids* that create the classic 'high' that the cats feel when sniffing these plants. The enjoyable feelings can stimulate the rubbing and rolling behaviour that transfers the oil from the plant onto the fur, where it is thought to help the cat repel mosquitos and other insects. This could be especially useful during a hunt, when the cat wants to keep still and not be interrupted by the urge to scratch itself.

The sometimes strong effects on cats make some people suspicious about using catnip. However, it is non-addictive and generally harmless in modest amounts. The effect lasts only 5–15 minutes, and it then takes half an hour to one hour or more before the cat can react again. You can provide cats with the dried leaves or extracted oil from these plants. The oil can be sprayed on toys or places to which you want to attract the cat, but avoid spraying it around the food bowl. Because it may cause contractions of the uterus, it is probably best to avoid using it around pregnant cats.

Guidelines for good cat care

Many governmental and non-governmental organizations provide guidance for cat care that you can find on the internet. The Norwegian Association of Pedigree Cat Clubs (NRR) has published some useful guidelines, based on the FIFe's guidelines (see Box 9.2).

Indoor cats and housing complexes

Sometimes, housing co-operatives or condominiums have rules banning cats. Others may allow indoor cats but prohibit residents from letting cats outdoors, or at least not to free-roam. This can be unfortunate as cats often thrive when they are allowed outdoors. They also help to keep the area free of mice and rats, which return after a cat ban is introduced.

Most cats that are used to roaming outdoors are stressed if subsequently confined indoors. The cat's behaviour develops through the experience gained during adolescence. They establish behavioural habits related to hunting, territorial defence, exploration of the environment and 'inspection rounds' in their home range. If we prevent a cat from engaging

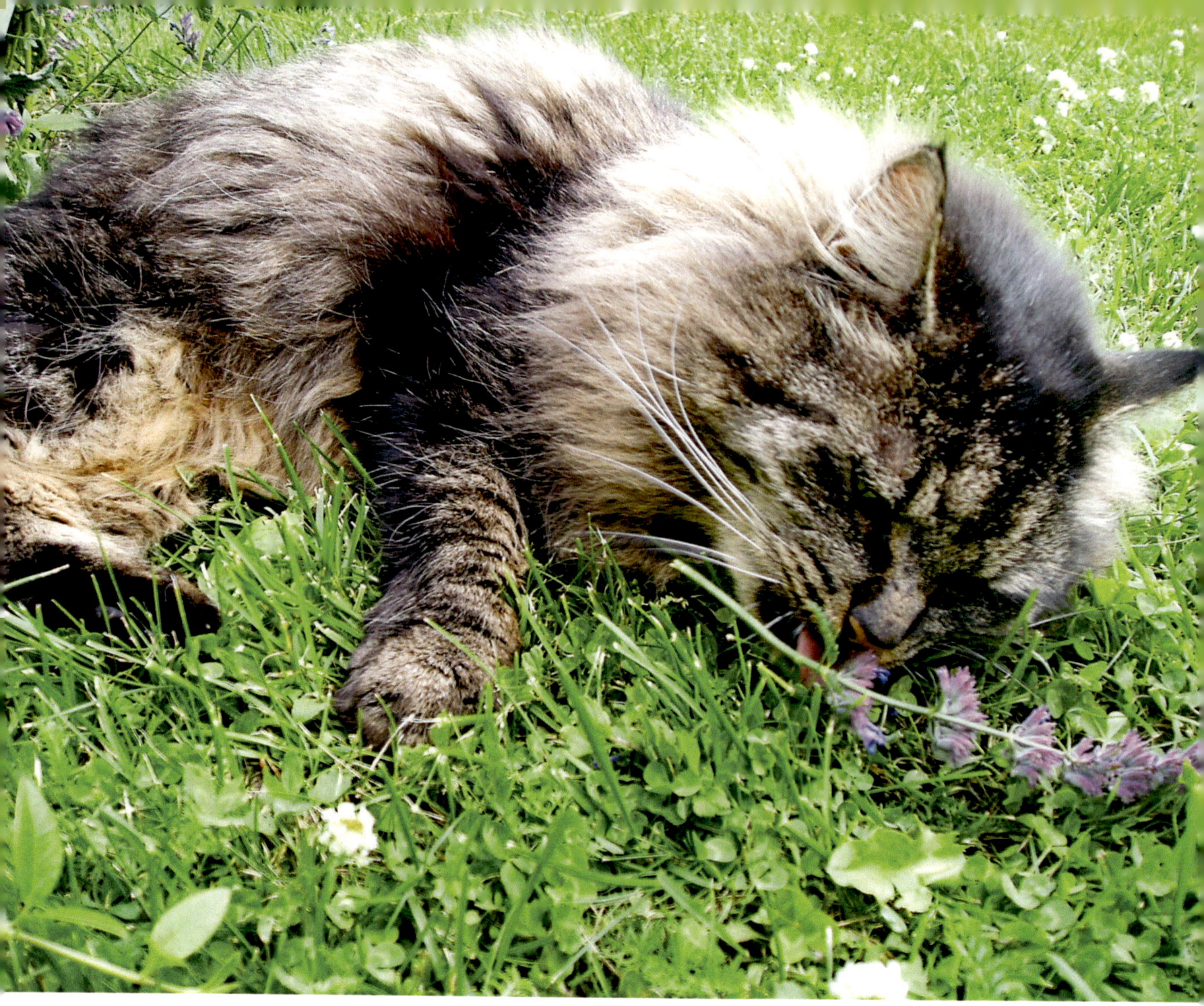

Fig. 9.7. A cat high on catmint, a less potent relative of catnip. (Photo: Nina Svendsrud, 2019)

in these habits, it may experience strong frustration. Therefore, the introduction of any prohibition on outdoor cats should only apply to cats that have never been allowed outdoors, as they will not miss what they have never known. If not, these cats should have free access to an enclosed outdoor area, a catio. While every area has different considerations, ideally, housing complexes would show tolerance towards cats and their responsible owners, allowing cats to accompany their owners outside on a leash, by facilitating construction of catios, or by letting cats free-roam. In this last case, it is recommended to require ID-tagging of the cats to allow recognition of which cats belong at the property.

The urge for sexual behaviour and reproduction cannot always be satisfied because of its adverse consequences, not least unwanted kittens. Housing complexes may, therefore, consider introducing requirements for neutering or use of birth control pills, though granting a dispensation for breeding cats registered in a pedigree cat club. Neutered cats tend to be territorial, keeping other cats from immigrating into the neighbourhood. Also, spayed females will not attract courting tomcats.

Cats that are tied up or on a leash

There have been cases where a housing unit has imposed a requirement that cats must be tied up if

Box 9.2. Guidelines for cat keeping. (Adapted from the Norwegian Association of Pedigree Cat Clubs (NRR) *Guidelines for Cat Keeping*)

General

Caring for the health and well-being of their cats is the most important task for every cat owner. The myth about the independence of cats and their ability to manage for themselves in nature have led to many tragic cat fates. Once you have a cat, you have taken responsibility for a living creature that is entirely dependent on its owners in order to live a good life. This not only involves ensuring that the cat's physical needs are covered. Cats have emotions and can feel strong affection for their owners. It is the responsibility of the cat owner to receive and repay this unconditional love. As general minimum requirements, cat owners must:

- be sure to provide living conditions that suit the cat's physical, behavioural and social needs;
- ensure that the cat always has access to food of a quality and amount that is adequate to maintain good health and fitness; fresh water should be available 24 hours a day;
- protect the cat from disease, stress and injury as far as possible; follow vaccination programmes according to your veterinarian's recommendations;
- inspect the cat daily to check that it has not received any wounds or other injuries, and that it has not been infected with parasites including fleas and ticks; and
- contact a veterinarian immediately upon suspected illness.

Indoor cats

To satisfy the cat's needs for physical activity, and social and predatory play, there are special requirements when cats are kept indoors. At a minimum, the cat owner must:

- Ensure that the cat has access to climbing frames and toys that satisfy its needs to climb, maintain claws and play, as well as having shelters and hiding-places to which it can retreat to be at peace. Sleeping places must be comfortable and adapted to the cat's preference for warm, soft surfaces.
- Avoid having too many cats gathered in a small area. Even though many cats value each other's company, avoid too dense a cat population as this can cause stress and aggression, as well as increasing the risk of disease.
- Set aside time for daily social contact with the cat, including play and petting. This applies regardless of whether you have only one cat or more. Each cat is entitled to receive attention and love from his owner. This also means that the cat owner must evaluate how many cats he or she has the capacity to take care of before acquiring more cats.
- Provide dry food pellets continuously or frequently, unless obesity or illness indicates otherwise. A cat, especially a female, eats an average of 15–16 times a day, and often prefers to eat at night. The digestive tract of the cat is suited to small meals at any time of day. Most cats will feel uncomfortable if they are fed only once a day.
- Place bowls of fresh water in several strategic places in the home where the cat usually passes. Cats will drink a minimum of 9–10 times a day, but only a small amount of water each time. Cats that only get dry feed may risk getting too little fluid, increasing the risk of diseases of the urinary tract and kidneys. When the cat passes a 'water hole' it tends to take a sip of water, reducing the risk of the cat drinking too little.
- Locate litter trays far away from the feeding area. If you have more than one or two cats, provide additional litterboxes. If the cats are not good friends, you may need one for each cat, plus an extra one. Because cats may prefer a place outside the litterbox rather than a dirty one, litterboxes must be kept clean. If the litter does not absorb urine into clumps, all wet patches should be replaced daily. If you use clumping litter, remove the clumps daily and replace with clean litter. Periodically, empty the litter box, wash it and provide fresh litter. Do this more frequently in households with multiple cats.

Outdoor cats

If you live in an area where you can let your cat go outdoors alone, you must be aware of matters relating specifically to the cat's welfare, while also being considerate of neighbours and the environment. Cat owners have a special responsibility to help raise the status of the cat in society. Responsible cat ownership therefore involves ensuring that the cat does not cause unnecessary discomfort to others or aggravate the living situation of other cats. As minimum requirements, the owner of cats going outdoors shall:

- be particularly careful that the recommended vaccination programme is followed precisely;
- regularly examine the cat for sores, wounds and parasites; if such are of a more serious nature, the veterinarian should be contacted immediately;

Continued

Box 9.2. Continued.

- ensure that male cats that are allowed to roam outdoors are castrated; this is because castration helps to protect the cat from fights and infection risks, taking long journeys away from home where the danger of being injured in traffic increases, and contributing to the birth of unwanted kittens;
- provide a sheltered place outside where they can seek refuge in bad weather (cold, rain, wind) if outdoor cats cannot move freely in and out of the house, for example through a cat flap. The refuge can be in the form of a 'cat house', a box or similar that provides protection against the weather and includes a soft sleeping place for the cat;
- adapt the diet to the increased energy demands of outdoor cats;
- set aside time for daily social contact, with petting and care of the cat;
- make sure that the outdoor cat is regularly dewormed.

Cleanliness

The more cats that live in the household, the higher the risk of disease. Homes with more than four cats must pay extra attention to cleaning. As minimum requirements, cat owners must:

- clean food bowls and water bowls before each replenishment with food and water;
- check the cat's sleeping areas, shake out cat litter, remove fur and keep them clean and dry;
- remove stools and urine daily (but do not remove all the litter); periodically, clean the litterboxes with soap and water; and
- make sure all cleansers are non-toxic/non-harmful to the cat.

Breeding cats

Responsible breeding is based on genetic principles, disease prevention and that every cat in the cattery receives the love and care that all cats are entitled to. All cats in the cattery must be vaccinated according to the current rules. Keep a record of health and breeding for all cats in the cattery. Here are minimum requirements for the breeder:

- Make a separate place or room for the pregnant female cat well in advance of birth. Here, the female shall have access to a suitable birthplace (e.g. a box), with which she can familiarize herself well in advance of the birth. The birth should preferably be supervised by the owner or another person with whom the cat is familiar and confident.
- If the breeder has a tomcat that is breeding cats outside the cattery, give him a separate room or cat house where he can be kept isolated from the other cats for a period after he is visited by a female cat, to avoid transferring any infection from visitors to the other cats in the cattery.
- Cats residing separately from the dwelling house shall have housing that at least complies with the following requirements:
  - a minimum of 6 square metres of floor space per cat, with a height of at least 1.80 metres;
  - more than one level (e.g. shelves, cat trees), and a sleeping and/or refuge area;
  - all areas are suitable for human access, and indoor areas are weatherproof; and
  - any outdoor areas provide sufficient shade to protect the cats from direct sunlight, and are constructed with good drainage. The cats have access to the indoors so they can remain dry if it rains or snows.
- A vet should be contacted immediately if a cat shows any of the following symptoms: fluids excreted from the nose or eyes, swollen and inflamed eyes, the third eyelid (nictitating membrane) is visible, repeated sneezing or coughing over time, vomiting without detectable cause, severe diarrhoea, especially if it contains blood, paralysis, nodules or swollen points on the body, extreme and abnormal sleep patterns, lethargy or fatigue, weight loss, especially if the cat loses weight quickly, apathy, blood in the urine, or difficulty in giving birth.
- Ensure that pregnant and lactating females receive a particularly nutritious diet. Breeding tomcats should also receive more nutritious food during mating periods.
- Kittens should suck milk from their mother until they are at least 6–7 weeks old. If cat mothers allow kittens to suckle longer, they should be allowed to do so unless the mother's health condition indicates otherwise.
- From the age of 3–6 weeks, while still sucking, the kittens should also be offered wet food at least two to three times a day. From six weeks to nine months of age, in addition to providing wet food, dry food (pellets) should be available continuously.
- The litter must be kept together, and the mother should be with them, until the kittens are at least 14 weeks old and ready for delivery to a new owner.

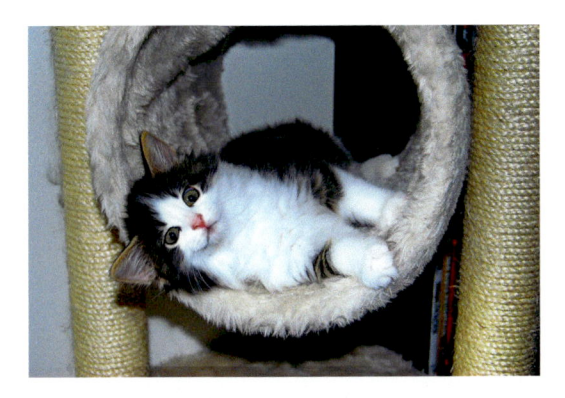

Fig. 9.8. Cats thrive in an environment that is adapted to their needs. (Photo: Veronica Opsahl, 2019)

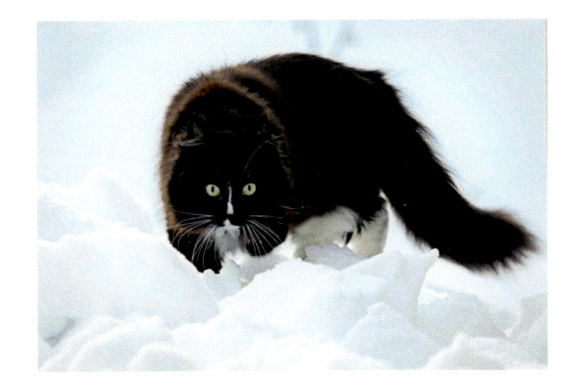

Fig. 9.10. Cats love to roam outdoors during winter. (Photo: Audun Braastad, 2019)

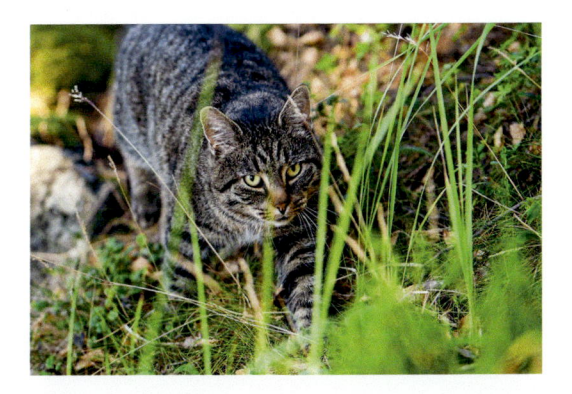

Fig. 9.9. A cat allowed outdoors can have a rich life. (Photo: Audun Braastad, 2019)

allowed outdoors. This is inappropriate for cats (and could be illegal depending on where you live). Cats have a need for exploration and activity in three dimensions. Cats examine scent marks from other cats and thus keep themselves informed about the movements of other cats in the neighbourhood. Such scent marks cannot be easily detected by humans unless deposited by an uncastrated tomcat. A cat will investigate rough terrain and hard-to-reach places where mice and rats are likely to be located. Here, the cat may have an important role in keeping harmful small rodents away from housing. During their walks in their home range, they also keep an eye out for available shelters in the event of an acute hazard: attack by a loose dog or harassing people.

Preventing cats from exploration leads to frustration and can result in behavioural disorders such as stereotyped behaviours, low aggression thresholds, and depressive behaviour. Sadly, we can observe this only too often in zoos where wild cat species are kept. Tying up a cat also presents a risk that the cat moves around such that the chain or rope gets wound around objects or the cat, so it gets shorter and shorter. If the cat tries to jump up and the rope gets snagged on something, it can end up hanging the cat. Clearly, this is no way to keep a cat!

Rather than walking on a leash with the owner, cats prefer to move around more independently of people. However, it is quite feasible to train a cat to walk on a leash if you start at an early age. If cats are not allowed to roam outdoors where you live, this can be an option.

What Are You Going to Do with the Cat during Holidays?

If you are going on a cabin trip during the holidays, it is often nice to bring the cat. However, if the cat gets lost, it can add to the stray/homeless cat problem. Perhaps the owners did not keep the cat sufficiently long indoors before letting it out of the cabin. If the cat gets spooked, it can take off and not return. While it may be hiding nearby in dense vegetation, it may not dare to come out even if hearing the owners calling (see Chapter 7).

If you don't take your cat on vacation, you must ensure adequate supervision by others. Care by good neighbours is ideal for cats that like to roam outside their home. Providing food and water and cleaning the litterbox are the most important tasks, but a social cat will appreciate it if the neighbour sits down and pets or plays with it for a while each day. A cat that accepts frequent contact with unfamiliar people and that is not too aggressive towards other cats can be comfortable at a boarding cattery. Although there are regulations for boarding catteries in some countries, the variation is great in terms of what cats get beyond the minimum requirements.

Requirements for Cat Boarding and Cat Shelters

In the past, cats were often boarded in cages, and guidelines for boarding catteries focused on the physical conditions (e.g. lighting, temperature), hygiene and making sure the cats could not escape. Nowadays, there is more focus on the behavioural and social needs of cats. For example, according to the 2015 Norwegian regulations covering cat shelters and temporary boarding, cats are required to have freedom of movement, regular activity and exercise suitable for their age and behavioural needs during their stay. Each cat must have sufficient space, and those that are hostile to each other must be kept separately. This also applies to shelters where the cats are often not well socialized to other cats.

If a shelter or boarding cattery offers outdoor areas for cats, they should be well drained to avoid becoming muddy and have areas of shade as well as free access to a sheltered indoor area. This will suit cats that are used to roaming freely outdoors. Indoor cats should be allowed to move around freely in a room indoors. Both indoors and outdoors, the cats should be able to move in three dimensions, with shelves at different heights, both to have a good view and to feel safer. For more information about how to design a boarding cattery, see the *Boarding Cattery Manual* published by the Feline Advisory Bureau (now called International Cat Care).

Cats must be fit for being held temporarily in a boarding cattery or shelter, and those kept at shelters must be fit to be sold or given to new owners without undue stress. Kittens born in animal shelters should be socialized to people and other cats

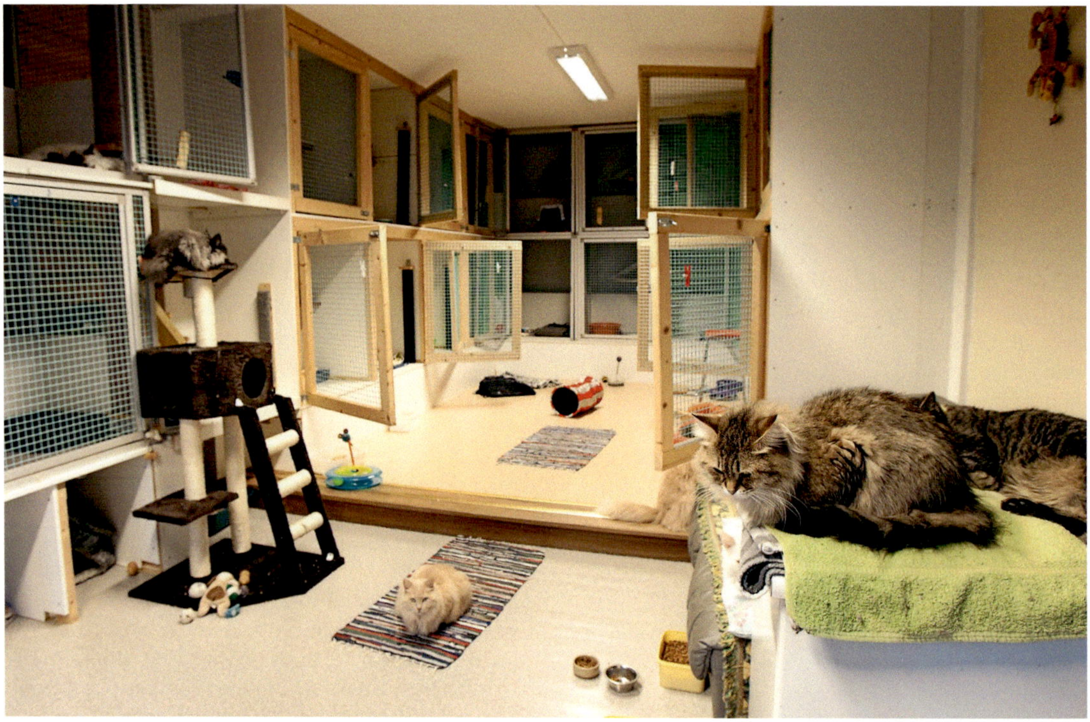

Fig. 9.11. There is no need to sit in a cage when you are at a boarding cattery or cat shelter. (Photo: Audun Braastad, 2019)

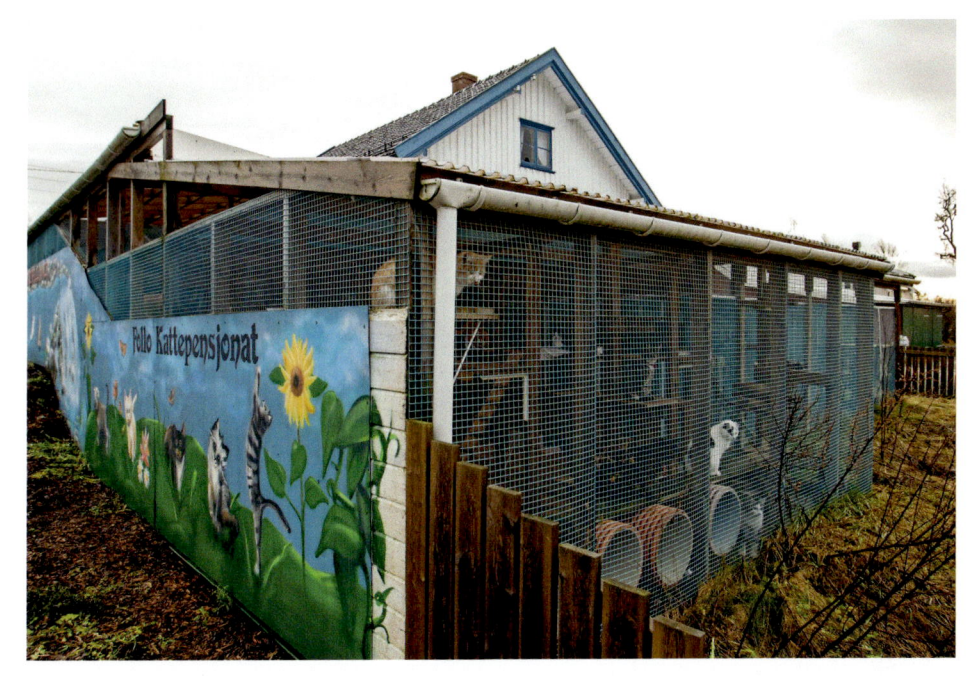

Fig. 9.12. Follo boarding cattery has a large covered outdoor area for the cats. (Photo: Audun Braastad, 2019)

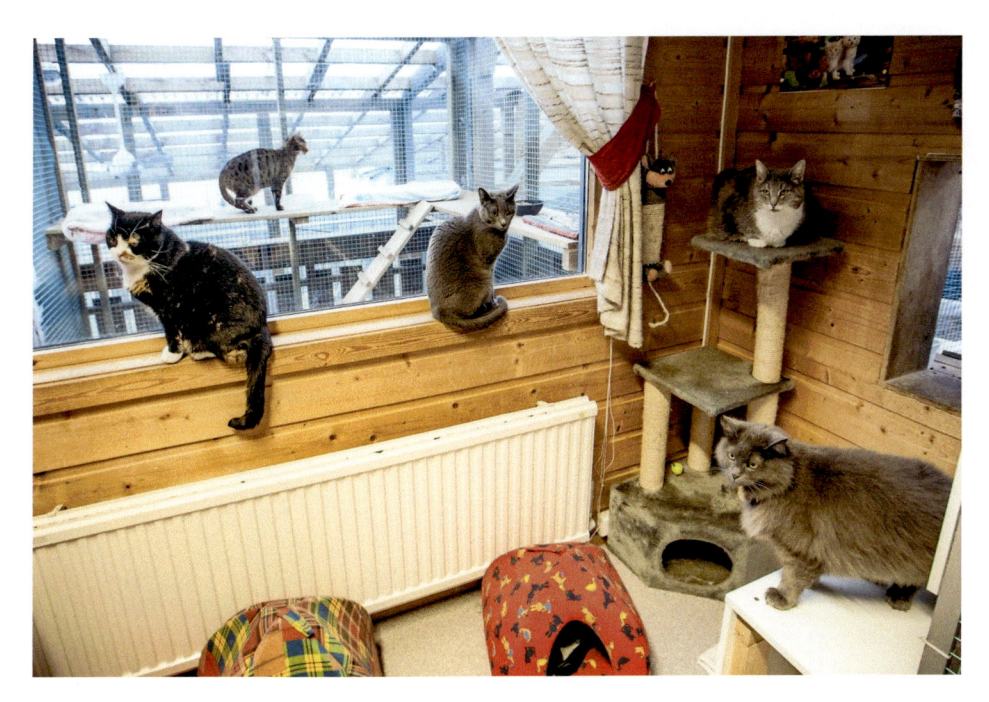

Fig. 9.13. In a boarding cattery, cats should be able to choose whether to stay indoors or in an outdoor fenced area. (Photo: Audun Braastad, 2019)

during the socialization period (see Chapter 2). Research in England shows that when kittens born in a cat shelter were given gradually more frequent and varied contact with different people over the period from 2–9 weeks, the kittens associated more strongly with their new owners and showed less fear of people after adoption. Cattery staff must have good competence and ensure that every cat's condition is monitored daily. Care is also needed to ensure that cats are returned to the correct owner.

Cat Assaults

The medieval witchhunts have their parallels today, often in the form of young people who torment cats. Many cats are tortured to death by hanging or crucifixion. Such behaviour might be seen in connection with the urge to control an animal that some people do not fully understand, or sadism towards weaker individuals. Research in the USA, reviewed by Petersen and Farrington, showed that young people who conduct such terrible acts may develop into adult offenders. Among prisoners convicted for rape, 48% had previously committed animal cruelty. Among those who committed sexual murders, 36% had abused animals when they were children and 46% had done so as adolescents. Among people treated for psychological disorders who showed aggressiveness towards humans, 23% had killed dogs or cats, and 18% had tortured them.

It is therefore extremely important to take this issue seriously when it occurs. You must not explain away this behaviour as mischief by children and hope they will grow out of it. Everyone – parents, teachers and neighbours – must act as soon as possible to notify police and school officials so that appropriate professional services are set in motion. This will help to prevent the torment of cats or other animals from being repeated and reduce the risk that such destructive behaviour is later directed towards people.

Further Reading

Baugh, S. and McBride, E.A. (2022) Animal welfare in context: historical, scientific, ethical, moral and One Welfare perspectives. In: Vitale, A. and Pollo, S. (eds) *Human/Animal Relationships in Transformation: Scientific, Moral and Legal Perspectives.* Palgrave Macmillan, London.

Bessant, C. (2002) *Boarding Cattery Manual.* Feline Advisory Bureau, Tisbury, UK.

Bessant, C. (2006) *Feral Cat Manual.* Feline Advisory Bureau, Tisbury, UK.

Broom, D.M. (2014) *Sentience and Animal Welfare.* CAB International, Wallingford, UK.

Kessler, M.R. and Turner, D.C. (1997) Stress and adaptation of cats (*Felis silvestris catus*) housed singly, in pairs and in groups in boarding catteries. *Animal Welfare* 6, 243–254.

McCune, S. (1992) Temperament and the welfare of caged cats. PhD thesis, University of Cambridge, UK.

O'Neill, D.G., Romans, C., Brodbelt, D.C., Church, D.B., Černá, P. et al. (2019) Persian cats under first opinion veterinary care in the UK: demography, mortality and disorders. *Scientific Reports* 9, 12952. DOI: 10.1038/s41598-019-49317-4.

Petersen, M.L. and Farrington, D.P. (2007) Cruelty to animals and violence to people. *Victims and Offenders* 2(1), 21–43.

Slater, M.R. (2007) The welfare of feral cats. In: Rochlitz, I. (ed.) *The Welfare of Cats.* Springer, Dordrecht, The Netherlands, pp. 141–175.

Steiger, A. (2007) Breeding and welfare. In: Rochlitz, I. (ed.) *The Welfare of Cats.* Springer, Dordrecht, The Netherlands, pp. 259–276.

Uenoyama, R., Miyazaki, T., Hurst, J.L., Beynon, R.J., Adachi, M. et al. (2021) The characteristic response of domestic cats to plant iridoids allows them to gain chemical defense against mosquitoes. *Science Advances* 7, eabd9135. DOI: 10.1126/sciadv.abd9135.

Supplementary materials entitled 'What can we do with homeless cats' and 'Why are kittens so different - individual variation' can be accessed at: www.cabi.org/the-cat-behaviour-and-welfare/

10 Learning and Training

There is an old English saying to warn the foolhardy, namely 'Curiosity killed the cat'. This and another declaring that 'Cats have nine lives' reflect their extremely inquisitive nature. As a relatively solitary species, it is particularly important to their survival that they know what is going on and how to react. Thus, it is no surprise that cats are very capable of learning from both their own experience and from watching others, and do so all the time. Cats cannot be trained, people say. This is not so, they can. Indeed, they can learn a cue and how to respond quite easily. However, being able to be trained (knowing what to do) and being obedient are not the same thing. To respond when a human asks for a behaviour, the animal must be motivated to co-operate with the person at that time. Cats are quite independently-minded creatures. As this is part of their attraction for us, we must not get frustrated if a training session is ended by the cat simply walking off, or once a behaviour is on cue, if the cat does not always choose to comply with our request. The cat should not be considered a biddable, obedient companion. If you want one of these, you have chosen the wrong species.

This chapter comprises a very short introduction to the basic principles of learning. These are the mechanisms that control how the cat learns from its own experience, both as a kitten and as an adult. Indeed, they apply to all animals, including us. It is useful for us to understand how animals (and humans) learn if we are going to have happy, relaxed and confident cats. It also means we are more likely to be aware of and avoid situations that will increase anxiety, frustration or fear, all of which can lead to problem behaviours. Importantly, if we understand how cats learn, we can use that knowledge to teach them useful things to help them live with us, such as to use a cat flap, to raise a paw on cue, and how not to be fearful of the carrying basket (carrier) or visits to the vet.

Learning is a major field of study, so here we describe and explain some important principles that everyone should know in respect of the three main types of learning – habituation, classical and operant. These apply to animals in general, not just cats. We also introduce latent, imitation and insight learning. As you read, we encourage you to think about just how important our behaviour is in the education of our cats. If you are interested in finding out more about how to train your cat, please see the Further Reading section.

Habituation

This is the most basic and weakest form of learning and is technically known as non-associative learning. In essence, the cat learns that if a stimulus occurs, say a noise, and there is no consequence, then it can ignore that sound. The cat is not learning a new behaviour, but its natural reflex behaviour is reduced. A reflex is an unconscious, unthinking response to an event. Habituation learning is important because it acts as a radar, filtering out unimportant information to allow the animal to concentrate on other things. Think for a moment about the sounds around you, the temperature in the room, the feel of the chair beneath you or the purring of the cat on your lap. You have been ignoring these while you were concentrating on reading – you have habituated to them. However, if anything changed, then you would be alert to it. In essence, the animal learns that if **Event A** (the stimulus) happens, then nothing of interest follows at this time, in this place. This means that habituation learning is very 'contextual', and therefore it does not transfer well to other situations. Hence its weakness as a form of learning.

Habituation can have long-term effects. Think of items around your home, such as pictures that you frequently walk past without consciously noticing them. You only become aware of them if something has changed – they have slipped and become crooked. You may also have noticed that your cat has learnt to ignore the sound of you opening (most) cupboards in your kitchen. The cat has habituated to the unique sound of each of these cupboards. Over repeated instances of you opening them, your cat has learnt 'if that sound occurs, there is no consequence of interest to me'. It hears each cupboard opening and will respond with a mild startle (perhaps an ear twitch) as its ears tell its brain that a new noise has occurred. But it will quickly habituate to the sound and seem as if it did not even hear it.

We can use habituation learning to help our cats cope with their world, which is full of various stimuli including movement, lights, objects, sounds and smells. For example, we may be thinking that we need to get our cat used to the sounds of babies and young children. We could do this by having a recording of their cries, laughter and chatter – which is usually louder and higher-pitched than the adult voices our cat is used to. If we played the recording frequently (in all rooms of the house), then our cat can become habituated to these sounds, as it does to the noise of the television or radio. This technique is also used to help cats and dogs become less concerned about fireworks.

It is essential to remember that the stimulus must be at a low enough level for the cat to learn that it is uninteresting, boring, neither pleasant nor unpleasant. At each stage, the cat must be relaxed before we slightly increase the noise level. You can help further by using your body language to signal that all is well and that you are not afraid in this situation. This is best done not by stroking but simply with gentle talk and 'cat-smiling with your eyes' – half-closing your eyes. Remember, only when your cat is ignoring the noise completely should you increase the volume, just a little – very little at a time.

If we increase the level of the stimulus too much or try to move on with the process too quickly, then your cat may become highly aroused (*sensitized*). When sensitized, the cat will be more susceptible to any repetition of the fear-eliciting stimulus, reacting more strongly and with greater fearfulness. In such a state, it is highly likely to make classical fear associations with other things around it at the time even though these things have nothing to do with the original stimulus – in our example the noise of children.

Sensitization

Sensitization interferes with your cat's ability to learn or perform behaviours it has already learnt, and makes it more alert to possible threats. An animal (or human) is sensitized when it is strongly physiologically aroused (stressed). This can be caused by any number of things, such as being too hot, tired, hungry, thirsty or anxious – as when in a new environment. This physiological stress is not just associated with unpleasant feelings – we can also be sensitized because we are excited. Regardless of why one is aroused, there is an optimum level for each behaviour we do, or new thing we learn. This is known as Yerkes-Dodson Law, and the general rule is: the harder the task, the lower the optimum level of arousal (Figs 10.1 and 10.2). This means the harder the task, we need to be less aroused so that the brain can concentrate, and we can maintain our performance. That is why we like music on when doing housework or cleaning the car (to keep us aroused and motivated) but prefer silence when we need to concentrate.

So when you start any session to use habituation to help your cat learn about noises, smells, sights or being touched, do make sure it is at a time when your cat is already nicely relaxed. This is also important when we are training animals using classical or operant learning, or asking them to do a behaviour that we have already taught them. While they need to be motivated and aroused, if too aroused, and thus sensitized, their performance will be impaired, yet too little arousal and they will not engage in the activity (Fig. 10.3).

Sensitization and habituation learning work together as the cat's radar system, keeping it informed of any changes in its world and 'unconsciously' alerting it to danger. Because of the weakness and the contextual nature of habituation learning, and the possibility of accidentally sensitizing the animal, it is advised not to rely simply on habituation to teach your cat to ignore harmless things. It is more effective to use a stronger form of learning, namely classical conditioning to form long-lasting pleasant associations. If the cat is already anxious about something in the environment, then the process known as 'desensitization and counter-conditioning' can be used. This process is also based on classical conditioning.

Learning by Association

Overview

There are two ways in which animals learn by making associations. These are known as *classical*

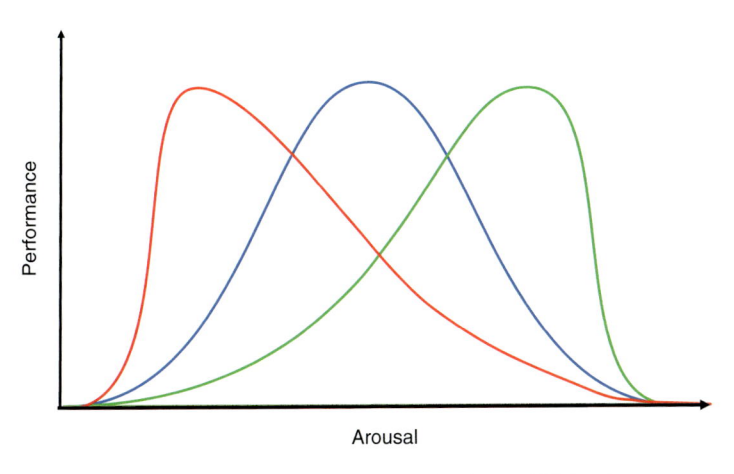

Fig. 10.1. The level of arousal needs to be lower when the task is harder, and higher for an easy task. Key: red = difficult task; blue = moderately hard task; green = easy task.

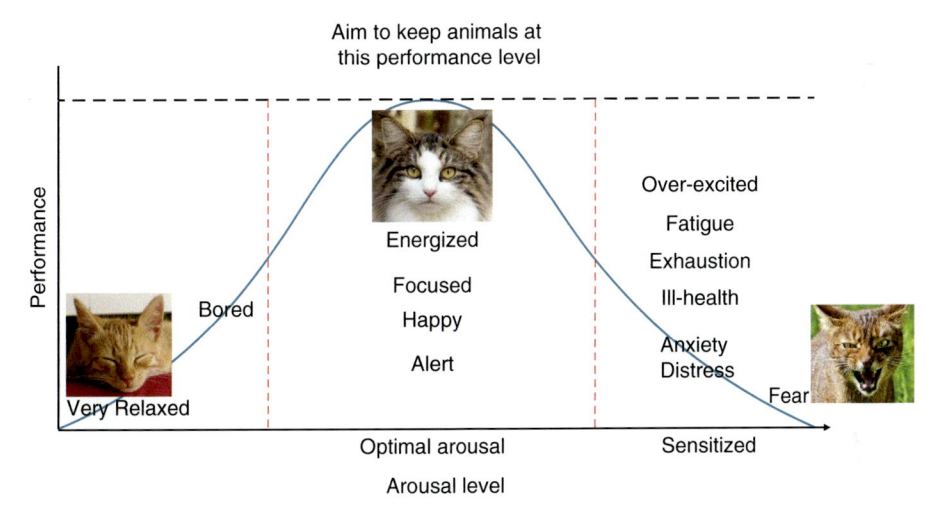

Fig. 10.2. Yerkes-Dodson law showing that performance is affected by the animal's arousal. Performance is the individual's ability to learn a new behaviour or to perform a previously learned behaviour.

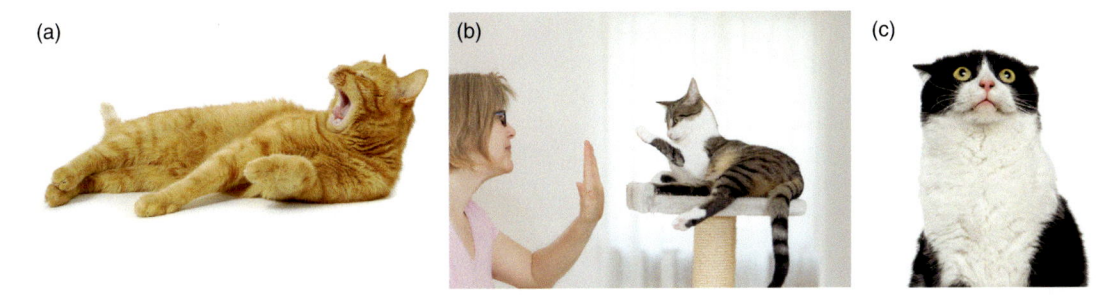

Fig. 10.3. Learning performance is influenced by the level of motivation and arousal. (a) the cat with too little motivation (https://depositphotos.com/13046468/stock-photo-sleepy-cat.html); (b) the cat that is just right, alert and engaged (Photo: iStock 956161022); (c) the cat that is too stressed – sensitized (Photo: iStock 483655165).

Learning and Training

and *operant* conditioning. The word conditioning simply means learning, and both terms are used interchangeably. The animal may learn through its own experience or by observing how others behave in different situations.

In classical conditioning, the animal learns to associate different stimuli with each other, and how it feels. The animal is not learning a new behaviour. It is learning that one stimulus predicts another. Your cat can learn that the sound of opening just one cupboard predicts food, regardless of what the cat is doing at the time. An originally negligible, neutral and uninteresting stimulus (the sound of the cupboard) is paired with a stimulus that is naturally important to the cat, an *unconditioned stimulus* (US), in this case the cat's food. When the cat smells or tastes the food, it will naturally start to salivate. Over several experiences of food following the (initially uninteresting) stimulus, the sound of that cupboard, the cat learns that the one predicts the other. The sound of that cupboard becomes what we call a *conditioned stimulus* (CS). The animal now reacts with what we call a *conditioned (learnt) response* (CR), starting to salivate just at the sound of the cupboard door and comes to you to see if you are going to give it some food. The noise of the cupboard door has also become associated with pleasant feelings. In essence, the animal learns that if **Event A** (stimulus A – the sound of that cupboard) occurs, then **Event B** (stimulus B – the food) will follow (irrespective of what the cat is doing) and it will respond with reflex behaviour (salivation) and will feel an emotion (in this example, pleasure).

Food is not the only pleasant stimulus for our cats; comfort, warmth, a toy or play partner, and access to the outside are others. Of course, your company (and strokes) are important. When you come home and your cat hears you opening the front door, it is likely that it will come to greet you. Just as with the food cupboard, it has associated the sound of the door with your return. It then will learn what predicts the door being opened and your arrival. This may be the sound of your car door being shut, and then it learns that this is predicted by the sound of you parking the car, which is predicted by the sound of your car's engine, which sounds different to all the other cars. Once these connections have been learned, the cat will get ready by the door when it hears your car coming down the street.

Of course, cats can learn unpleasant associations, too. These may be mildly unpleasant, frustrating or scary. Fear is learnt through classical conditioning. It is vital that animals learn about potentially life-threatening events and the events that came immediately before. They need to do so very quickly as, after all, they may not get a second chance. Scary events are very salient, that is they are obvious and very important to the animal, more so even than food. We and our cats can learn fear-related associations after only one experience, a single exposure to the scary stimulus. The information that preceded the scary stimulus is in the cat's memory, and the brain takes that information and makes associations. The cat will start to feel anxious when these predicting stimuli occur. For example, the experience of visiting the vet may have been frightening for all sorts of reasons: the smell of antiseptic, the sight and smell of dogs and unknown cats, being handled by unknown people, having an injection, and so on. The cat's brain processes all the unusual events that preceded these, right back to when you put the carrying basket on the floor before leaving home. It now runs and hides as soon as it sees the basket!

Of course, cats are small, relatively solitary creatures and having a cautious, basically anxious approach to novelty is very important for their survival. As we shall see in Chapter 11, anxiety and fear are the emotions that underpin most problem behaviours.

Operant conditioning is how an animal learns new behaviours, and it is the type of learning we use to train them to do behaviours on cue (command). The animal learns the association between its actions and the consequences of that behaviour. It is called operant learning because the animal is 'operating on' the environment through its behaviour to get the good things in life (reinforcers) or avoid unpleasant things (punishers). That is, it learns which behaviours work. In essence, the animal learns that if **Event A** occurs and **IT Does** something, then **Event B** will occur, and it will feel an emotion. When we train an animal, we are guiding it to discover the behaviour we want, the behaviour that will be successful in getting the animal something nice – the association between 'it does something and Event B will occur'. Once this is learnt, we can then introduce the cue and teach that the behaviour will only be successful if Event A (the cue) occurs.

Of course, an animal also learns by itself, through trial and error. It tries different behaviours, different possibilities. When, more-or-less by chance, it finds a favourable solution, it is rewarded, and that specific behaviour is reinforced. You may have watched this in action as your cat has taught itself how to use the cat flap or open a door. Event A was the closed cat flap and your cat learnt to do something, push with its head, for Event B to occur – the cat flap opening.

To recap, in classical conditioning, the animal learns that a previously uninteresting stimulus now predicts something important. It has learnt to associate one event with the other. In operant conditioning, the animal has learnt to associate its own behaviour with an outcome, in the presence of a particular stimulus (Event A). So it is learning that Events A and B are associated and connected by its behaviour.

There are some general points that apply to both classical and operant learning which we shall now examine.

For associations to be made there are three important rules that must be kept:

1. The events must be obvious and important to the cat.
2. The events must occur together, frequently, in the same order – so that the association whereby A predicts B is clear; otherwise, from the cat's perspective, there is no connection between these events and it will not learn the association.
3. The events must occur close together in time – within a few seconds. (In operant learning, this also means that Event B must closely follow the behaviour.)

There is one important exception to this last rule and that is *taste aversion*. This unique type of classical learning is widespread among the animal kingdom, and you may have experienced it yourself. Taste aversion is when an animal learns to avoid a specific, usually novel, food that has made it feel sick. Clearly it is advantageous to learn this quickly and a single experience can lead to lifelong avoidance of the food. However, the animal may not feel sick until several hours, or even a day, after eating the food. Even then, it can still learn this 'taste = feeling sick' association and refuse that food in the future. Cats are naturally quite reserved about new foods and will only try a small portion to start with, just in case it makes them feel nauseous.

There is also an important exception to the second rule that we have already mentioned; namely that learning a fear association can happen with just one single exposure.

Sometimes the associations made seem to be odd, superstitious even. But this is explained when you understand the power of association. For example, imagine the cat jumped into a chair in the living room and just then the smoke detector started screeching nearby. The cat would not realize the connection of the noise with smoke from the cooker in the kitchen. Rather, the cat will associate the scary noise with the chair, and now has the superstition that this chair is dangerous. Consequently, it will choose a different chair in future. Likewise, a cat may have learnt to shake its paw before pushing the cat flap open with its head. It is likely that it did this when it first succeeded in opening the flap, as perhaps it had a bit of dirt on its foot. The cat now has the superstition that the required behaviour is 'shake paw and push with head'.

Extinction

If rule 2 is broken – when Event B does not follow Event A or does not do so reliably enough – then *extinction* occurs. In extinction, the response weakens and may seem to disappear. It appears that the animal has forgotten what it had previously learnt, but that is not the case.

Extinction in classical learning

Let us imagine you have moved the cat food to a different cupboard. For some time, your cat will continue to respond to the sound of the original food cupboard and get up to see if you are going to feed it. Gradually, it learns that this is no longer a relevant piece of information and will stop responding to that noise. Its response has undergone extinction (Fig. 10.4). Instead, the cat is learning the new association – the noise of the new cupboard predicts food. But it has not forgotten the previous association. Research has shown that your cat has learnt that 'for now, the original association is not relevant'. You may notice that, sometime later, the cat responds to the sound of the original cupboard. This is known as spontaneous recovery of the response. It will soon extinguish again. If you were to move the food back to the original cupboard, it would recover its previous response very quickly.

Likewise, a fear association is never forgotten, and this means that fear cannot be cured. However, we and our cats can learn to manage fears by the

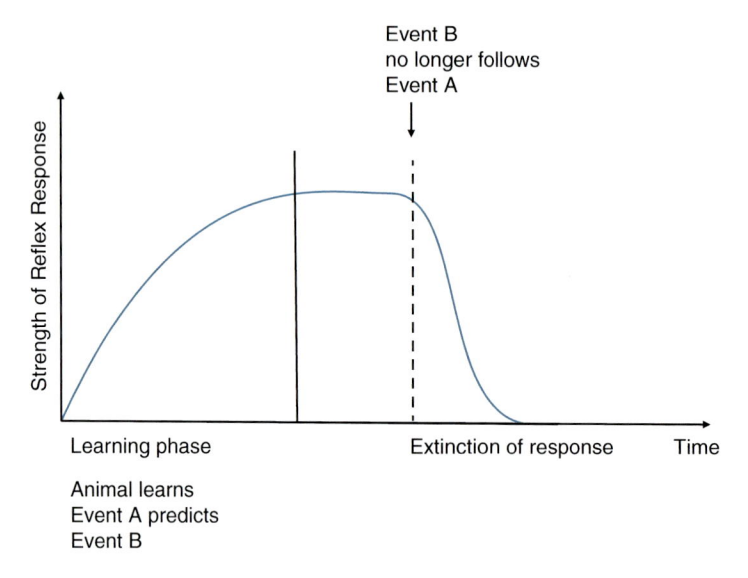

Fig. 10.4. Classical conditioning: diagrammatic representation of the learning phase showing that learning reaches a point where the animal has nothing more to learn about the association between Event A and Event B, and the extinction phase when Event B no longer reliably follows Event A. Note: extinction is not the same as forgetting, and if the association occurs again in the future, the animal's learnt response will reappear.

extinction of old associations and learning new associations. This is achieved through *desensitization* and *counter-conditioning*. This is the process of teaching new associations with the stimuli. The least scary predictors of the scary event are introduced and associated with pleasant things, such as favoured food or play. To know which are the least scary, slightly scarier and very scary predicting events, we will need to have carefully watched to see at what point the cat starts to show even slight anxiety and identify the relevant least-scary stimulus. This, then, is the starting point. It is essential to keep the cat's anxiety levels as low as possible so that it is calm and not sensitized. For, as we know, if sensitized, the cat will be less able to learn a new, pleasant association. Once the cat is no longer showing anxiety with this stimulus, it has learnt the new association.

Only then is it time to introduce further stimuli that were associated with the fearful event. This is done gradually, one or two at a time, in order of increasing importance (scariness) to the cat. These stimuli may be sounds, smells, sights or touch. We are unlikely to know every single stimulus in the environment that the cat has learnt to be worried about, but the aim is to make pleasant associations with as many as possible of the things that made up the original jigsaw of conditioned stimuli. The cat then learns to associate these with something pleasant and relax in their presence. Again, it is important to do this very gradually. You need to be constantly aware of your cat's communication throughout as you need to be careful not to reward anxiety or the actual fear response. If you do, this is likely to exacerbate your cat's fear. It is also essential to reinforce the new learning every so often – quite frequently – throughout the cat's life so that it does not extinguish. This will help prevent the fear resurfacing in the future.

Take the example of the vet and the carrying basket. To prevent the chance of a fear association being made, we could have used habituation learning by having had the carrying basket always out as part of the cat's normal environment. Even better, we would have deliberately used classical conditioning to teach the cat that the basket was a safe and pleasurable place to be. Ideally, we would have done this long before it ever went on its first car ride or visit to the vets. This is where a good breeder can really help. The breeder would have had a carrying basket in the kitten's pen, ideally the one that will go to the new home with the kitten. If that cannot happen, it is helpful to leave the basket brought by the new owners with the mother and kittens for a few hours before taking the kitten home in it. It is also important to put some bedding material that the mother and kittens have used into this basket. This material will smell of the queen and littermates, smells that are calming as they are associated (through classical learning) with 'home, family and feeling safe'. The use of familiar bedding is also important when adopting rescue cats, as the rescue shelter has been their home.

At the new home, owners should keep the carrying basket in a favoured resting area with the familiar travel material and a comfortable blanket inside, and frequently put titbits in there that the kitten/cat considers delicious. When the kitten/cat is happy to go in to eat, then move on to the next stage in its learning, namely that being shut in the basket is OK. Frequently, but not every time, briefly shut the basket door while the cat is eating, opening it as soon as the cat finishes. This enables pleasant associations to be made, namely that this basket is a safe and good place to be. Gradually, increase the time the cat is in the basket with the door shut. Post in more of its favourite treats whilst it is in there. When the cat can relax in there for a few minutes at a time with the door shut, then start to lift the basket off the ground, just for a few seconds and put it back down again. Let the cat out and give it another treat. Increase the time you are carrying your cat around your home in the basket and treat it when you let it out, back at the place where the basket is kept. It is important not to make your cat feel 'basket sick'. We often forget to think about how we carry the basket. If we carry it in one hand, our arm may swing as we walk along and this can be quite unsettling, rather like being on a fairground ride or a bad car ride. Keep the basket as steady as you can when you lift it, when you walk and when you put it down.

If the cat is already fearful of the basket, then smaller steps will need to be taken. Now we will need to use the process of desensitization and counter-conditioning described above. Desensitization means keeping the animal calm, that is, attentive but not anxious or fearful. Remember the Yerkes-Dodson Law – avoiding a high level of stress is necessary for learning. Counter-conditioning occurs when the cat learns an opposite association, so what was unpleasant will now be associated with pleasant events. In essence, we are putting the original association on extinction – it is not forgotten but weakened.

Let us presume the carrying basket has been kept in a cupboard and has only been used for the trip from breeder to home, and to the vet. The cat is now anxious as soon as it sees the basket and runs away. We want to change this behaviour. However, we do not want to contaminate a favoured (safe) resting place with that anxiety. So the first step is to leave the basket in a neutral part of the house, with a comfortable blanket inside and the door off or secured open. Frequently, put some favourite treats in the vicinity of the basket, far enough away that your cat feels safe and relaxed enough to eat them.

When the cat is reliably eating the treats, gradually, over several days and only a few centimetres at a time, place treats closer to the basket, eventually just inside the basket and then further in. Once the cat is happy to go all the way into the basket to get the treats and stay in to eat them, then discreetly (when your cat is not around) move the basket 4–6 centimetres towards where you are planning to keep it long-term. Even this move may be too much for the cat to cope with and it no longer will enter the basket to get the treats. In this case, you will have to go back a few steps in the process, placing food near the basket, before your cat will feel confident to enter again. Over time, with these gradual steps, you will get the basket to its final position. Then you can (gradually) start to close the door for very short times whilst your cat eats, letting it out as soon as it has finished. As described above, slowly increase the time between it finishing eating and opening the door, initially by just a second or two. Eventually, you will be shutting the door and lifting the basket. Do not rush the process and be prepared that it may take several weeks.

Extinction in operant learning

Extinction also occurs in operant conditioning, but it does so slightly differently. In classical learning, the association that is disrupted (extinguished) is between two stimuli, Events A and B (e.g. the sound of the cupboard opening and food) and consequently the cat's reflex response (e.g. salivation) wanes away. However, in operant learning, the association is between the cat's conscious behaviour and the outcome. When this is disrupted, there is a short-term increase in both the strength and variety of behaviours the cat shows. This is known as the *extinction burst* and reflects the cat's frustration at not getting what it wanted (Fig. 10.5).

For example, a cat has learnt that if it sits and miaows in a certain way its owner gives it a tasty snack. Should the owner decide not to do this any longer (as the cat is getting quite demanding and chubby), then the cat will become frustrated and

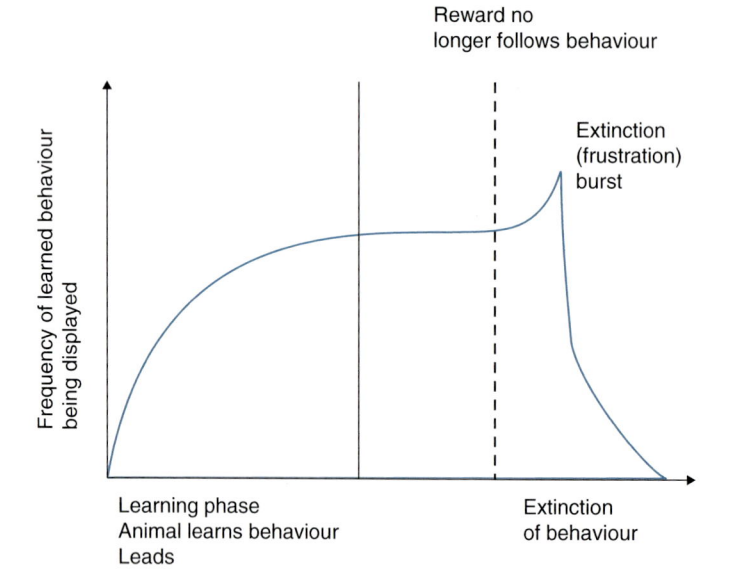

Fig. 10.5. Operant conditioning: diagrammatic representation of the learning phase showing learning reaches a point where the animal has perfected its behaviour to gain the desired outcome, and the extinction phase when the reinforcer no longer reliably follows its behaviour. This shows the frustration burst where the animal will show an increase in strength and variety of behaviour, until it learns that this is no longer successful. Note: extinction is not the same as forgetting, and if the reinforcer follows the behaviour in the future, the animal will start to show that behaviour again.

try harder. It will miaow louder, get up and walk in front of, and paw at, its owner. This is the extinction burst. Only when it realizes none of this is working will these behaviours decline, and extinction occur. As an aside, if the owner gives in during this extinction burst and feeds the cat, the cat simply will have learnt that it must do all these extra behaviours to get that tasty treat and will do so in the future. This was not the owner's intention. Likewise, once extinction has been successful, should any of the original undesired miaowing behaviours be rewarded in the future, the cat will repeat them, for, as we know, extinction is not the same as forgetting.

The careful engendering of mild frustration, and thus the extinction burst with its variety of behaviours, is used by trainers to guide the animal to understand which is the desired behaviour they are wanting it to learn. This technique is called *shaping*. It is important that the cat or other animal is only mildly frustrated as, otherwise, it may simply walk off or otherwise disengage and stop co-operating with the trainer, or even show its strong feeling of frustration through aggressive behaviour, known as 'extinction-induced aggression'.

Generalization and discrimination

Two more aspects of learning that help explain our cat's behaviour are the principles of generalization and discrimination. These apply to both classical and operant learning and are a key part of the process of training an animal to perform a behaviour on cue.

Animals can easily *generalize* their learning across stimuli that are similar. They also can *discriminate* between stimuli that are clearly different, realizing that what they have learnt about one is not applicable to the other. For example, an outdoor cat can learn to discriminate between different bird species, and between young or injured birds that are easy to hunt as opposed to others that are more likely to get away.

A kitten, rescue cat or ownerless (stray) cat that is not used to humans will eventually learn that the person who cares for it is harmless and indeed associated with pleasant events (e.g. food) and pleasant emotions. If this is the only person the cat has met, or the only one who makes it feel this way, then it will only have this person's characteristics to focus on; for example, an adult woman who is blonde, does not wear glasses and smells of a particular anti-perspirant/soap/perfume. The cat may become anxious and hide if another person enters the room – perhaps a man or a child or even another lady – but with dark hair, glasses and/or a different scent. It has *discriminated* between them and the original person it knows.

In contrast, if the cat has met many different people, having only pleasant experiences with all of them, the cat will *generalize* its learning about people and be more confident when meeting new people in the future. This is important for cat breeders to think about, as we saw in Chapter 2. If the owner/breeder does not have lots of people who can visit and help socialize the kitten, then they can imitate others by changing their appearance; wear different clothes, different scent, change their voice and actions to give the variety of experience the kittens need – all associated with nice things such as food, play and gentle stroking. After all, one does not have to be a child to behave in a childlike manner, or old to behave as an elderly person.

Discrimination learning is used when we train our cats, and they also use it to learn about their world. For example, you may decide that your cat should not have access to the outside at night. The cat flap has a red slide – in one position it means the flap can be opened, and in the other position it means that the flap is locked. While the red colour is only apparent to us humans, the cat will notice the clearly distinguished positions. Your cat will soon learn to discriminate between them and learn what they mean. The cat can now avoid becoming upset and frustrated at trying to get out of a locked cat flap.

We must apply the same principle of clarity when we train our cat to do a particular behaviour on cue. It is important that each cue, be it a hand signal or a word, is easy for your cat to discriminate from any others it has learnt. Once learnt, the cat should respond to the cue even when it is used by other people, or if you say the word when you have a cold or sore throat. As long as it sounds similar enough to the original, the cat will be able to generalize its learning.

Operant Conditioning

As we have seen, in operant conditioning the animal learns to associate its behaviour with the outcome, that is, Event B. It learns that its behaviour has a consequence. The outcome can be something pleasant or unpleasant. In the cat flap example, the cat learnt that if the slide is on the left, Position 1 (the cue), and it pushes the flap, there is a pleasant outcome of the flap opening. It has also learnt that if the slide is on the right, Position 2, then pushing behaviour results in the unpleasant outcome of the flap remaining shut and the cat feeling frustrated.

Pleasant outcomes are known as *reinforcers* as they reinforce or strengthen the preceding behaviour. That behaviour is more likely to occur again. If miaowing in a certain way when in the kitchen causes the owner to feed the cat, then the food becomes a reinforcer for this miaowing. The cat will miaow in this way more readily next time it wants a snack, and it will generalize this to other rooms.

Unpleasant outcomes are known as *punishers*. They reduce the likelihood of the preceding behaviour occurring in the future. If now the outcome of the initial miaowing is no food, or being chased out of the kitchen, then the cat is less likely to miaow in the future, though there is likely to be an extinction/frustration burst. Miaowing has been punished.

Operant learning is essential to survival and to having a happy life. It enables the cat to learn how to get the good things in life (e.g. food, somewhere safe and comfortable to rest, to be a successful hunter, to know its way around its territory) and how to avoid or escape from the bad things in life (e.g. the neighbour's scary dog). This is the type of learning that most people have heard about as it is the basis of training. Of course, animals do learn by themselves, but training is when humans guide that learning in ways that we want. In training, we use both reinforcement and punishment. What is important is to understand how we use these so that we maintain a trusting relationship with our cat and are less likely to accidentally teach it behaviours we do not want.

Reinforcement and punishment

We use the concepts of reinforcement and punishment to describe the outcomes of behaviour expressed by the animal. In the case of reinforcement, we want to increase the likelihood that a certain behaviour occurs. Using punishment, we want instead to weaken the tendency of the animal to exhibit a behaviour. We can either add (+) a stimulus (positive) or take away (-) a stimulus from the animal (negative). We then get four different situations which are linked in pairs. These are *positive reinforcement* and *negative punishment*, and *negative reinforcement* and *positive punishment* (Fig. 10.6).

Positive reinforcement and negative punishment (reward/no reward pairing)

The 'pleasure–frustration' method of training

Positive reinforcement is when the outcome of a behaviour is a pleasant, 'appetitive' stimulus, often called a reward. The cat will do more of that behaviour. For example, when the cat is sitting quietly in the kitchen, its owner gives it a reward. The reward might be food, a stroke, a look and a smile, praising it, dangling a toy to play with, having a door opened, or basically anything else your cat likes/has an 'appetite' for at that moment in time (Fig. 10.7). The associated emotion is pleasure, and the cat will learn that sitting quietly in the kitchen is a behaviour to be repeated.

Negative punishment occurs when a behaviour causes the removal or withholding of a pleasant stimulus (no reward). The behaviour will be less likely to be repeated in the future. In the previous example, sit was rewarded but all other behaviours such as miaowing, weaving around the owner's legs and jumping on the worktops did not get a reward. All these behaviours were negatively punished. The associated emotion is frustration. If these behaviours have been rewarded before, the cat is likely to feel rather more frustrated, to a greater or lesser degree. Frustration will be greater if the cat has had lots of experience of these behaviours being rewarded. The cat will show an operant extinction burst, such as louder miaowing and more circling around the legs, before it 'gives up'. This behaviour must be ignored. The owner must be aware of this extinction burst and hold firm. As described earlier, if they give in 'to keep him/her quiet' by giving a reward when the cat is miaowing more insistently, then all they have done is to teach the cat that quiet miaowing does not work but yelling at its owner does. Similarly, the child who is standing quietly in the store is the one who should get the cake or candy, not the one who is misbehaving or screaming. If the cat sits down quietly, then it should be rewarded immediately.

Another example is when your kitten is playing excitedly with a toy and, in the heat of the 'battle', bites or scratches you. If the toy is taken away immediately when this behaviour starts, then the kitten will learn that the biting or scratching when playing is punished (negatively); the fun ends and this behaviour will be less likely to occur in future. It is important to try to do this right from the start, so that it does not learn that biting and scratching are part of the game – prevention of problems is the much better strategy.

The simple rule is to reward the behaviour you want and ignore (negatively punish) the behaviour you do not want. It is also why it is sensible to decide how you want your new kitten or cat to behave as soon as (or before) you get it. Then you

	Reinforcement	Punishment	
Positive	Positive Reinforcement Add nice Emotion = pleasure, joy	Positive Punishment Add nasty Emotion = fear	Positive
Negative	Negative Reinforcement Take away nasty Emotion = relief	Negative Punishment Take away nice Emotion = frustration	Negative

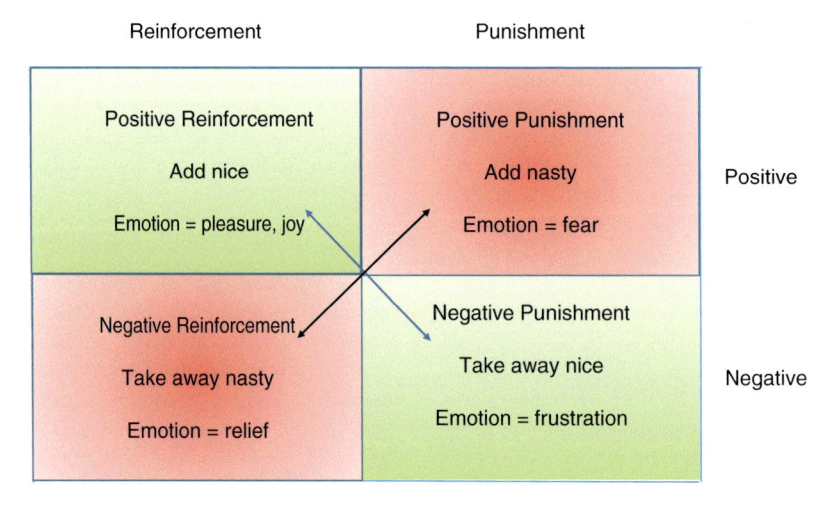

Fig. 10.6. Showing the positive reinforcement and negative punishment (reward/no reward) pairing and the negative reinforcement and positive punishment (fear–relief–anxiety) pairing.

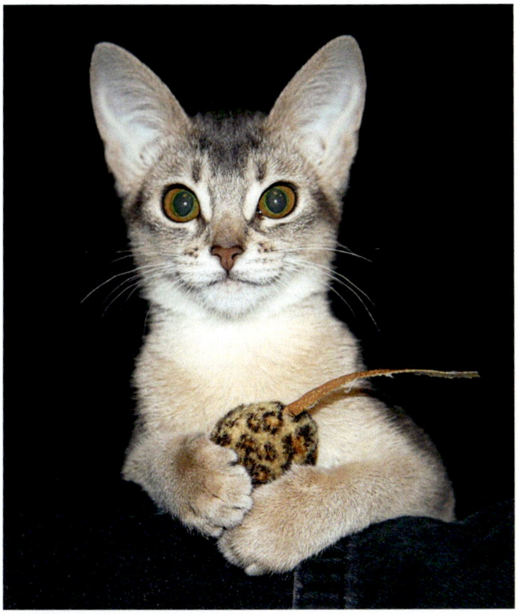

Fig. 10.7. You can give your cat its play mouse as a reward (reinforcer) when it behaves as you wish. (Photo: Heide Kvaløy, 2019)

can teach the correct behaviours right from the start, rather than try to undo its learning later, which is more difficult, will cause your cat anxiety and risks that the previously unwanted behaviour will re-emerge in the future. We all know from our own lives that learnt habits are difficult to change. The same is true for our cats and other animals.

Negative reinforcement and positive punishment

The 'fear–relief–anxiety' method of training

Negative reinforcement occurs when a behaviour causes the removal or withholding of an unpleasant stimulus. The associated emotion is relief, and the result is that the behaviour will be more likely to occur again in that situation. For example, let us assume your cat bites you and is hanging on to your hand with its teeth. If you pull hard on its collar, you cause uncomfortable, even painful, pressure on its throat. If you release that pressure as soon as the cat takes its teeth away from you, the cat will learn that letting go leads to relief. The cat will learn to let go when you pull the collar slightly or go to touch the collar – it has learnt how to avoid/escape the pressure. The cessation of an unpleasant stimulus acts as a kind of reward – the animal feels relief, a very powerful emotion. However, for this to occur, something unpleasant must occur first. This is positive punishment.

Positive punishment is when the behaviour causes an unpleasant stimulus to occur. The associated emotion is fear, and the animal learns not to do this behaviour and so avoids the fear. In the above example, the positive punishment, the unpleasant stimulus, was the pressure on the cat's throat when it started biting. The cat will learn that certain stimuli predict the positive punisher, which helps the cat avoid it in the future. This learning how to avoid positive punishers can be important for its survival. In our example, the cat will learn to stop biting when it feels the owner touch its collar, or even reach towards it. Our aim is to teach the cat not to bite. We may think this is a fine method, and indeed the cat may stop biting. However, we may not realize that now the cat feels anxious when its collar is touched. This may become generalized, so your cat becomes anxious about being touched and stroked. It may start to avoid not just your hands but you. The bond you had with your cat is damaged.

Positive punishment and negative reinforcement form the basis for 'cat scarers' that make a loud noise when a cat is near, for example when a cat jumps into a neighbour's flowerbed to use it as a toilet. The cat is positively punished for jumping into the flowerbed and feels relief when it jumps out again, as the unpleasant noise stops. The idea is that the cat will learn to avoid the positive punishment by not jumping into that flowerbed in the future. Of course, it may still jump into other flowerbeds which it discriminates as different. After all, there is no 'scarer' machine there. There may also be unintended consequences of using a 'scarer'. What if a person is around, say a child playing in the garden, when the 'scarer' is activated? The cat may make a fear association with that child. Such an association may generalize to other children. Regardless of this possibility, the cat has been scared. Owners may wish to consider other ways to provide their pet with outdoor access without upsetting the neighbours, such as a catio or walking on a leash (see Chapter 11).

Should we use positive punishment? Are there other ways of training our cat?

The simple answer is 'No'; we should not use positive punishment, and 'Yes'; there are other ways of training your cat. They involve using the reward and no reward pairing, namely positive reinforcement and negative punishment.

There are several reasons for this. The most important is that positive punishment can permanently damage the relationship between the cat and the person, especially if the animal does not fully understand why it is being punished. Remember that this method relies on making the cat feel anxious.

A damaged relationship can easily happen if the positive punishment is not applied consistently, every time the behaviour occurs, day or night. It will also happen if the animal does not know which behaviour will keep it safe from this frightening or painful outcome. Either way, the result is an animal that is increasingly anxious, and which generalizes this anxiety to aspects of the owner (e.g. certain movements) and/or the environment that it has (classically) associated with the unpleasant, frightening experience. Remember the cat that associated the chair with the sound of the fire alarm. What about the cat who was chased out of the kitchen for miaowing? This cat may become anxious about the kitchen and learn nothing about its miaowing behaviour, especially if sometimes it is chased away and sometimes not. Unpredictability is confusing and makes us all feel anxious.

In extreme cases, the animal acts as if it considers that almost everything it does is wrong and results in unpleasant outcomes. This makes the animal so anxious that it does not dare to do anything when the owner is nearby or when in a particular room or situation. The animal is suffering from depression and chronic stress, a state known as *learnt helplessness*. This may be displayed by the cat being very passive, or simply hiding when the owner is around or tries to touch it. It would be like living with someone who is very unpredictable and likely to be aggressive with no warning. You would be very anxious in their presence and prefer to avoid them.

Likewise, if the positive punisher is too strong the cat is extremely likely to make a fear association, not with its behaviour, as intended, but with aspects of the environment, including the owner. This, too, is a classical association and may mean the cat avoids the owner or strikes out with its claws or bites when touched. This is because the classical learning of the fear is stronger than any operant learning. Remember that fear associations can be learnt from a single exposure and are never forgotten. How do you know what will be too strong a punisher for any individual cat? The answer is that you don't. Each animal is an individual, and what may be a mild punisher to one may be extremely scary to another.

However, even milder forms of positive punishment can have unfortunate consequences. Many owners use a spray of water from a water gun or a spray bottle as a 'gentle' punisher for cats that scratch furniture or curtains. Mildly unpleasant outcomes are often not effective, and the cat continues the behaviour. It becomes habituated to the mild punishment and experiences it as 'somewhat uncomfortable, but soon over'. Though the owner repeats the spraying often, it does not stop the unwanted behaviour. Consequently, the owner becomes increasingly exasperated, maybe to the point of rehoming the cat. Alternatively, the owner turns to ever more severe punishers and the cat becomes fearful of the owner.

Clearly, positive punishment is not at all helpful and can lead to unintended and very damaging consequences. It is not recommended as a method for teaching your cat or any animal or human. It is far better to reward the behaviour we want, and thus teach the cat to choose to do these behaviours so that we can live together in harmony. Rewards put the animal in a positive mood and strengthen the social bond between you and your cat.

The alternative method – reward-based training

Cats can be trained using the same positive reinforcement (reward) method as we use for training dogs, birds and animals in zoos. It is based on the reward/no reward pairing described earlier and is known as *shaping*. Sometimes, as in 'clicker' training, a specific sound is used to mark the desired behaviour.

In brief, 'clicker' training is used to help shape a new behaviour. First, a noise, the click of a clicker, is classically associated with food. We can use that noise in our operant training to *mark* the behaviour we want at the precise moment it occurs. The clicker itself is not obligatory. Instead, some people mark the behaviour using a word such as 'good' or 'yes'. There are two advantages to the clicker. First, it is a neutral sound, so our emotions do not interrupt the cat's learning and the sound is consistent in all training sessions. Secondly, we tend to be slightly faster at the physical movement of clicking the clicker than saying a word. Therefore, our marking of the behaviour we want is likely to be more accurate. By the way, if your cat is deaf, a visual signal – a flash of a torch, or a touch on a certain part of its body – can be used as a marker instead of a clicker.

Shaping is the rewarding of any behaviour the cat offers and incrementally rewarding behaviours that are increasingly closer to the final desired behaviour we want to teach. These incremental steps are 'engineered' by withholding the reward and engendering a little bit of frustration – a small extinction burst. This causes the cat to offer another form of the behaviour that is slightly closer to the final behaviour (Fig. 10.8).

Only when the behaviour has been shaped to the desired form and the cat is offering it reliably, do we move to the next stage. That is, we add a unique visual or verbal cue (command) just before the behaviour occurs. With repetition, the cat will learn that this cue predicts its behaviour and thus the reward. We then must teach it that the cue is a signal of when to perform the behaviour. We do this by using its ability to discriminate. This is done by only rewarding the trained behaviour *if* the cue is given. Now the cat has learnt the full operant sequence: if Event A (the cue) occurs and I do the behaviour, then Event B occurs (the reward) and I feel pleasure.

Once the behaviour is learnt on cue, the clicker is no longer used, though, of course, we continue to reward the animal for responding correctly to the learnt cue (Fig. 10.9). The clicker is simply a means for clearly communicating with the animal during the teaching (training) phase.

We can teach our cat a range of behaviours including to touch a target (very useful for moving it from one place to another), to sit, to lie down, to walk on a lead or by your side, to do an agility course that you have designed in your living room, to touch different named objects, and even to retrieve toys. Some people may consider these as 'tricks' and think they demean the cat in some way. In fact, training provides mental stimulation and physical activity for the cat and enhances its relationship with you (Fig. 10.10). Also, many 'tricks' can be extremely helpful in looking after your cat's general care and health. This is often called husbandry training. It is only us humans who worry about what we call it, as from the cat's point of view it is all interesting and rewarding.

Training your cat to be touched all over helps it to be more relaxed when examined by the vet. Your

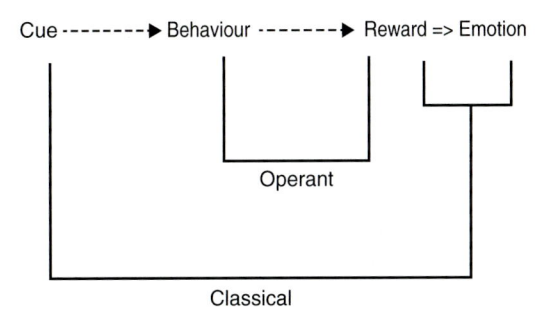

Fig. 10.9. What the animal finally learns – if the cue occurs, and I do the behaviour, then there is a reward. This diagram also shows how operant and classical conditioning work together when we train a new behaviour.

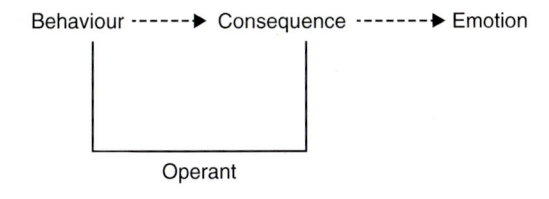

Fig. 10.8. What the animal learns first – its behaviour has a consequence – the operant part of operant learning.

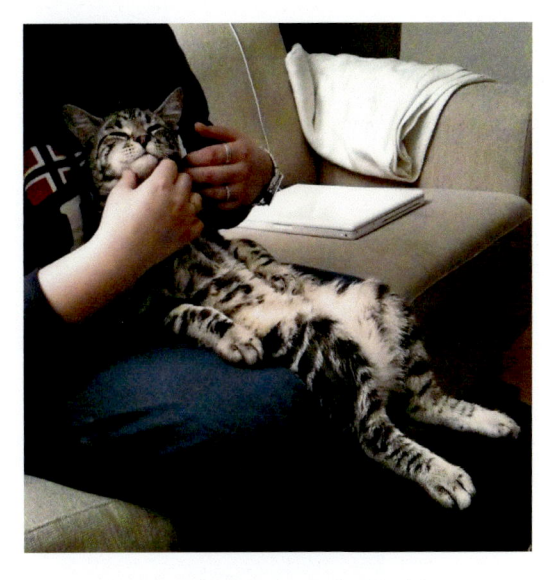

Fig. 10.10. Using pleasant methods of training reinforces the trust and bond with your cat. (Photo: Grete Nakling, 2019)

Learning and Training

119

cat giving a paw, lying on its side and opening its mouth when asked are useful for health checks, by you or the vet. Giving a paw lets you check claw length and asking your cat to lie on its side is an opportunity to look for ticks or to brush it. You can train 'lie on right' and 'lie on left' as two different behaviours with two different cues. Likewise, teaching your cat to open its mouth on cue allows you and your vet to look for any teeth issues and facilitates oral administration of medicine.

A very useful behaviour to train is 'leave', also called 'look at me' or 'boring'. This is teaching your cat to move its nose away from things. If we move the cat's nose, we can move its head and thus its body. This is a useful behaviour for when you want to ask your cat to stop biting or scratching you or any object, or to stop it from getting into a cupboard or box you would rather it left alone.

Another helpful cue is to get your cat to sit in a particular place, such as on a little blanket or mat, while you get its meal ready. This avoids the cat walking around your legs and being a trip hazard or getting up on the work surfaces. You can use the same training to teach it to sit in a particular place on your desk or on a stool beside you while you are working (Fig. 10.11).

Guidance on training these and other behaviours can be found in the books and video links listed in the further reading section.

Reinforcement schedules

When we teach a cat to sit and wait, we start by rewarding every time it sits. This is called a *continuous reinforcement schedule*. Once the behaviour is performed on a cue word, 'sit', and the cat is reliably responding to the word, then we can start to lengthen the time it will remain sitting before we give the reward. We do this in gradual stages, by just withholding the reward by a second, then increasing it a few seconds at a time. This is called an *interval reinforcement schedule*. Basically, we are teaching the cat to gamble. It learns, 'If I wait just a little longer, I may get the reward'. Likewise, if we are teaching our cat to walk beside us, initially we reward every step, then gradually increase the number of steps before it gets the reward. This is known as a *ratio reinforcement schedule* because we reward only every X times the behaviour occurs. In this case the behaviour is a single step. So the cat is now gambling that 'If I take just another step, I may be rewarded'. Gradually, we can build up from one step to three steps, five steps, eight steps – before the reward arrives. Varying when or how often the cat is rewarded can strengthen the behaviour, but it is important to build up gradually, otherwise the delay to reward may be too long and the behaviour starts to extinguish and the cat walks off. Another way to maintain your cat's co-operation is to vary the reward – for example by using a variety of different-flavoured food treats.

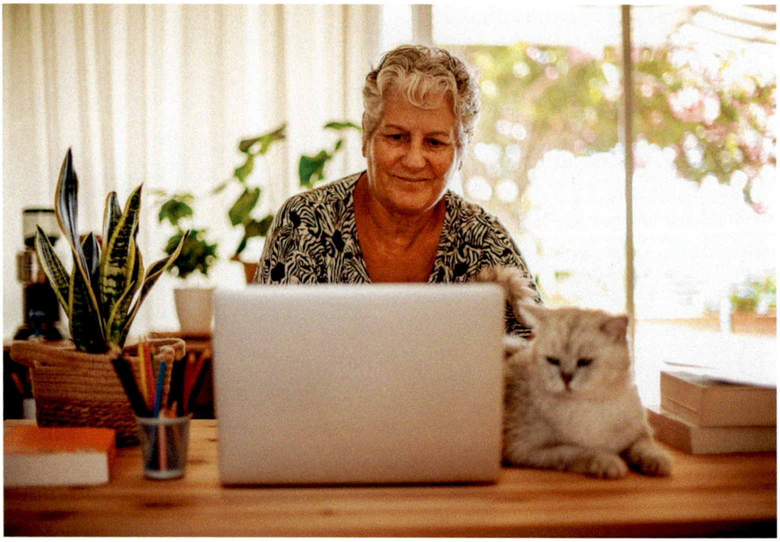

Fig. 10.11. Teach your cat to sit beside you when you are on your computer. (Photo: iStock 1271670507)

Similarly, when your cat is naturally doing a behaviour you like, remember to reward it. This might be rewarding your cat for being relaxed. Doing this every so often will put the cat in that gambling frame of mind – 'If I lie here a bit longer, I may get a reward'. Whether the behaviour has been taught to be on cue, or is just occurring naturally, it is important to remember to reward every so often, to avoid extinction.

All cats learn and all owners can teach, so do not be afraid to explore this further through the suggested reading. If you are unsure, ask a dog trainer or cat behaviourist who uses clicker training to teach you how to teach your cat. This may be face-to-face or online. A huge advantage of the internet is that many trainers and behaviourists can help cat owners remotely. When it comes to training, you and they will obviously have to work on 'cat' time rather than 'dog' time – cats like short sessions and, being rather more independent than dogs, may not always wish to have a training session when you do. There is no reason why cats cannot be taught new behaviours (tricks) throughout their lives; the limitation is our time and imagination.

Training and practising cues that the cat has learnt is fun for both the cat and for the owner. It should be continued throughout the cat's life and can fit into your daily routine. For example, while you are waiting for the kettle to boil or need a break from the computer, use the time for a fun practice session. Cats like multiple little meals throughout the day and we can use that to our advantage to have lots of short training sessions. In each, we can use a portion of the cat's daily food ration (along with some non-fattening special treats like small pieces of fresh, cooked chicken or fish). Apart from strengthening and maintaining a wonderful bond with you, practising all the 'tricks' it has learnt improves your cat's physical and mental welfare. This is a form of enrichment. As with people, maintaining physical and mental exercise throughout life helps delay mental deterioration, known as cognitive dysfunction (senility). It also helps keep your cat physically fit and can indicate when there may be a health issue. For example, you have taught your cat to roll over on cue, but one day it is more reluctant to do so or tries but fails. That may be a sign of some pain, perhaps due to arthritis, and tells us that a trip to the vet is needed.

As we shall see in the next chapter, some cats do display behaviours that are problematic for their owners. The majority of these will have an aspect of inappropriate learning as part of the problem, requiring rehabilitation (re-learning) as part of the approach to modifying the undesirable behaviour.

Latent (Hidden) Learning

Exactly when an animal has learnt something is not always obvious. Both we and animals can learn things without changing our behaviour at that time. We have learnt relevant information and, when needed, we demonstrate this by the behaviour we display. Until then, what we have learnt remains 'hidden', hence the term *latent learning*. For example, when the cat arrives at a new home, it will explore the surroundings carefully. Afterwards, it will regularly check for any significant changes in the environment. Such exploration gives the cat knowledge that it does not need now but may need later. When needed, the cat will know where there are places to hide, rest in the sun or watch the birds.

Social and Imitation Learning

Part of growing up is learning basic survival skills. For kittens, these include learning what are threats and how to avoid them, and what is good to eat and how to catch and kill it. As described in Chapter 2, when her kittens are only five weeks old, the queen will bring back live prey to the nest to demonstrate and give them opportunities to practise and hone their killing skills. Known as social learning, researchers have studied the ability of kittens and adult cats to observe and learn from other cats how to access food from puzzle boxes. Certainly, those who had the opportunity to observe an experienced demonstrator cat tend to solve the problem more quickly than those who had to work it out all by themselves.

This may not be so surprising. More recently scientists have confirmed what many an astute owner already suspected – cats can observe and learn from a completely different species, humans. For example, cats will look to their owner for information, especially if there is something in the environment that may be a threat. They will follow our gaze to look where we are looking and will follow our gestures as when we point at an object.

In 2021, Claudia Fugazza and her colleagues showed that cats are capable of even more than this, that they can imitate a human's novel actions. This has been demonstrated in other species and you may have heard of it in reference to dogs as 'do as I do', perhaps better called here as 'be a copycat'. This is of interest to scientists because it indicates that animals have an understanding that our arms are like their legs, our hands are like their paws, and our heads are like their heads – albeit we are upright and two-legged. This requires the animal to have a mental representation, a map of its body and ours and recognize what would be a similar action. Eibsu is the 11-year-old cat that has enlightened us to this ability. When asked, she will copy her owner in a variety of novel behaviours - using her mouth to pull on a piece of string, touching a box with her paw or face. See the link below to a video of Eibsu showing her skill.

Learning by Insight

Finally, one last example of learning shows just how clever our cats are. When a problem arises, cats do not always have to physically try out different solutions. Like us, cats and other species of mammals, birds and reptiles can think out different possible solutions in their mind. When they arrive at an idea of what would work, they perform that behaviour. This is termed learning by insight. The animals are using mental representations to work out a solution. There are several scientific studies and anecdotal examples of this.

In one, the scientist hung a piece of meat on a string so that it was higher than the cat could reach, even if it jumped up. Also in the room was a small box on wheels. The researcher had previously taught the cat to use its mouth to pull this box by the handle. When the cat was released into the test room, it naturally tried to jump up after the piece of meat. When that did not work, the cat sat down, licked its paws for a while (displacement activity) and seemed to be thinking. After a while, the cat suddenly went over to the box, pulled it so that it was beneath the piece of meat and then easily jumped onto the box and got hold of the meat.

Summary

Cats learn throughout their lives. Even our older cats keep learning. Understanding how our cats learn means we can better prepare them for living in our human world. Training them to perform a variety of behaviours on cue can help prevent anxiety and fear. It also enhances the bond between cats and humans. Just as for us, learning new things and solving problems can lead to better mood, and less boredom and frustration. Providing enrichment toys and puzzles, practising behaviours they have learnt and training new ones throughout their life will help make our cat's later years as enjoyable and mentally stimulating as their earlier ones.

Further Reading

Bradshaw, J. and Ellis, S. (2016) *The Trainable Cat: How to Make Life Happier for You and Your Cat*. Basic Books, New York.

Fugazza, C., Sommese, A., Pogány, Á. and Miklósi, Á. (2021) Did we find a copycat? Do as I do in a domestic cat (*Felis catus*). *Animal Cognition* 24, 121–131. DOI: 10.1007/s10071-020-01428-6.

Houston, K. (2014) 21 Days to the Perfect Cat. Hamyln, London.

McCoy, D.E., Schiestl, M., Neilands, P., Hassall, R., Gray, R.D. and Taylor, A.H. (2019) New Caledonian crows behave optimistically after using tools. *Current Biology* 29(16), 2737–2742.

Pryor, K. (2003) *Getting Started: Clicker Training for Cats*. Sunshine Books, Waltham, Massachusetts.

Videos

Fugazza, C., Sommese, A., Pogány, Á. and Miklosi, A. Did we find a copycat? Imitation in a domestic cat (the video of Eibsu). Available at: www.youtube.com/watch?v=-BU4tmyidpg (accessed 21 April 2022).

Linda Ryan, a UK cat behaviourist, has some helpful videos on how to train your cat:

Cat carrier training https://www.facebook.com/watch/?v=297576148513494&_rdr

Handling training: https://www.facebook.com/watch/?v=244803293382860

Oral handling basics: https://www.facebook.com/watch/?v=729445687996613

11 Problem Behaviours in Cats

Introduction

All behaviours have two fundamental causes – a genetic blueprint which sets the stage for personality traits and characteristics; and, secondly, the environment, which provides all the experiences an animal encounters throughout life. A particularly important time in terms of experience is during development from conception to social maturity and adulthood. The behaviour patterns used by the individual cat in any given situation will be the result of its genetically predisposed characteristics *and* its experiences throughout life. The extent to which genetics combine with the environment to create different behaviours will be unique to that individual, reflecting his/her personality. Of course, later experiences in adulthood and the ageing process itself will also influence behaviour, but these will still reflect the individual's personality.

Three feline personality types have been described, and for each the behavioural response to a situation will vary. This is illustrated in Table 11.1 when a neighbourhood cat peers in through the window of the home of a cat, who is inside (Fig. 11.1). Remember also the description of ear signals in Chapter 4.

As we saw in Chapter 8, behaviour is affected by external stimuli such as temperature or the surface on which you are sitting or walking; and by internal stimuli, including thirst and hunger. Another set of internal stimuli that influence behaviour are hormones. These may be those involved in reproduction or development, e.g. thyroxine, or the stress hormones cortisol and adrenaline that prepare the cat for action. The extent to which any given behaviour is shown is driven by motivation – how much the cat wants to achieve a given outcome from its behaviour, based on how important the outcome is at any given time.

Combining all these behavioural drivers leads to each individual cat showing a range of behaviours – some of which are desirable to us humans and some of which are less so. We call behaviours we do not want 'problems' and often take a variety of actions to try to change those problems or unwanted behaviours. However, if we are going to be successful in restoring human–cat harmony, we need to understand why the cat is doing what it is doing.

What Is Problem Behaviour in Cats?

There are two main categories of problem behaviour. First are those that are defined as problematic by the human but are normal cat behaviour. The second type is those that reflect that the cat has a problem, which may have a medical or genetic cause.

Cats often show unwanted behaviours if they have had an impoverished environment during the crucial stages of development, or if they are under high levels of stress and anxiety due to inadequacies in their current physical or social environment. Social issues are due to the other living creatures in their lives. For cats, these other living beings are usually us humans or other cats. Of course, they may have been socialized as a young kitten to other species, such as rabbits and parrots, which also form part of the social environment. However, owners need to remember that these and other small pets, e.g. rodents and reptiles, are potential prey and any cat may be tempted. The owner has a responsibility for their safety and welfare, too.

Changes in behaviour will occur as a normal part of development and growing up – kittens often play more, both with objects and socially, than do adult cats. The frequency and duration of play behaviour may decline, but not disappear, as the cat ages, particularly in the later stages of life.

It is key when we take on the responsibility of becoming a cat owner that we manage our own awareness and understanding of what a reasonable expectation of a cat's behaviour is. This is true for any pet we decide to own. Then we can avoid

Table 11.1. Examples of responses of a resident cat to another outside the window.

Personality type of the cat inside the home	Potential behavioural responses to the neighbourhood cat peering in through the window
Sociable, confident, easy-going Samantha	Shows some signs of being alert, with somewhat dilated pupils, erect ears and interest in the other cat and moves slowly towards the window for a better look
Timid and fearful Tabitha	Runs away from the window into another room, hissing, with hair raised, widely dilated pupils, ears flattened towards the skull; hides behind the door frame and peeks around the corner to check where the other cat is
Active, aggressive Arnie	Struts up to the window, showing signs of defensive aggression and confrontation; pupils only somewhat dilated, ears partly backwards and partly low, focused stare

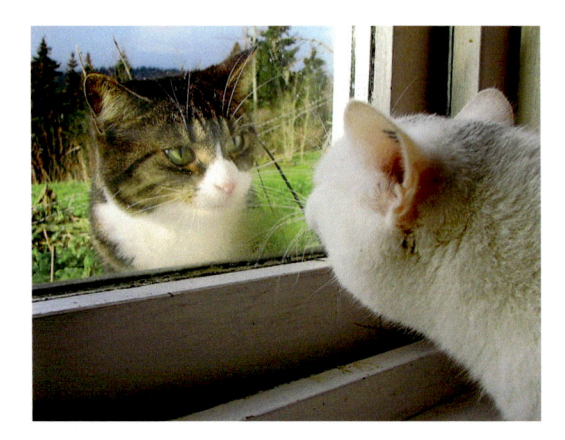

Fig. 11.1. Neighbourhood cat looking through the window into the home of the resident cat. (Photo: Ann Kristin Solvang, 2019)

problem behaviours, spot any that may be developing and take steps to remedy the situation as soon as possible. Once an adult, any significant or sudden changes in the behaviour of our cat will have a cause. What that cause is requires thorough investigation and analysis before any attempts are made to try to modify the behaviour (see types of behaviour problems and solutions sections below).

Who Is the Behaviour a Problem for – the Cat or the Human?

It is important to realize that, often, the problem behaviour is not a problem for the cat, but it is unwanted or unacceptable, and, therefore, problematic for us. Many behaviours described as problems by people are normal behaviours that the cat shows at the wrong time, in the wrong place, or directed in the wrong way, as we humans see it.

It is like when we call native plants in our garden weeds simply because we have decided they are growing in the wrong place at the wrong time. Examples of normal cat behaviours we may find problematic include toileting, scenting or marking, defending territory or resources or bringing back prey. They are simply being a cat. Categorizing these behaviours as problems is often related to our human perception of our home setting in which cats now live as our companions. However, there are ways to ensure that even these behaviours do not ruin a perfect human–cat relationship.

Owners may wish their cat would not bring back dead, or living, birds, mice, voles, frogs etc. into the home, depositing them in the kitchen or, worse, on the owner's bed! It is a behaviour we find disgusting and distressing, especially as we would prefer to see and hear the birds in the garden and let the mice, voles and other wildlife live their lives in peace outside. As explained in Chapter 6, these 'presents' represent only about a fifth of the animals your cat kills. This problem can be considerably reduced by using a CatBib®, a Birdsbesafe® collar cover plus a bell, or by providing your cat with an outdoor enclosure, a catio.

Like us, cats relax more at home when they have given their surroundings a personal touch. We put up pictures and display ornaments, cats leave their scent and scratch marks at important places around the home. We would prefer that they didn't choose the corner of our sofa as one of these places, or use it for doing a cat 'manicure' as their new claw nails grow through! This latter behaviour may have started because there were inadequate resources available – no scratching posts, or the posts were not located in 'cat-suitable' places.

Likewise, the cat may be toileting in an unacceptable way, outside the litter tray. There will be a reason for this. It may be because there is only one litter tray which is in an unsuitable location for the cat, or it contains too little cat litter or litter of a type the cat does not like to use. Alternatively, this toileting behaviour may indicate a medical issue such as feline urinary tract infection.

Illness can lead to unwanted behaviours, including inappropriate toileting. Sometimes these have an emotional component, such as idiopathic cystitis, which may be caused by stress or anxiety. This can lead to further problem behaviours as the cat learns to avoid stimuli that are fear-provoking, namely the litter tray or the type of litter.

As another example, consider the cat that is losing weight and not eating as much as usual. It may have dental problems making eating painful, or the location of the food may be less accessible if it has some pain. Alternatively, this reduced eating may be indicative of anxiety and stress. Perhaps the cat is concerned about the presence of another cat in the home that is restricting its opportunities to eat, as we saw with Missy and Tommy in Chapter 8. Fear and anxiety are major causes of problem behaviours in cats.

Lack of socialization, poor handling or inadequate resources can all result in anxiety or fear. Problematic behaviours can result from a poor early environment. If the cat lacked adequate socialization and stimulation, it may be frightened and stressed by being around people or in a human home (Fig. 11.2).

It may be that the cat was not handled appropriately or by enough people as a kitten or was not properly educated by the breeder about the domestic setting of a home – the noises and smells, and the presence of other pets (Fig. 11.3).

There may also be difficulties created through the ways in which we communicate and interact with our cat. Perhaps we over-handle the cat, or pick it up too often without warning it that is what we are going to do; or we may be using a type of brush for grooming which it does not like as it is rather painful. Using a softer brush, or a rubber type, such as a Zoom Groom, can be effective and less painful; and if your cat is long-haired, use an untangler comb with teeth that swivel. Ideally, all grooming sessions will be short and end with a special treat.

Our cat's response to being handled, picked up or groomed may change with age due to conditions such as arthritis, or to injury or illness, which can occur at any age. Older cats may also be more sensitive to touch and generally less tolerant of being handled or groomed. You should ask your vet about pain relief.

Less frequently, unwanted behaviours are caused by or compounded by the cat's individual personality. As we saw with Tabitha (Table 11.1), some may be more generally anxious and timid, whilst others, like Arnie, have character traits that may predispose them to show aggression.

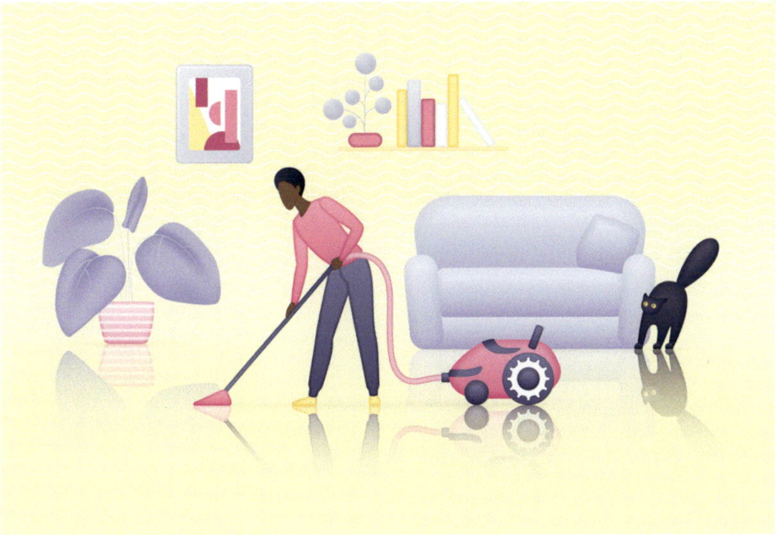

Fig. 11.2. The human home has lots of potentially scary noises and machines. (Photo: iStock 1389681805)

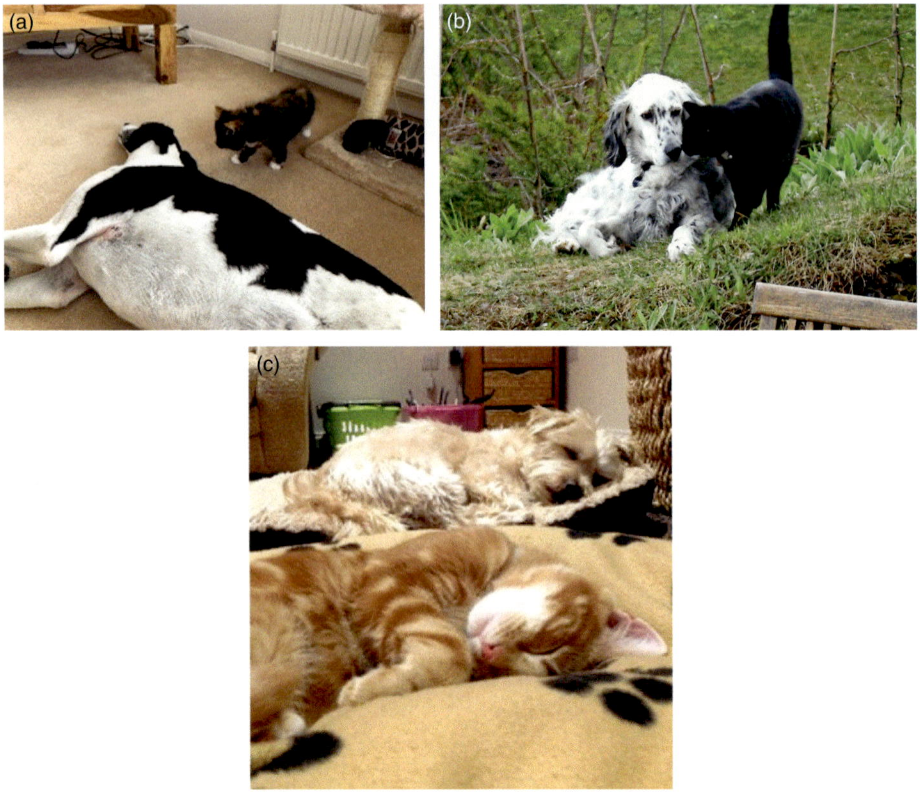

Fig. 11.3. Socialization of kittens to a calm, well-behaved dog can lead to a life-long friendship. ((a) Photo: Jane Williams, 2022; (b) Photo: Jorun Margrete Elvestad, 2019; (c) Photo: Jane Williams, 2022)

These examples illustrate why it is important to investigate the reasons why the cat is showing the problem behaviour. Not doing so can lead to the problem worsening and widening as the cat tries to find different ways to feel as relaxed and happy as it can. So for each case, we need to understand the cat and its life history and lifestyle.

The rest of this chapter describes some of the more common problem behaviours and reasons why these may occur. Also provided are some suggestions to help address the situation. As outlined above, any change in behaviour may be the result of injury or illness, so you should always have your cat seen by a vet first.

Taking steps to address problem behaviours relies on us, the cat's owner and caretaker, changing our behaviour, too; even if only to be more diligent in cleaning the litter trays. Changing our cat's behaviour can be very successful but is never a 'cure'. Behaviour can reappear should future circumstances trigger it. This may be because we have returned somewhat to our old ways, e.g. not always cleaning the trays when needed, or because of some other factor beyond our control, such as the cat being frightened by something when it is outside.

Clearly, providing for our cats in ways that reduce the likelihood of problems developing is preferable. Prevention is always best. Previous chapters have provided much information from which we can decide how we can give our cats the best quality of life. This chapter suggests approaches that can be used to address problem behaviours that have arisen, many of which can also be used by owners as preventative measures. The exceptions are where veterinary involvement is essential, namely anything relating to illness or other physical concerns, and use of drugs.

When looking for help for any unwanted behaviours shown by your cat, you should seek advice from a vet and/or a qualified, assessed, regulated (QAR) behaviourist. In the UK, the Animal Behaviour and Training Council is the organization recommended as having suitably informed, ethical behaviourists using humane methods (www.abtc.org.uk). In North America, you can contact an Animal Behavior Society Certified Applied Animal Behaviorist. The American Veterinary Society of Animal Behavior and the American College of Veterinary Behaviorists are suitable sources for information about veterinary specialists. In Europe, the European Board of Veterinary Specialisation has a College of Animal Welfare and Behavioural Medicine which identifies behavioural specialists.

Excellent behaviour counsellors come from different backgrounds, including biologists, animal scientists, psychologists and veterinarians. Whatever their background, they will have undertaken further education in behaviour modification, which includes cats. Many, such as those in the UK, will ask that the cat is referred by its vet. Even if this is not the case, always ensure they have some co-operation with the vet so as to check for medical causes of behaviour and if any medication is appropriate as part of the behaviour therapy.

In all cases of problem behaviour, the first stage is for the cat's usual vet to rule out any medical causes. For example, undiagnosed pain may be causing stress and anxiety which, in turn, will impact behaviour. Without resolving the pain through veterinary intervention, the source of the stress and anxiety will remain and any behaviour modification attempts will not be successful.

Preventing and Addressing Problem Behaviours – General Principles for All Cases, for All Cats and for All of Life

Punishment

Positive Punishment is to be avoided at all costs. This means not shouting at the cat, telling the cat off, pushing the cat away, or using any other aversive techniques. These include water sprays, products with aversive scents, shaking cans of stones, chasing the cat, or throwing something at the cat. All of these can be very frightening for a cat and are more likely to exacerbate the problem behaviour. Whatever the original cause of the behaviour, making the cat more fearful or upset will only increase the likelihood of more unwanted behaviours. In addition, all attempts to punish the cat for unwanted behaviours will have a negative impact on the animal's emotional health and therefore its welfare. This is also why the use of positive punishment is not advisable for any animal, or child.

Cats have little if any understanding of why their owner might be angry with them and why they are displaying these behaviours towards them. Positive punishments also damage the bond between owner and cat. From the cat's perspective, the owner is now unpredictable and a potential threat. The development of trust – being able to be relaxed and calm in the presence of that person – is likely to be lost.

Consistency, predictability, stability

It is true that problem behaviours that have underlying causes relating to the cat's genetic make-up or medical issues can occur regardless of the environment. However, to both prevent and address problem behaviour, we need to create a human- and cat-friendly home environment. We have a major impact on the environment in which the cat exists, and we are responsible for creating a home that promotes its physical and emotional health and welfare. This is one which is:

- **consistent** – we always interact with the cat in a kind, pleasant way;
- **predictable** – our responses are always the same in any given situation; and
- **stable** – the environment is relatively static and not too stimulating or frightening.

These are fundamental to a pleasant, safe environment for our cat(s) and relate to our interactions with them and the resources and lifestyle we provide for them. The safer the cat feels, the calmer and more relaxed it will be and the less likely it will be that we see unwanted or problem behaviours.

Interactions

To interact in ways that our cats find pleasant, we need to understand how cats like to interact with us. This can help prevent problems developing around stroking, handling and grooming. Cats like to have many short interactions with people and other cats – hello…goodbye; hello…goodbye; and so on. Body contact through rubbing and marking against people and other cats is a greeting, a form of communication and social gesture. Cats like to be touched gently and calmly – not with sudden movements or vigour. They like to be able to see what people or other cats are going to do – no surprises (except when playing)!

Owners need to be aware of this and allow the cat to choose when to be touched, stroked or picked up. Generally, cats prefer not to be picked up. If they *choose* to jump up onto your lap, that is fine, but they are usually less keen on being *taken* off the ground. Being lifted makes them nervous as they have lost their ability to use the surface they should be standing on as a platform from which to take off and run. Your cat will like gentle strokes around the shoulders and chest, maybe along the sides, but seldom on its belly as this is a body part that is vulnerable to being bitten by a predator. They may head-rub you but would prefer that you did not rub their head in return; rather, hold your hand still for them to rub against it, or move your fingers slowly and gently over their head, neck, cheek or under the chin. If the cat walks away, they should be allowed to go – this is not the moment to try to hold onto the cat for a hug or a cuddle; it will come back in its own time.

Resources

As with our interactions, we can increase predictability within the environment by making access to specific areas very predictable. For example, doors are always either open or shut depending on whether a room is always or never an available space for them. If you do not want your cat in the guest room, keep the door closed whether you have guests staying or not. Likewise, you may decide that the cat flap is always locked when the cat comes in for its evening meal so that it is indoors at night.

When considering resources, the aim is to provide the cat with as much choice and as easy access as possible to available resources. This is key to improving health and emotional well-being and reducing problem behaviours. It is particularly important in multi-cat households, where resources and access to them may be limited due to the presence of other cats. Whilst it is sad for the owners, rehoming one or more cats may be the better option if the environment does not allow provision of sufficient space for a core area with resources for each cat in the home (see Case Study 1).

As discussed below, resources are essential in preventing problem behaviour arising out of

---

Case Study 1: Multi-cat household case involving aggression

Four male cats – Toby, Jimmy, Neville and Ted; and three female cats – Betty, Jemima and Lily, all neutered

Problem: aggression from Ted towards some of the other cats

Ted has injured Betty, Jemima and Lily. Ted and Neville have also had fights where both cats have been injured.

These seven cats live together in a house with access to a garden in the daytime but not at night. At night they must come indoors, although Neville will often refuse and stays out. One male cat (Ted) is a bully and is often aggressive towards Jemima and Lily who are both young, timid cats. Jemima and Lily spend time together, often sleep in the same place and will groom each other. Ted will also bully Betty but rarely gets the opportunity as she leaves as soon as he appears.

Toby is sociable with all the cats – he is a friendly 'uncle' to them all – even Ted gets along with him. Toby will groom any of the other cats when they are around, but this rarely happens with Ted or Neville. Ted and Neville do not groom Toby. Jemima and Lily only groom each other.

Betty spends most of her time on a chair under the dining-room table. She is not seen very often, and never when Ted is around. She can be around Jemima and Lily, but they tend to ignore her. Toby will groom Betty, and she will spend time with Toby if none of the other cats is around. She will groom him as well.

Jimmy is Toby's friend, and they spend a lot of time together. Toby seems to look after Jimmy. They often sleep together and groom each other.

Neville is an independent cat who does not spend much time in the home. He spends most of his time outdoors and is known to be a hunter. If at home, it is not unusual for him and Ted to have 'unfriendly' conversations, which can lead to fights.

Clearly, the welfare of *all* these cats needs to be improved.

First, we must identify the social groups these cats have formed:

- Those in the same social group can share the same space (or core area) and the resources within it.
- Those in separate social groups need their own space with the full set of available resources – food, water, sleeping/hiding-places, litter trays, toys, enrichment, their own catio, etc.

Continued

The social groups are:

- Ted (on his own)
- Toby + Jimmy
- Toby + Betty
- Jemima + Lily
- Neville (on his own)

These five social groups need their own space and resources. They can time-share sleeping and resting places. The places in the house where they choose to spend time, feed and sleep are their core areas. While there may therefore be some overlap of space used, it is essential that in each identified core space each of the groups needs:

- feeding stations
- water
- sleeping and hiding-places
- litter trays for overnight

In addition, pheromones are needed 24-7 throughout the home. Ted needs more mental stimulation through games, puzzles and training. Indeed, it should be considered that the best solution for the welfare of all the cats is that Ted is rehomed to a place where he is the only cat in the household.

boredom or frustration. We would be wrong to think that only young cats and certain very active breeds get bored. Boredom and frustration can and does occur in any cat whose environment lacks enrichment, or who does not receive sufficient opportunities for mental stimulation. It can also occur in cats that need more social interactions with their owners who are not present enough, perhaps because of work commitments, or who do not engage sufficiently through training or play to meet the cat's needs. Common behaviours resulting from boredom and frustration include attention-seeking behaviour aimed at the owner, such as meowing or continuously rubbing the owner or patting at them to try to engage with them. This could also be seen as kneading with claws while sat on the owner's lap. The cat may show inappropriate play or even mounting behaviour towards the owner or another cat or pet in the home. As we see later, inappropriate play and attempts to practise the hunting sequence with the other as the 'prey' item involves teeth and claws and is certainly not to be encouraged as part of cat–human interactions.

Resources include, but are not limited to, litter trays, hiding- and resting-places (Fig. 11.4), activity toys, puzzle feeders, and games. Additional mental stimulation is acquired through regular sessions of reward-based training. Additional provision of space with a catio (Fig. 11.5), and taking your cat for excursions in your garden on a leash (Fig. 11.6), will provide safe, daily experiences in an outdoor setting, whether the owner is at home or at work.

Lifestyles

There are two common social scenarios for cats living in homes as our companions. Either the cat is a single cat living alone in the home with humans, or the cat lives with the human family and other cats. The problem behaviours which might be commonly seen will be greatly affected by this one aspect of home life – single- or multi-cat households. Often, cat lovers are keen to give more than one cat a home. However, the consequences of this should be carefully weighed; a feline friend can become a feline foe.

Single cats in a home are more likely to be able to live their lives in a way that suits the ethology of the domestic cat – as a solitary hunter. They do not have to share their core area with another cat; they do not have to compete with another cat for essential resources such as food, water, resting and sleeping places or litter trays. They have their humans all to themselves. While they may still develop problem behaviours, they will not have the potential stresses associated with sharing their home with other cats.

Several cats living together in a home will almost always be more challenging for each of them. Cats trying to live in harmony with other cats often find

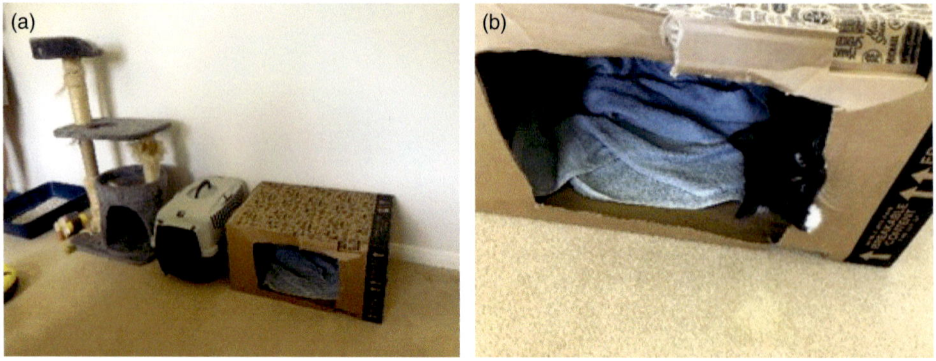

Fig. 11.4. Boxes, beds, activity centre and a litter tray. Note (a) the carrying basket is part of the normal environment, and (b) that boxes can also be toys. (Photos: Jane Williams, 2022)

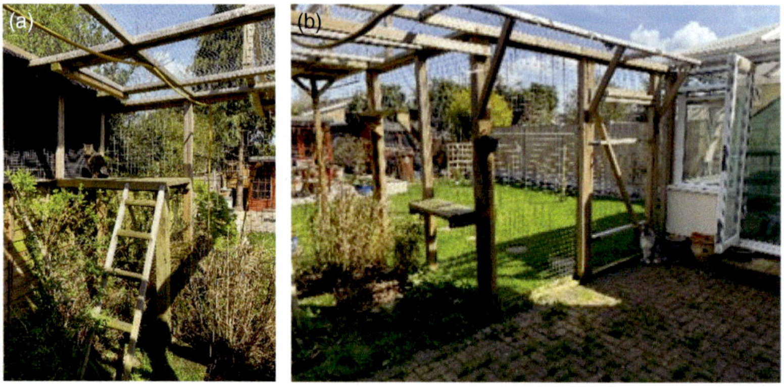

Fig. 11.5. Catios can be the perfect playground and do not need to be expensive to build. They should contain hiding-places, activity options, ropes, ladders, boxes, plants and perhaps a space for the owner to sit. (Photos: Jane Williams, 2022)

this very stressful. Frequently, they end up time-sharing resources or trying to carve out their own territory in an inadequate space, or with too few resources. As we have mentioned, when it comes to resources, cats always need choices – where they are, when they are available, whether they are suitable. The more cats there are in any given space the more difficult it becomes to create sufficient choices to meet the needs of each cat.

The other main difference in lifestyle concerns the indoor/outdoor life. It is whether the cat, or cats, are kept fully indoors, or indoors with access to a safely enclosed outdoor area (a catio or cat-fenced garden) or indoors with free-range access to the outdoors. All three types of management have pros and cons in respect of the cat's welfare (Table 11.2; Box 11.1), as well as for the development of problem behaviour and thus owner welfare (Table 11.3).

Types of behaviour problems and approaches towards solutions

It is worth remembering that emotions drive behaviours (Chapter 8). Anxiety, fear and frustration are the emotions that underlie 99% of behaviour problems (Table 11.4) in cats as well as other species. Additional drivers include pleasure, as in learnt attention-seeking from owners; boredom, which is often linked to frustration; and underlying medical problems, which may cause pain, as in dental pain, or just feeling unwell. All of these can have a negative impact on a cat's emotional state.

There are various ways in which problem behaviours can be grouped. We have chosen to do so from the perspective of the emotional drivers that cause them. We shall then look at how these emotional states manifest themselves, in terms of different types of problem behaviours they may cause or contribute to.

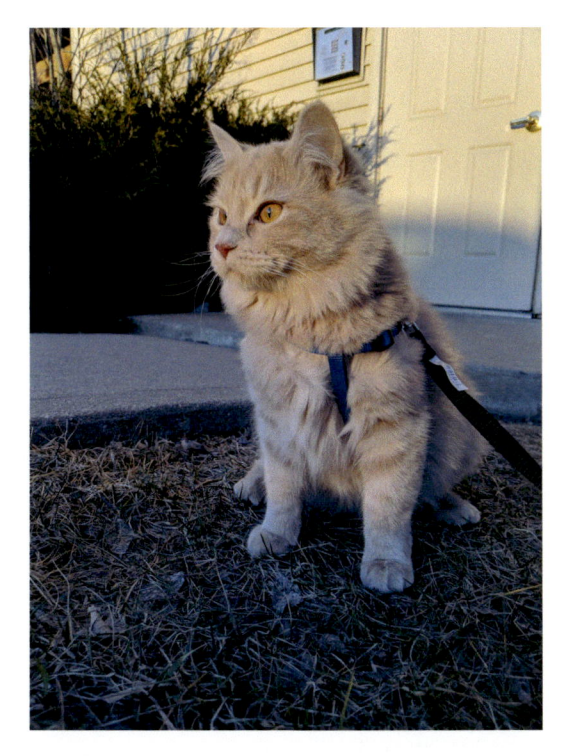

Fig. 11.6. Cat on a leash enjoying the outdoors. (Photo: Rbreidbrown, CC BY-SA 4.0 – https://creativecommons.org/licenses/by-sa/4.0 via Wikimedia Commons)

At the end of the chapter is a 'Summary of approaches mentioned to Prevent and Address Problem Behaviour'. Amongst other things, this contains information about pheromones, nutraceuticals and drugs, which are referred to below in respect of various problem behaviours. Please note, these are based on names used in the UK.

Emotional States

Anxiety 1: generalized anxiety

This is where the cat is anxious for much of the time. There will be many triggers in life to create anxiety, including environmental stimuli, people, other pets in the household and neighbourhood cats. Often undesirable toileting and/or aggressive responses are the behaviours seen when the underlying emotional state is anxiety or fear. Anxiety and fear, or distress, can develop either because several factors come together to create a situation in which the cat is fearful, or the cat can become more generally anxious or fearful if it is anxious for a significant proportion of the time.

Explanation

Often the cat's genetic make-up will mean that it is predisposed to anxiety and feeling anxious. Those, like Tabitha, who are timid or shy, have less resilience to recover from potentially frightening situations. Early life experiences can also contribute to increased anxiety, for example due to limited socialization as a kitten, as we saw in Chapter 2. This can lead to fear and anxiety around people. Lack of exposure of 3–12-week-old kittens to environmental stimuli that are a normal part of domestic life can lead to fear of those stimuli in later life.

Although predators, cats are small, delicate and fragile, and when outdoors they too can fall prey to larger predators. They are aware of the very important need not to get caught or injured. This aspect of cat ethology leads them to readily feel stressed or fearful, as there are many situations in life which may be potentially harmful and are to be avoided.

Solutions suggested for generalized anxiety

To reduce generalized anxiety there are several approaches and techniques that can be employed. These allow the cat to cope with the multifarious triggers that lead it to experience increased feelings of anxiety. The use of cat pheromones is one such approach. As the manufacturers describe them, these act to increase feelings of happiness and harmony. In some cases, the use of anxiety-reducing drugs can be of help. Regular kind handling by owners may be required, always on the cat's terms, at times and in places the cat enjoys. Reward-based training is often beneficial as this creates a favourable association with the people doing the training, engendering feelings of pleasure. Once behaviours are being performed on cue (and rewarded), they should be practised in various places around the home. This can help build the cat's confidence and reduce anxiety. Then the behaviour can be asked for and rewarded in the presence of previously worrying situations, such as when the washing machine is on or a visitor is sitting quietly in the same room.

Anxiety 2: specific anxiety and fears

These can occur even in generally happy, contented cats. Their personality type may be one of general confidence and assertiveness, as in Samantha and Arnie, but one or two unexpected events or situations may cause a cat to be frightened. For most of

Table 11.2. Welfare benefits by cat lifestyle.

Benefits	INDOORS ONLY SINGLE CAT	INDOORS ONLY MULTI CAT	INDOOR + CATIO SINGLE CAT	INDOOR + CATIO MULTI CAT	INDOOR + FREE ACCESS OUTDOORS SINGLE CAT	INDOOR + FREE ACCESS OUTDOORS MULTI CAT
Reduced likelihood of injury from other cats	✓	X	✓	X	X	X
Reduced likelihood of injury from other animals/cars/or unknown persons	✓	✓	✓	✓	X	X
Reduced likelihood of cat infectious diseases	✓	✓	✓	✓	X	X
No neighbourhood disputes	✓	✓	✓	✓	X	X
Beneficial for local wildlife	✓	✓	✓	✓	X	X
Reduced likelihood of cat being lost, locked in a building, or stolen	✓	✓	✓	✓	X	X
Avoidance of physical/thermal discomfort by not being able to access indoors	✓	✓	✓	✓	✓	✓
Cat can have access to sufficient resources for a good/excellent quality of life through which they can show normal behaviours, including hunting artificial prey (toys)	✓	✓	✓	✓		

Key: ✓ = benefits of lifestyle. X = benefit is unlikely to occur due to lifestyle.
Indoor cats – may be more likely to lack the full range of resources required to provide a stimulating enriched environment. However, this can be improved significantly through provision of activity play centres, activity feeding toys, regular short reward-based training sessions with owners.
Indoor + Catio cats – more space for the cat can be achieved through the use of catios – outdoor enclosures often attached to the house which allow outdoor access in a controlled way. This can be very beneficial for indoor cats and has the advantage of being safe and secure.
Indoor + Outdoor cats – may lack some resources and an outdoor lifestyle may be detrimental in terms of the relationship with the owner, particularly if access to indoors is restricted and the cat is forced to be outside when s/he would prefer to be indoors.

> **Box 11.1.** Outdoor Cats
>
> **Secret life of the cat: What do our feline companions get up to?**
>
> Armed with GPS tracking devices and micro-cameras, a team from BBC 2's *Horizon* programme in collaboration with the Royal Veterinary College set off to a Surrey village to find out what cats do when their owners are out.
>
> Meet Ginger, Chip, Sooty, Orlando, Hermie, Phoebe, Deebee, Kato, Coco and Rosie. They are 10 of the 50 cats studied in the village of Shamley Green, Surrey, for *Horizon*'s 'The Secret Life of the Cat'.
>
> As part of one of the largest ever research projects into domestic cat behaviour, the *Horizon* team, aided by the Royal Veterinary College and Lincoln and Bristol Universities, tracked dozens of cats over several 24-hour periods using specially designed collar GPS devices and tiny 'cat cams'. The result: scientists discovered the cats appeared to timeshare territories to avoid confrontation with neighbouring felines and visit each other's houses. However, the cat cam footage also revealed that squabbles over territory remained.
>
> See more at:
>
> https://www.bbc.com/news/science-environment-22567526
> https://www.bbc.co.uk/programmes/b02xcvhw
> https://www.bbc.com/news/science-environment-22821639
>
> ***The 'catscape' in a Norwegian village***
>
> The largest such study published so far was conducted in 2021 by scientists from the Norwegian University of Life Sciences. They GPS-tracked 92 owned cats that had free access to the outdoors. All the cats lived in the 1.1 km^2 (0.4 square mile) residential area of the university town of Ås, 30 km south of Oslo. The 92 cats represented 73% of the cat population in this neighbourhood. On average, the researchers gathered 168 hours of data per cat (21 days at 8 hours a day). In the gardens of 47 of the cats, they also placed a wildlife camera that detected movement and recorded behaviour for ten seconds each time it was triggered. All these data were used to produce the 'catscape', the use of the landscape by the cat population including the intensity of use of each spot.
>
> The results revealed that cats spent 79% of their outdoor time within 50 metres of home. The average maximum distance a cat strayed from home was 352 metres, but some travelled less and some ten times further, with the range being between 48 and 3384 metres, which is about two miles! The catscape showed that this, quite typical, residential area experienced very full cat presence. There was little space, or safe places (terrestrial refuges), for wildlife to avoid potential cat predation.
>
> (Bischof *et al.*, 2022)

the time, these cats are calm and relaxed, but they will be anxious when they predict that the frightening situation will reoccur – as they will have learnt through classical conditioning about those predictive stimuli (see Chapter 10). The cat may have had a frightening experience at the veterinary practice – some pain or a dog barking at it. The cat will now feel anxiety when a vet visit is about to take place – as when the carry basket is taken out of the cupboard – and fear when they are at the practice. Another common specific fear is that of loud or sudden noises that are infrequent and unpredictable such as bangs from car doors or fireworks. This can then generalize to other sudden noises, even quite quiet ones.

Explanation

These anxiety-based responses to specific stimuli may have their origins in early life. For example, insufficient early exposure to some types of humans, e.g. children or men, may lead to fear in their presence or create anxiety in anticipation of them being present. There is also an element of operant learning involved in how the cat learns to cope with these anxieties and fears. Some may learn that running away does not work – the person still strokes it or picks it up. It then shows fear-induced (defensive) aggression, which makes the person go away. As this strategy is successful, it will be reinforced and will be seen more frequently, and may even become the cat's first response in such a situation. Indeed, the cat may learn to 'attack' the person, or anyone similar, just for approaching.

Solutions suggested for specific fears

Taking this last example, let us imagine that the specific fear-provoking stimuli are men. The methods outlined above for general anxiety can be helpful. In addition, a carefully constructed desensitization

Table 11.3. Likelihood of problem behaviour by lifestyle.

PROBLEM BEHAVIOUR GENERAL	PROBLEM BEHAVIOUR DETAIL	INDOORS ONLY SINGLE CAT	INDOORS ONLY MULTI CAT	INDOOR + CATIO SINGLE CAT	INDOOR + CATIO MULTI CAT	INDOOR + FREE ACCESS OUTDOORS SINGLE CAT	INDOOR + FREE ACCESS OUTDOORS MULTI CAT
ANXIETY/FEAR	Anxiety/Fear of specific stimuli	✓	✓	✓	✓	✓	✓
ANXIETY/FEAR/MEDICAL	Toileting (defecation/urination)	✓	✓	✓	✓	✓	✓
SCENTING/MARKING/ TERRITORIAL BEHAVIOURS	Spraying	✓	✓	✓	✓	✓	✓
	Clawing/Scratching	✓	✓	✓	✓	✓	✓
AGGRESSION TO PEOPLE	Defensive	✓	✓	✓	✓	✓	✓
	Redirected	✓	✓	✓	✓	✓	✓
	Inappropriate play	✓	✓	✓	✓	✓	✓
AGGRESSION TO OTHER CATS	Defensive	X	✓	X	✓	✓	✓
	Redirected	X	✓	X	✓	X	✓
	Inappropriate play	X	✓	X	✓	✓	✓
OTHER TYPES OF AGGRESSION	Maternal	✓	✓	✓	✓	✓	✓
	Inter-male						
	Medical						
	'Despotic' personality						
HUNTING	Hunting	X	X	✓	✓	✓	✓
SOCIAL BONDING	Attachment to owner-related problems	✓	✓	✓	✓	✓	✓
	Attachment to cats-related problems	✓	✓	✓	✓	✓	✓
ABNORMAL	Pica	✓	✓	✓	✓	✓	✓
	Self-mutilation - overgrooming	✓	✓	✓	✓	✓	✓

KEY: ✓ = Commonly seen   X = Not likely   ✓ = Less likely

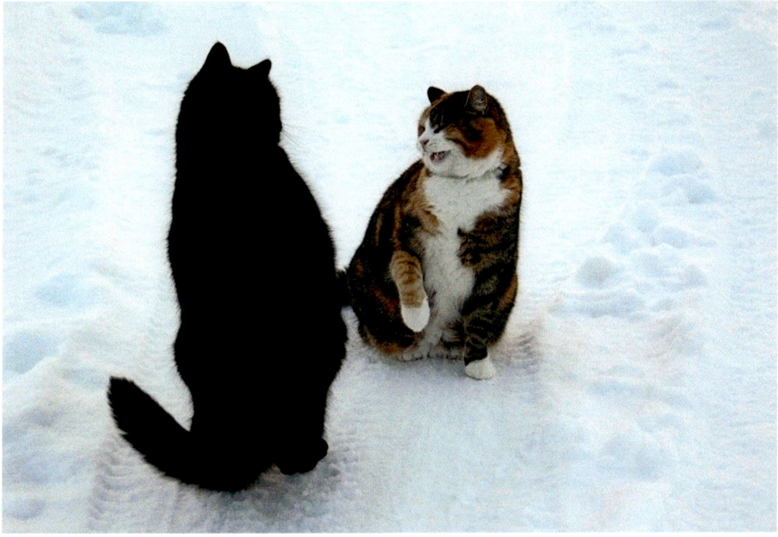

Fig. 11.7. Social aggression between neighbouring cats is more common than cat owners appreciate. (Photo: Janne Helen Lorentzsen, 2019)

and counter-conditioning procedure will be needed (see Chapter 10), first to the presence of men, so that the cat can ignore them rather than attacking. Reward-based training, using previously learnt 'tricks' as part of the counter-conditioning, can really help. Now the cat learns not just that men can be ignored but that their presence may be a good thing because it is linked with pleasant experiences and pleasant interactions with men, namely responding to a cued behaviour and receiving a reward. Depending on the depth of fear and other factors, for example the amount of time the owners can dedicate to this, there is the potential that, eventually, the cat will feel relaxed enough to be touched by men.

Frustration

Frustration is an emotional state which can easily lead to problem behaviours such as attention seeking, aggression and repetitive behaviours.

As we saw in Chapter 8, frustration arises when the cat wants something it cannot get. That may be because of physical or social barriers; the bird cage is out of reach, or Tommy's prevention of Missy getting to the food, or the cat wants to get off your lap and no longer be stroked but is not able to do so. Alternatively, the cat wants something to go away but it repeatedly refuses to do so, such as the person who insists on pestering the cat to play or be stroked.

Another cause of frustration is boredom due to lack of stimulation (physical and mental).

Explanation

Let us take the example of the bored cat that is seeking pleasure through play, hunting or other mentally stimulating activities and is attempting to find opportunities for these. In this situation, the cat may well show attention-seeking behaviours towards the owner, e.g. patting them continuously with a paw, meowing incessantly or rubbing around their legs. Frustration can also occur if the cat becomes over-stimulated and tired and is seeking rest but is being repeatedly woken up by the children who want to play. It may resort to aggression to make the humans go away.

Solutions suggested for frustration issues

These types of situations are generally resolved through the owner learning how to avoid the circumstances that cause the cat frustration. These either require more input of the right sort from the owner, e.g. reward-based training for mental stimulation, voluntary play sessions and other sources of enrichment; or less input, such as by providing the cat with resting places where it is assured of being left in peace, even in a busy household with young children.

Table 11.4. Problem behaviour by possible related emotion.

PROBLEM BEHAVIOUR GENERAL	PROBLEM BEHAVIOUR DETAIL	AVERSIVE, UNPLEASANT EMOTIONS				APPETITIVE, PLEASANT EMOTIONS		
		Anxiety	Fear	Frustration	Anticipation (Hope)	Pleasure	Relief
ANXIETY	Generalised anxiety (personality/extreme poor socialization)	✓	✓				
	Anxiety/Fear of specific stimuli (learnt)	✓	✓	✓			✓
ANXIETY/FEAR/MEDICAL	Toileting (defecation/urination)	✓	✓	✓			✓
SCENTING/MARKING/ TERRITORIAL BEHAVIOURS	Spraying	✓	✓	✓			✓
	Clawing/Scratching	✓	✓	✓			
AGGRESSION TO PEOPLE	Defensive	✓	✓				
	Redirected			✓			
	Inappropriate play			✓	✓	✓	
AGGRESSION TO OTHER CATS	Defensive	✓	✓				
	Redirected	✓	✓	✓			
	Inappropriate play			✓	✓	✓	
OTHER TYPES OF AGGRESSION	Maternal	✓	✓	✓			
	Inter-male			✓			
	Medical						
	'Despotic' personality						
HUNTING	Hunting	✓	✓		✓	✓	
SOCIAL BONDING	Attachment-related problems	✓	✓		✓		
ABNORMAL (MALADAPTIVE)	Pica	✓	✓	✓			
	Self-mutilation - overgrooming	✓	✓	✓			

We shall now examine how these emotional states manifest themselves as different types of problem behaviour in different circumstances related to the cat's lifestyle (Tables 11.3 and 11.4), with some thoughts on how to address these. Initially, we shall look at a normal cat behaviour which is often problematic for owners – scent marking – and then three problem behaviours that are anxiety based – toileting issues, attachment issues and over-grooming and pica. Finally, behaviour that is often simply called 'aggression' is considered. Aggressive behaviour is complex as it may be caused by anxiety, fear, frustration or pleasure.

Scenting or Marking Behaviours

As we saw in Chapter 4, rubbing, scratching or clawing objects are all natural behaviours which allow a cat to leave its scent behind. This is a way of informing any other cats that this is where the cat lives and it defines their core area, with all the vital resources it needs to survive. Such marking is also done in important hunting and relaxation areas outdoors away from home, as part of the cats' time-sharing system. Maintaining these resources in space and time is vital, so scent marking is very important. Scratching and clawing also leave a clear visual marker, as many owners will testify, their furniture or door frames bearing witness (Fig. 11.8).

Cats may also signal their presence by spraying on vertical surfaces, or eliminating urine, or sometimes faeces, at specific sites. Indoors, this is often on objects that are warm and so release more of the cat's odour, e.g. the radiator, TV or other electronic device which is switched on much of the time.

Whilst this is likely behaviour aimed at increasing the cat's self-confidence, there may also be medical causes of excessive urination or spraying. There can also be sexual drivers if the cat is entire. Finally, spraying may be exacerbated where there is insufficient space or resources accessibility in a multi-cat household.

Solutions suggested for scent marking and scratching

As for all problem behaviours, it is important to stop any positive punishment. You may need to restrict your cat's access to some areas where it has been marking. Scratching and clawing can be directed onto more appropriate scratching posts located in the multiple places the cat considers suitable for leaving its own scents – where it has been scratching is a good indicator. The owner can also regularly use synthetic cat pheromones – facial (Feliway® Classic) to make the cat feel at home and

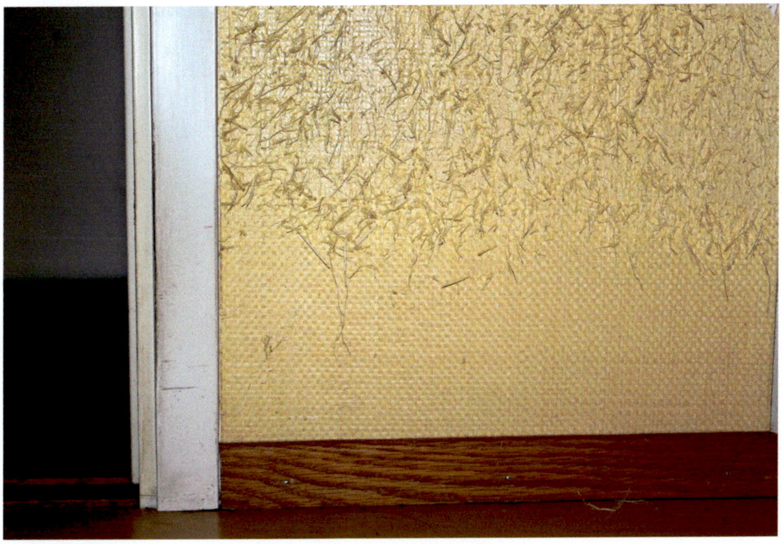

Fig. 11.8. Wall scratched by a cat. (Photo: Bjarne O. Braastad, 2012)

reduce scratching at inappropriate places and inter-digital (Feliscratch®) to attract scratching at scratching posts. The facial one provides the cat with reassuring scents that will make it relax and can be disseminated via a diffuser, while the inter-digital one entices the cat to deposit its own scents as a territory marker. See more about these products below, in the section 'Summary of approaches to prevent and address problem behaviour'.

The cat's anxiety about insufficient resources and/or its territory being at risk from intruders needs to be addressed. Make sure all cats in the household have good access to the resources they need, in separate places for each social group (see Case study 1), and keep the neighbours' cats out (see Case Study 2). Go to your friend's home to look after their cat while they are away rather than bringing it into your home, and consider showering and changing your clothes when you come home after interacting with cats elsewhere.

In spots where the cat has sprayed or urinated, the area needs to be cleaned appropriately. First rinse the area and its immediate surroundings with plenty of cold water, and pat it dry with a clean cloth. Then clean the area either with a commercial enzyme-containing product sold for this purpose or by using a 10% solution of biological laundry liquid, which you let dry and then wipe off with surgical spirit (rubbing alcohol); but do colour-test the surface *before* using the alcohol. These same cleaning regimes need to be used where the cat has defecated in an inappropriate location.

Inappropriate Toileting

Any change in toileting behaviour, be it urinating or defecating in inappropriate places, should mean a trip to the vet to rule out any medical cause, e.g. diseases in the urinary system or constipation due to hair balls. From a non-medical perspective, unacceptable toileting is due to anxiety or fear, or inappropriate provision of resources. Often the issue is the type and depth of litter provided and the location of the litter tray. In multi-cat households there may be an insufficient number of litter trays. In essence, your cat may be toileting outside the litter tray for any of several reasons:

- The substrate may be unacceptable.
- The litter trays may be in unsuitable places, e.g. in busy hallways or near doors, making the cat anxious and therefore unwilling to use the tray.

After all, a cat is particularly vulnerable when toileting.
- Owners may have told the cat off for unacceptable toileting, thus creating further anxiety and exacerbating the problem, making urination not just outside the litter tray but in other rooms more likely – often somewhere hidden.
- The kitten may not have been taught by its mother to identify and use the tray as the acceptable indoor toilet area. It may not have had access to a tray at this important time (for example, if you adopted a homeless cat).
- Indoor cats have no option to toilet outside and they are entirely reliant on their owners for suitable provision of litter trays. Cats are clean animals and do not like to use a dirty area and usually like to cover their faeces. If there is only one tray and it is not clean enough, or there is not enough litter in the tray, or it is a non-preferred or unfamiliar litter type, then the cat may toilet somewhere else.
- In multi-cat households there should always be at least one more tray than there are cats – for choice to be available and in case a tray has been soiled and not yet cleaned.
- As your cat enters old age it will become less mobile as joints stiffen due to conditions like arthritis. This may mean your cat is less able to get into or squat in a lidded litter tray so you will need to be creative to provide it with the privacy it needs but with easier access. One way is to cut a cat doorway into a large cardboard box which you then place over the unlidded litter tray. The extra height of the box will mean your cat will be able to sit more upright to toilet. This is a preferred position for many cats, so the higher cardboard box can be preferable for cats of any age who want privacy and more comfort.
- Some older cats may develop feline cognitive dysfunction (see below) and have increased anxiety and difficulty in locating the litter tray.

Solutions suggested for inappropriate toileting

- Address causes of nervousness or anxiety by considering the cat's physical and social environment as discussed throughout this chapter.
- Increase predictability within the environment by making access to resources very predictable, e.g. doors always open or shut so that. specific

rooms are either always or never available. Make sure that doors to rooms with litter trays are always open.
- The type of substrate may need to be changed to a non-clumping type, or one which feels softer on the cat's paws. The depth of the substrate should be at least 3 inches (7 cm). When introducing a new litter type, offer both until the cat is used to the new type.
- Consider the type of litter tray. Some cats prefer open trays (Fig. 11.9) and others prefer enclosed, lidded litter trays, or climbing into a larger box containing the tray so they have privacy but can always get out and never feel trapped.
- Increase the number of litter trays and put them in quiet, secluded locations (Fig. 11.10).
- Stop any punishments for unacceptable toileting.
- Increase confidence and sense of well-being through activity toys, play and reward-based training.

Feline Cognitive Dysfunction

Some geriatric cats will develop feline cognitive dysfunction. This is a degenerative disease due to the normal ageing process. It can manifest in several ways including: inappropriate toileting, confusion and spatial disorientation, changes in sleeping habits and increased anxiety and irritability (see also Chapter 3).

As advised for us humans, keeping your cat mentally and physically active throughout its life will provide a buffer to this disease developing and the rate of its degenerative progress.

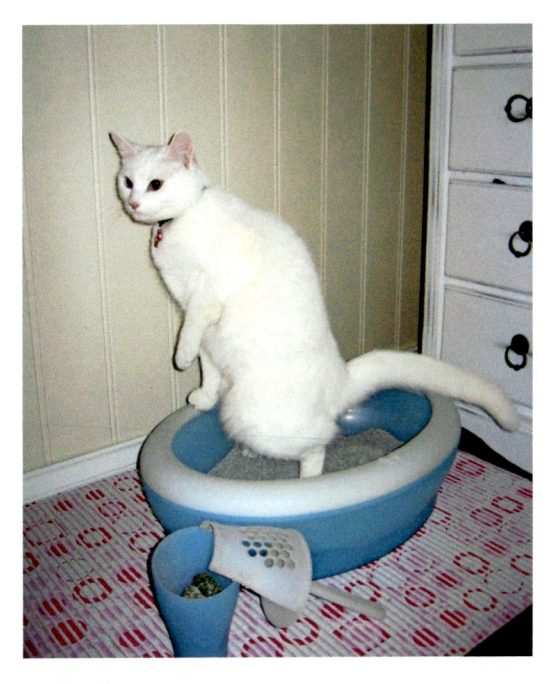

Fig. 11.9. This is how to use an open litter tray! (Photo: Janne Helen Lorentzsen, 2019)

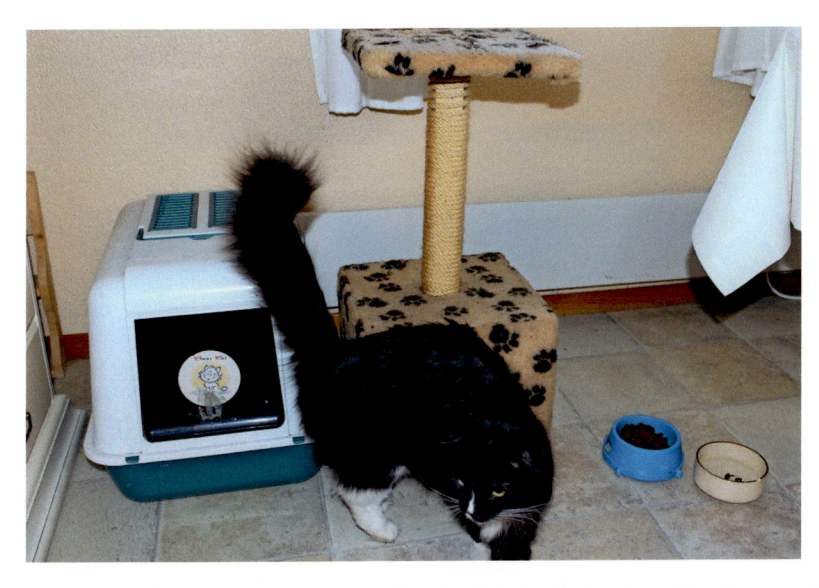

Fig. 11.10. 'No, I will not use that!' Place litter trays away from food and water bowls, resting places and disturbances. (Photo: Bjarne O. Braastad, 2012)

Problem Behaviours in Cats

Solutions suggested for feline cognitive dysfunction

Reducing anxiety and supporting the active brain is key to help slow any decline and help restore previous desired behaviours.

This can be achieved through providing mental stimulation, appropriate play (adjusted to the cat's physical abilities, e.g. moving the toy more slowly), gentle grooming and social interactions with owners. Pheromones and nutraceuticals can help, including Feliway, Zylkène, Aktivait and Cystophan, as can anxiety-reducing medication.

Attachment-related Problems

These occur when the cat is unable to establish or maintain a normal relationship with one or more of the most significant humans in its life.

Some will show over-attachment to and over-dependence on one owner. To keep the chosen carer to themselves, the cat may show aggression towards other people, including visitors and other members of the household. Alternatively, the cat may totally ignore other people and any attempts by them to interact. If people force the issue and try to push the cat into unwanted interactions, again aggression may result.

In other cases, the cat will be under-attached, be socially independent and shun all interactions with humans. This can be problematic if the owner was hoping for a cuddly cat which likes to sit on their lap and interact with them in other friendly ways, such as rubbing the owner's legs and arms or engaging in play with them.

Solutions suggested for attachment problems

OVER-ATTACHMENT. This involves the cat always wanting to be near the favourite owner so the solutions will involve teaching the cat to cope with being separated from that person – very small steps at a time. This may need to start with the use of a lidded indoor pen to teach the cat that it can cope with being in the same room as the owner, but not in physical contact. As with introducing the carrying basket (Chapter 10), the indoor pen must be introduced gradually and made to be a place of comfort, relaxation and where nice things occur, such as favourite foods. It is helpful to put a sleeping box and a raised platform in the indoor pen to help the cat feel safe (Fig. 11.4). The pen should be in a room where the owner spends most of their time so they can intermittently reinforce the cat's relaxed behaviour with a piece of food dropped in or a gentle word.

Increasing pleasant interactions with other people will also be of benefit to restructure relationships. Other family members and visitors can prepare the cat's dinner, play with fishing-rod toys, be involved in training the cat and practising the cues it has learnt. Of course, if the cat is aggressive to other people, then this must be done with caution (see aggression section). Initially, using the indoor pen and, later, the use of a harness and lead, is often needed to extend opportunities for safe interactions.

UNDER-ATTACHMENT. This may develop in cats who have been under-socialized to humans and therefore need to develop more pleasant associations with people. The best way to do this is through food. This can be done by the owner talking in a gentle soothing voice while preparing the cat's food and putting the bowl down, handfeeding, and employing a feeding regime which includes activity feeding toys to extend the feeding process whilst indirectly engaging with the owner who is in the same room.

The owner must not attempt to pick the cat up. Indeed, stroking may be too much of a test for its anxiety and may lead to a defensive aggressive response. Slowly, a programme of desensitization and counter-conditioning is needed, as described below (Defensive aggression).

Pica and Over-grooming

Both pica and over-grooming, also known as self-mutilation, are repetitive behaviours that have become pathological – a stereotypy. As was discussed in Chapter 8, these behaviours are rooted in anxiety and/or frustration caused through exposure to strong or prolonged distressing circumstances. These include environments that are relatively barren and under-stimulating (boring and frustrating), or are causing anxiety by being too busy, over-stimulating and thus threatening. Or it may be that the cat is living in a stressful social situation.

Pica is when the cat sucks, chews and even swallows items that are not food, but which can damage the cat's intestines. Predominately, this behaviour is directed at fabrics such as soft toys, blankets, towels or clothing. Regrettably, pica is often not recognized as a problem by owners but perceived as a cute behaviour.

In addition to being an indicator of anxiety or stress in general, pica can originate from the kitten having had a traumatic weaning experience, resulting in an abnormal missing of suckling from the mother while lying in a huddle of soft, warm fur (Fig. 11.11). This can happen if the kitten is separated from the mother and littermates too early, before the kitten's digestive system is fully adjusted to eating only solid food. There can also be medical reasons for this behaviour, including a lack of a dietary component if the cat is not eating a balanced diet. Some breeding lines may be more genetically predisposed to develop this behaviour than others. Whatever the root, anxiety will be the emotion associated with pica.

Another pica-like, behaviour is when a cat takes small, often woollen, objects as a substitute for prey, e.g. woollen socks. Sometimes a cat can be seen entering the room carrying such an item and emitting the type of miaowing call a mother will use to inform their kittens that she has brought home a prey animal and it is mealtime. This is not pica but occurs in relation to predatory behaviour. It is best addressed through ensuring your cat has plenty of opportunity to satisfy this behavioural need through playing with appropriate toys and puzzle feeders.

Over-grooming/self-mutilation is another manifestation of extreme anxiety or distress. This is where the cat licks, chews or pulls out its own fur, even to the point of biting itself (Fig. 11.12). There

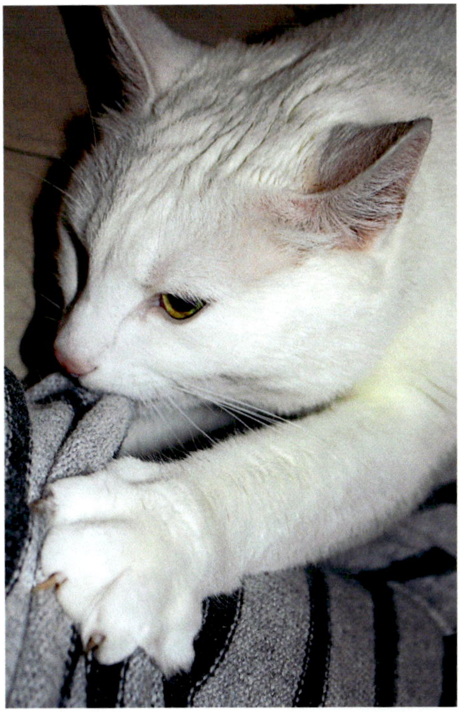

Fig. 11.11. Sucking and chewing on a sweater is especially common in cats taken prematurely from the mother cat, though this is not always the cause. (Photo: Janne Helen Lorentzsen, 2019)

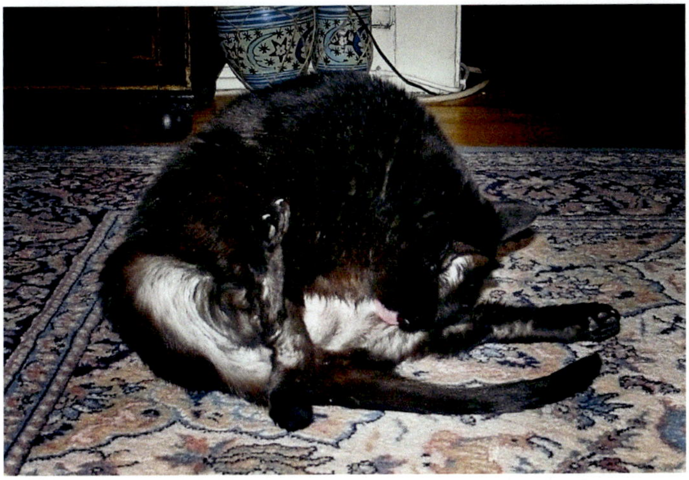

Fig. 11.12. After extensive over-grooming, a cat may have large hairless body parts. (Photo: Steve Browne and John Verkleir; Creative Commons Attribution 2.0 Generic license CC BY 2.0., https://commons.wikimedia.org/wiki/File:Feline_psychogenic_alopecia.jpg)

may be medical conditions contributing to this, e.g. skin irritation due to parasites, allergies, pain or a neurological condition. Indeed, these may have been the original trigger for the behaviour. Over-grooming may also be caused by a strong frustration, e.g. after having lost a companion with whom the cat allo-groomed – that is, they groomed each other. So the cat started over-grooming itself as a substitute for this social grooming.

As with pica and other extreme responses to anxiety and stress, over-grooming can have a learnt component. These repetitive behaviours cause the release of endorphins in the brain which give the cat some temporary relief, hence reinforcing the behaviour. The behaviour then becomes a learnt coping strategy to help the cat cope with its anxiety.

Another aspect of learning that can contribute to these abnormal behaviours is the response of the owners. We may unwittingly reinforce (reward) the behaviour by giving attention to the cat, such as telling it how cute it is for sucking its blanket or trying to distract it by offering a treat or toy when it is over-grooming.

Solutions suggested for pica and over-grooming/self-mutilation

It is essential to discover and address any medical conditions, allergic reactions or parasites. If that is not done, then any means of addressing the associated anxiety will not be successful. As with all anxiety-based issues, it is imperative to ensure that the cat's physical and social environment can meet its needs and address any shortcomings. Further help to reduce anxiety may come from nutraceuticals such as Zylkène and pheromones, e.g. Feliway Classic or Feliway Optimum. For some, drug therapy may be needed.

It is important not to punish or accidentally reward the pica or self-mutilation. This means these behaviours must be ignored. However, increasing opportunities for pleasant activities throughout the day, including play sessions and training new behaviours, will increase your cat's confidence in being able to cope with its world.

Aggression

We can categorize aggressive behaviours as clawing and biting. The intent to aggress is usually preceded by warning behaviours including growling, hissing and spitting (see Chapter 4). Aggression may be intra-specific, that is between two cats, or inter-specific, that is between a cat and a different species. In most cases, that different species is either the human or some other pet in the home.

Both inter-specific and intra-specific aggression can be the expression of one of several possible emotions, notably anxiety, fear or frustration. These arise from various motivations. The cat may be anxious/fearful and be defending itself, its kittens (maternal aggression) or its resources (e.g. inter-male aggression) from a perceived or actual threat. It may be frustrated at not being able to fulfil its desires, as in redirected aggression, or, in the case of inappropriate play/predatory behaviour, find the behaviour pleasurable. Aggressive behaviour will reflect the cat's character, as in the despotic personality of a bully cat like Ted (Case study 1). Aggression can signal that the cat is in pain, is ill or has a neurological disorder. In all cases of aggression, the cat will have been learning about the situations that led it to show the behaviour and the outcome of doing so.

Thus, as with all problem behaviours, any behaviour-modification programme will need to address potential medical issues, the environment and the cat's learning.

Defensive aggression

This is rooted in fear or anxiety and usually occurs when the option to run away and hide is not available. If the cat is trapped and frightened, then aggression is the only option to make the other cat, person or animal move away, and therefore reduce the perceived threat. Other causes could be pain/medical issues, and defensive aggression will be shown by a queen protecting her kittens or a cat protecting a resource that is limited, such as the only food bowl in a multi-cat household.

Defensive aggression towards people

This is usually linked to the person stroking, handling or grooming a cat that may be frightened due to previous poor experiences. For example, a long-haired cat whose fur had become matted experienced pain when the knots in the hair were pulled, or a cat may have been restrained for grooming or have experienced pain when handled or being picked up due to illness or a medical condition. All these experiences would lead to a classical association being made with people's hands and possibly generalized to non-grooming interactions of being stroked or handled. The cat's response is to defend itself.

Social behaviour problems leading to anxiety and so possible aggression will include communication issues with owners. Cats prefer frequent, low-intensity interactions and to initiate them themselves. They come to see their owner, say hello by rubbing their face on the owner's legs and move away again, and repeat this sequence a few times. If the owner attempts to handle, stroke or pick up the cat when the cat just wants to say a brief 'hello', this may cause anxiety.

Likewise, if the cat is picked up without warning, it will be startled and likely to show aggression (Chapter 8). This is not surprising if we consider it from the cat's perspective. They are rapidly lifted several feet (a metre or more) in the air, some six times their own height, often held around their abdomen. They have no feeling of support under their legs and might feel pain from the person's fingers putting pressure on their internal organs. Imagine if that was you suddenly swung up 30 feet (10 metres) with no warning at all! This would be a completely different experience from the thrill you get from 'scary' fairground rides. We still experience the fear-related neurotransmitter 'adrenaline rush' as our body prepares us for the worst – that is the thrill. But it is only a thrill because we are strapped in and have been told the ride is built to be safe. We have also been 'warned' of when it will happen and, importantly, we have chosen to take part. If none of those things were in place, you likely would be very frightened and resist (show defensive aggression) if someone tried to put you in a similar situation again.

Solutions suggested for defensive aggression to people

It is important to redirect social interactions with humans to those that are less intrusive, through play and training. To begin with, an indoor pen may be appropriate to use for safety purposes. It is essential that people desist from behaviours that cause the aggression, for example, persisting in trying to stroke the cat or hold on to the cat when it would clearly prefer to be left alone or not picked up. Instead, the cat should be taught to associate handling or holding with something pleasant – soft, gentle speaking by the owner or favoured food treats. Begin by briefly touching the cat on its flank and immediately giving it a treat. Gradually increase how long you touch, and where on its body, always rewarding each time. In terms of picking the cat up, start with just enticing it onto your lap for food and let it move away when it wishes. Slowly increase the time before you reward it (the interval reinforcement schedule described in Chapter 10).

For all cats (and small dogs and other small animals), we need to let them prepare to be picked up, rather than simply scooping them up without warning. This is easy to do through classical learning – choose a word that is going to tell your cat it is about to be lifted. Anne uses the word 'carry'. When the cat is comfortable with being on your lap and stroked over its body, then say your 'carry' cue and gently lift its front legs just a couple of centimetres (an inch) by putting your hand between them so the cat's chest is supported. Put the cat back down and reward. The next stage is to do this whilst running your hand around the cat's rump. Eventually, you will be picking the cat up in a way that it finds safe as you are providing support under its chest and rump (Fig. 11.13).

As described earlier, in the example of a cat frightened of men, it may also be necessary to desensitize and counter-condition the cat to the presence of a particular person with whom there is a frightening association. This involves the cat learning to cope with the presence of that person and linking that person with something that the cat finds very enjoyable and pleasant (see Case study 2).

Defensive aggression towards other cats

This occurs in response to an actual attack or aggressive signals from another cat. This could be a cat in the same household, or threatening behaviour from a neighbourhood cat. This can be due to competition for resources that both cats desire at the same time, or because one cat is in the space of another, including the local 'bully' who may have entered another cat's home, as in the case of Tarzan and Beryl (Case study 2).

Solutions suggested for defensive aggression towards another cat

As we saw with Ted in Case study 1, if the aggression is between cats in the same household, then an important part of the solution is to create more space for each cat. This is so that sufficient

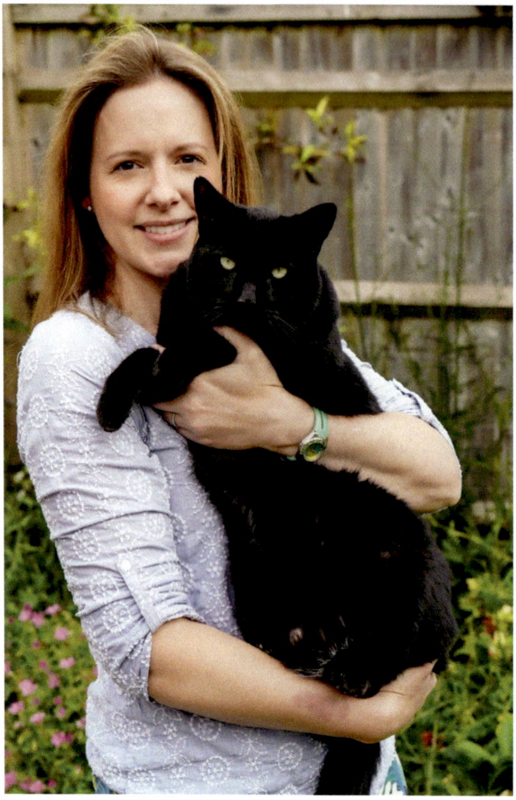

Fig. 11.13. Holding Kaeto in a safe and supported way. Note how the fingers of the hand gently restrain the front legs close to the body, so the cat cannot leap forward, whilst its body weight is fully supported under the hind legs. (Photo: Nicky Trevorrow and Anneleen Bru)

resources – food and water bowls, litter trays, sleeping and resting places, enrichments and toys – can be provided for each cat. This reduces competition for resources and allows each cat to feel more secure in its own core area.

While cats generally avoid trouble, there are 'bully' cats, like Ted and Tarzan, who seem to have quite despotic personalities. These cats are often very confident, active and will not restrain from showing offensive aggression to get what they want. Where the problem is a local 'bully' cat, fitting a magnetic- or microchip-triggered cat flap that only lets your cat into the house will help. However, this will not stop any issues outside, including the bully making your cat anxious by spraying the cat flap and declaring ownership, or waiting to ambush your cat when it goes outside. It is difficult to deter bully cats. A catio, or other form of cat-proof fencing, is usually the best solution. If using cat-proof fencing, you must ensure that it not only keeps your cat in but also keeps other cats out. The last thing that you want is other cats, especially the local bully, getting in and being trapped in your cat's space.

Redirected aggression

This is when the cause of the original aggressive response, e.g. another cat, is not the actual target of the aggression which follows. It may be that the cat that is the actual focus of the aggression is too threatening to challenge, so an easier target is the unfortunate recipient of the aggression. The aggression is redirected at another nearby – a person, a different cat or another pet – simply because they are more accessible and happen to be in the wrong place at the wrong time. We do the same. Consider being annoyed with your boss but you cannot challenge them directly. You are angry and frustrated at not being able to express your feelings, and so are likely liable to be grumpy, even shout at the next person you speak to. You have redirected your aggression.

Redirected aggression may occur when a person tries to handle a cat that is already in a heightened state due to a previous aggressive exchange with another cat. For example, if the owner tried to pick up Arnie whilst he was confronting the cat on the other side of the window, they may well have been scratched. Alternatively, the person could try to intervene in a cat fight and be injured as a result. The focus of one of the cats can quickly change from the feline foe to the nearest available target.

Whilst redirected aggression arises out of the situation of the moment, it can result in a classically learnt association being made with anxiety and the recipient target. This will increase the likelihood of aggression being directed towards the same individual in the future. Likewise, the recipient is likely to become anxious in the presence of the aggressor in the future. After all, from their perspective, the aggressor is now clearly unpredictable.

Solutions suggested for redirected aggression

First, we have to consider what caused the situation and try to prevent it occurring again.

Teaching your cat to 'leave' things or look at you and to come when called are all helpful. These cues can be used to reinforce the cat to come away from

> **Case study 2:** Aggression towards people
>
> This case involves two cats, Tarzan and Beryl, and Beryl's two owners, Dan and Lisa. Tarzan is a cat that lives in the neighbourhood. He is confident and has a rather aggressive, despotic personality and has often been seen in cat fights locally. Beryl had got on well with her human family. She is an indoor cat, who had previously been described as content, calm and quite friendly with her owners and keen to interact with them, but timid with other cats, and unfamiliar people. Then there was the incident.
>
> One day, Beryl's owners were decorating the kitchen door which led to the garden. The door was open, and Tarzan decided this was the moment to visit Beryl's place to check out her home for food. Lisa was painting in the kitchen with Beryl sitting near her on a chair when Tarzan flew in like a tornado. Chaos followed, with Beryl being chased out of the kitchen by Tarzan; Lisa was unable to get him out of the house for a good ten minutes. Beryl was terrified and hid behind the living-room sofa.
>
> As a result, Beryl started to show aggression towards Lisa. She would no longer be touched, stroked or handled by her. She had previously sought out both Lisa and Dan for social interactions. It transpired that, at times, both Lisa and Dan had been over-handling Beryl. Now she refused to have any interactions with Lisa, who was naturally upset by this. Beryl's association between the frightening invasion of her territory by Tarzan was now classically associated with Lisa's presence.
>
> Beryl was now anxious in Lisa's presence and especially so when Lisa tried to touch her. Indeed, this had now escalated to Beryl showing defensive aggression. There had been several incidents where Beryl had frightened Lisa by aggressively clawing at and biting her legs. The relationship and trust had become so broken on both sides that now Lisa was afraid to be in the same room as her beloved cat.
>
> Explaining why and how this sad state had been reached enabled Lisa to understand more and feel confident in taking part in a behaviour modification programme to restore her previously harmonious relationship with Beryl. She was also aware that this would be a slow process and that how fast it progressed was dictated by how comfortable Beryl felt.
>
> This programme included several of the suggestions outlined in this chapter. These included Lisa stopping trying to initiate (force) Beryl to be touched or stroked but waiting for Beryl to learn that she was not a threat. This, combined with several sessions of reward-based training and linking Lisa's presence with much more pleasant experiences, soon meant that Beryl started to be more relaxed in her presence and was learning to tolerate Lisa again.

the emotional situation that is making it feel anxious or frustrated, for something much more pleasant, like a favourite titbit, or a game. This should be practised (frequently) when the cat is calm, and then in the area where the redirected aggression occurred and in increasingly similar situations. All this will help prevent emotional escalation in the future.

Where the cause relates to tension between cats, then, as ever, the physical and social environment must be assessed and steps taken to reduce the tension and thereby reduce any anxiety or fear which may be driving aggressive reactions. This may include use of pheromones, additional space, and providing each cat with all the resources they need as and when they need them. If the initial cause of the frustration was an external neighbourhood cat, then, ideally, it should be prevented from entering the home – as in the resident having a catio. If, as with Arnie, the problem is a cat looking through the window, then the sight of the other will need to be blocked. This may mean drawing blinds or denying the resident cat access to the room with those windows.

If an anxiety association has been made with the person who was the target of the redirected aggression, then steps, as described for defensive aggression, will need to be taken.

If there has been a breakdown in the relationship between the cat that redirected its aggression and the cat that was the recipient, with one or both now being anxious in the other's presence, then pheromones can help, as will ensuring there are places to be out of sight in each room that the cats can access – places of safety in all rooms. There will also need to be desensitization and counter-conditioning training. This is so that each learns to associate the presence of the other with pleasant feelings, with good things happening, such as gentle interactions with owners or special food treats that are only available when both cats are in the room. To begin with, this may mean having the cats in separate indoor pens or each restrained on a leash so that attacks are prevented. As with defensive aggression, restoring a degree of trust and relaxation in the presence of the other can be a slow process.

Offensive aggression

Rooted in frustration, or underlying anxiety/fear, this is often seen during stroking, handling or grooming. It is when the cat apparently instigates aggression and appears angry for no obvious reason, at least from the owner's perspective. The aggression seems to be unpredictable in that it does not always show itself in what appear to be similar situations. The cat may be using this type of aggression to stop the unwanted stroking, handling or grooming, especially if its earlier signals have not been noticed. It may also occur when the cat is frustrated by not being able to access desired resources.

Offensive aggression is also seen as part of sexual competition between male cats near females in heat. Emotionally, this is a mix of anxiety/fear at the potential loss of a resource and frustration at the other cat's dismissal of earlier signals advising it to go away.

Finally, predatory behaviours are often labelled as offensive aggression if directed to non-prey individuals, particularly if they involve humans (e.g. human hands, wrists and ankles). In fact, this is not aggression and is more accurately described as inappropriate play.

Solutions suggested for offensive aggression

As with other aggression issues, it is important to consider the environment and ensure that your cat has sufficient space and resources. Pheromones may also be appropriate. This is to address issues causing frustration and any anxiety or fear which may be driving the aggressive behaviour. Preventing neighbourhood cats from accessing the core home area, outdoors and indoors, will reduce the need for territorial disputes.

Inappropriate Play

This is considered a form of aggressive behaviour only because it includes biting and clawing. It is not a form of social play, but object-oriented 'predatory' play. It comprises the predatory behaviours of stalk, pounce, bite and claw. Unlike true aggression, this behaviour is motivated primarily by pleasure and possibly some frustration if there are limited opportunities for these activities. Ideally, the motivation for this natural behaviour is satisfied through playing with suitable toys. It is inappropriate when it is directed towards people, or to other pets which also find this distressing. It is often seen in younger cats but is not restricted to any age group. In many cases this inappropriate play/predatory behaviour has been encouraged by owners who played with the kitten using their hands or feet (Fig. 11.14). Now the cat has learned that hands

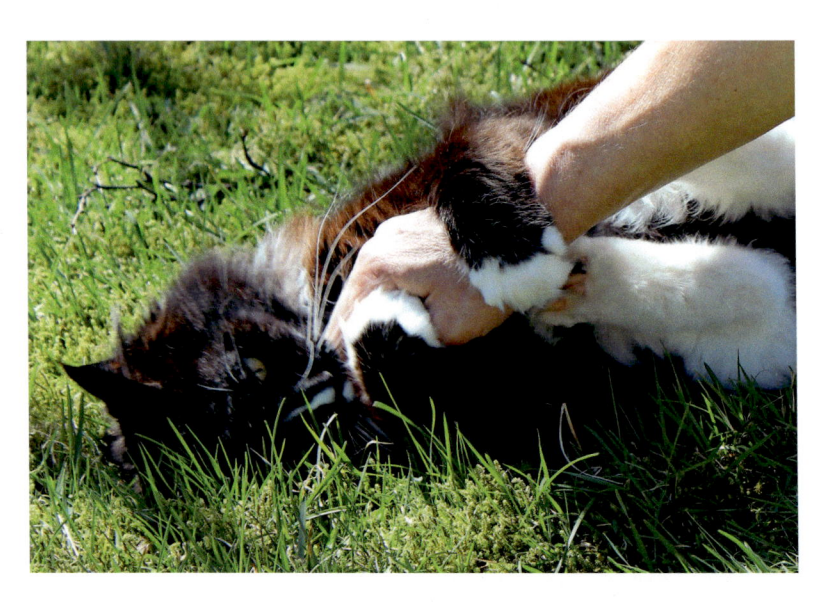

Fig. 11.14. Cats can learn that hands are toys to be bitten and scratched. (Photo: Bjarne O. Braastad, 2012)

and feet are toys and tries to interact with them accordingly by stalking and hunting them and then jumping on them and grabbing them with extended claws in a pretend 'kill' attempt. This is painful, especially if you are only wearing slippers. Additionally, the cat may learn that this is an excellent way of getting its owner's attention if it is bored – it certainly gets attention, and owners may accidentally reinforce it by distracting the cat with food.

Solutions suggested for inappropriate play

Playing with a person's hands or feet must be replaced by plenty of opportunities to play with appropriate toys. This means people must not respond to the cat's attempts to play with their hands/feet and this unwanted behaviour is put on extinction. As we saw in Chapter 10, it is likely that the cat will have a frustration burst and will initially try harder to instigate the inappropriate play. It is important that family members do not react, so they will probably need to wear protective clothing such as rubber boots and leather gardening gloves.

The owner needs to be proactive in initiating play sessions – redirecting the cat to a suitable toy. Starting games instead of waiting for the cat to do so will quickly help the cat learn how to get a fun time. The types of appropriate toys are fishing-rod toys, including those with food parcels at the end of the string rather than a toy. These allow the cat to catch the 'prey' item and eat it and thus complete the hunting sequence. There are also modern versions of the clockwork mouse, namely remote-controlled toy mice. Some toys do not necessarily need a person present and include puzzle feeders and toys on elasticated string that are hung from doorhandles or beams (Fig. 11.15). This means your cat can satisfy its desire to play at any time it chooses.

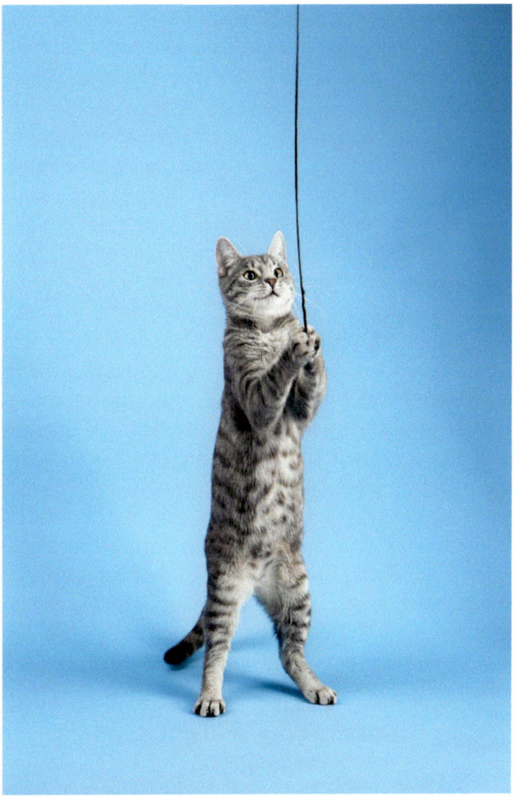

Summary of Approaches to Prevent and Address Problem Behaviour

Knowledge and understanding

To both prevent and address all cases of problem behaviours, owners need to have a good understanding and awareness of the world from the perspective of their cat. They need to be able to recognize the ways in which their cat is seeking to communicate with them and how best to respond to those communications and the cat's environmental and social needs.

Fig. 11.15. A cat playing with an elasticated string attached to the ceiling. (Photo: Depositphotos 9431729)

Resources

The home must provide sufficient resources, ideally an excess of resources for each cat. The cat needs to be able to make choices, e.g. between locations of food; litter trays; scratching posts; lookouts; resting, hiding- and sleeping places. Providing food in several locations can be helpful for the single cat and is essential in multi-cat households. For litter trays, a minimum of one per cat plus one extra will avoid trouble.

Change of diet or feeding regime

Cats eat little and often. Provide frequent or free access to food (*ad libitum* feeding). As explained in Chapter 6, a high-meat diet and object play seems to help satisfy cats, nutritionally and psychologically, reducing the need for outdoor cats to predate on wildlife. Unlike food that is always presented in a bowl, using activity (puzzle) feeders or hiding

Problem Behaviours in Cats

food parcels makes food and eating more interesting and can be psychologically more satisfying, as long as the cat does not find the challenges too difficult and gives up. Providing at least part of the cat's daily diet in this way has another advantage in that the cat is less likely to become obese, especially if it is an indoor cat. Activity feeders, commercial or homemade, imitate the natural aspects of eating (hunting), namely seek, obtain and consume. They do not need to be expensive; for example, a cardboard box full of scrunched-up paper with dry food pellets scattered inside, or the cardboard centre of a toilet roll folded up with a few pellets inside, are perfect pretend 'mice' that your cat can 'kill', then dissect and eat the contents. You may need to start with something the cat particularly likes – a few pieces of cooked chicken to get your cat interested in working out this new puzzle. Providing food in various ways, with some in a bowl, is beneficial for cats whether they have access to outdoors or not, but perhaps especially for those kept indoors. They are beneficial for cats of all ages, including for older and geriatric cats.

Increase mental and physical stimulation

Such stimulation needs to be provided throughout the cat's life and should include activities that the cat can do alone, e.g. puzzle feeders, hanging toys, etc., as well as human interactions. By providing for several short sessions each day that give our cats the opportunity to engage with us in pleasant, rewarding ways, we can improve their quality of life immensely. This also reduces boredom and frustration and the behaviours these emotions may lead to. Appropriate interactions are playing games; short, gentle grooming and stroking sessions; training and practising some simple cues; even working up to see if your cat, like Eibsu, can learn to be a copycat (Chapter 10).

Outdoor access

Outdoor access can often improve welfare but must be balanced with other considerations. These include local wildlife and your neighbours, and, importantly, the safety of your cat. Are there high numbers of neighbourhood cats? Is there a bully cat? What is the danger posed by traffic, or of becoming accidentally trapped in someone's garden shed or garage? Could your cat be stolen, or simply decide to move away from home? A catio is the safest way to provide your cat with accessible access to the outdoors, via a cat flap. If you live in an apartment, this could mean simply enclosing the balcony. No matter how small or large the area you have, a catio can be made into a stimulating playground, as well as a safe place where your cat can relax and watch the world go by, enjoy the sun, or choose to play with raindrops and snowflakes.

CatBib®

If your cat is going to be free-roaming, or you have used cat-proof fencing in your garden but still wish to enjoy the birds and other wildlife, then the CatBib® is an effective answer. Research conducted at Murdoch University in Australia by Michael Calver and colleagues showed that the CatBib® stopped 94% of cats from catching all types of birds (not just songbirds), 45% of cats from catching mammals, and 33% of cats from catching amphibians and reptiles. The CatBib® is attached to the cat's collar and hangs loosely over the cat's chest. Cats quickly adapt to wearing it in less than a day. The CatBib® works by gently interfering with the precise timing and co-ordination a cat needs for successful bird catching. It does this by the simple principle of coming between the cat and the bird prey just at the last moment, as it is pouncing. Importantly, it does not interfere with any of your cat's other activities. The CatBib® only affects your cat's ability to catch wildlife. A cat wearing a CatBib® can run, jump, climb trees, eat, sleep, scratch and groom. Using the CatBib® is part of being a responsible pet owner to control your pet's impact on wildlife.

Keeping your cat indoors at night will also help reduce predation on small mammals and other nocturnal wildlife needing protection, such as frogs and toads.

Birdsbesafe® collar cover

An alternative is to use a Birdsbesafe® collar cover. These are attractive and help warn birds of the cat's presence, as verified by several scientific studies. Combined with a reasonable-sized bell, this can help protect nocturnal animals, too (Chapter 6, Fig. 6.4).

Thundershirt/body wraps (Mekuti®, Anxiety Wrap®)

These can have some benefits for some cats in reducing anxiety and distress by creating a sense of body pressure and support for the fearful cat.

Pheromones

These can be purchased as synthetic analogues of naturally occurring cat pheromones. They have three main effects regarding messages the cats receive, which can be explained in a simple way like this:

- Friendly messages: cats mark their home area as familiar by rubbing their face against corners, furniture, people or other cats. This is thought to release a 'friendly message' that provides reassurance to the sender cat and its companions.
- Calming maternal messages: after the mother gives birth, it is claimed that she sends calming pheromonal messages to her kittens. These are released from the area around her nipples, in the mammary zone, and seem to have a relaxing effect.
- Business card messages: like graffiti, cats inform others of their presence within their home range or at least their core area, and have their own way of telling other cats 'I am here'. They scratch in visible places leaving visible marks and pheromonal messages, the latter coming from glands between their toes. If another cat detects this message within its home range, it will be likely to scratch there too – as if they were exchanging business cards.

Feliway® Classic – the analogue of facial pheromones deposited when rubbing, the product claims to send friendly messages to cats, reducing behaviours such as hiding, scratching or spraying.

Feliway® Friends (Felifriends) – this diffuser/spray contains a synthetic copy of 'cat appeasing pheromone' (CAP), the maternal pheromone described above. (This use of the word 'appeasing' by the manufacturer refers to its calming effect, not anything to do with social hierarchies as discussed in Chapter 4.) Produced by a queen cat after giving birth, it is supposed to help nursing kittens feel secure, content and relaxed in each other's company. Feliway® Friends is advertised as sending 'harmony messages' that help restore harmony between adult cats living together. It is asserted to help with aggression towards people in frightening situations, and aggression between cats. It is also proposed for use preventively, e.g. before and after a trip to vet and when introducing a new cat if there is already a resident cat.

Feliscratch® – this is a synthetic copy of the pheromone deposited by the interdigital glands between a cat's toes when it scratches on objects. It has a blue colour that provides a visual marker to the cat and is proposed for enticing cats to scratch in desirable locations, namely the provided scratching posts.

Feliway® Optimum – this feline pheromone complex is a combination of several synthetic cat pheromones and is claimed to provide cats with a message of enhanced serenity. This holistic message is proposed to help all cats feel more comfortable and secure in their home by providing reassurance, thereby also reducing stress between cats living in a multi-cat household. It may help with indoor spraying, inappropriate scratching and reducing anxiety in the veterinary environment or cattery.

Nutraceuticals

These are designed to supplement the nutrients in normal cat food. They contain ingredients which provide the building blocks for calming or relaxing neurotransmitters, e.g.:

- Anxitane™ – active ingredient is L-Theanine
- Zylkene® – active ingredient is alpha-casozepine, which influences the opioid systems and may increase GABA activity
- Solliquin® – active ingredients: L-Theanine and plant extracts *Phellodendron amurense* and *Magnolia officinalis*
- Cystophan® – support for feline idiopathic cystitis (FIC), proposed to lower urinary tract disease by supporting healing of bladder wall; contains Glucosamine, Hyaluronic acid, L-tryptophan
- Aktivait®Cat – proposed to help reduce age-related mental function loss by supporting brain function, improving metabolism and signalling. Contains fatty acids/phospholipids and antioxidants Vitamin C and E, selenium.

Drugs

This area is entirely the remit of your vet. No owner should attempt to decide how to medicate their cat, or buy drugs from a source that has not been advised by their vet – it may not be reputable and could harm your cat. Any decision regarding suitability of any drug and its dose is *entirely* a decision for the professional.

There are types of drug therapy that can be used in conjunction with behaviour modification approaches to reduce fear, anxiety and distress. In the UK and many countries, the drugs mentioned below are only available through a veterinarian. They may be used to help with feline cognitive dysfunction and to support a variety of behaviour modification programmes where the behaviours are severe, having a significant impact on welfare, or are deep-seated, long-term and resistant to change. Their action is for short-term or long-term treatment. The examples given are purely for the types of behaviours for which they *may* be used. They do not represent the full and increasing range of medications available:

- analgesia for pain relief, e.g. dental or arthritic pain;
- anxiety, pica – tricyclic anti-depressants (TCA), e.g. Clomipramine, Amitriptyline;
- stereotypies/compulsive behaviours – TCAs, e.g. Clomipramine, Amitriptyline; Selective Serotonin Reuptake Inhibitors (SSRI), e.g. Fluoxetine, Fluvoxamine; and
- fear-related aggression – monoamine oxidase inhibitors (MAOIs), e.g. Selegiline.

Please note that reference to specific nutraceuticals, pheromones and drugs are based on names used in the UK.

Conclusion

In this chapter, a range of the more common problem behaviours seen in cats has been described and possible underlying causes explained. This, and the information given in the previous chapters, will help owners take appropriate steps to provide a suitable physical and social environment for their cat which will help prevent problem behaviours occurring. Where problems do arise, it is essential to understand that each cat is an individual, as are the people and other animals with whom it lives. Where it lives and how its environment is managed will also be different. Thus, throughout this chapter, we have only provided suggestions for approaches to addressing undesirable behaviour. There is no such thing as the definitive recipe book for resolving problem behaviour. Having said this, we reiterate that in *all* cases, the first step is for the vet to rule out any medical causes.

Further Reading

Bischof, R., Hansen, N.R., Nyheim, Ø.S., Kisen, A., Prestmoen, L. *et al.* (2022) Mapping the 'catscape' formed by a population of pet cats with outdoor access. *Scientific Reports* 12, 5964. DOI: 10. 1038/s41598- 022- 09694-9.

Bradshaw, J. and Ellis, S. (2016) *The Trainable Cat: How to Make Life Happier for You and Your Cat.* Basic Books, New York.

Bru, A. (2019) *I Love Happy Cats - Guide for a Happy Cat.* Schiffer Publishing, Atglen, Pennsylvania.

Ellis, S. and Sparkes, A.H. (eds) (2016) *ISFM Guide to Feline Stress and Health: Managing Negative Emotions to Improve Feline Health and Wellbeing.* International Cat Care, UK. Available for purchase at: https://icatcare.org/shop/isfm-guide-to-feline-stress-and-health-pdf (accessed 14 July 2022).

Horwitz, D.F. (ed.) (2018) *Blackwell's Five-Minute Veterinary Consult Clinical Companion: Canine and Feline Behavior*, 2nd edn. Wiley, Ames, Iowa.

Houston, K. (2014) *21 Days to the Perfect Cat.* Hamlyn, London.

McMillan, F.D. (2020) Mental health and well-being benefits of personal control in animals. In: McMillan, F.D. (ed.) *Mental Health and Well-Being in Animals,* 2nd edn. CAB International, Wallingford, UK, Ch. 6.

Pryor, K. (2003) *Getting Started: Clicker Training for Cats.* Sunshine Books, Waltham, Massachusetts.

Walker, B. (2009) *The Cats' House.* National Cat Protection Society, Newport Beach, California.

Supplementary materials entitled 'Fear and anxiety in cats', 'Aggression in cats', 'What can you do when the cat bites', 'When the cat scratches furniture', 'Urine marking in cats', 'The cat's toilet preferences' can be accessed at: www.cabi.org/the-cat-behaviour-and-welfare/

12 People and Cats

To say cats are popular is an understatement. Japan is noted for its cat cafés; and its 'cat island', Tashirojima, is a popular destination for cat-loving tourists. Istanbul is called by some the City of Cats, or 'Catstanbul', while the cats of Rome have a special status as part of the city's bio-heritage. Americans own the largest number of cats, with cats being found in about one in every three households. In the UK, it's one in four. Cats are more popular as pets than dogs in Canada, Argentina, northern Africa, much of Europe and most of Asia. In 2020, some 27 million urban Chinese households owned one or more cats. See Chapter 1 for a brief presentation of numbers of cats around the world.

So, we may ask, who are cat owners? What kind of relationship do people have with their cat? How do people keep their cats and what sort of restrictions are placed on keeping cats in various parts of the world, or types of accommodation, and why? Scientists have been interested in these questions since the 1980s and the main method used to gain insight has been by sending surveys to cat owners. This chapter looks at a few studies to illustrate what we know, and there are some suggestions for further reading if you wish to explore further.

What Characterizes Cat Owners?

In 1998, two Master's students, studying with Bjarne – Ingrid Westbye and Agnethe Sandem – sent surveys to Norwegian cat owners, receiving a combined total of 934 responses. In 2014, Silja Eriksen, another of Bjarne's students, surveyed 1212 Norwegian cat owners. Some of the information in this chapter comes from the work of these three students. Westbye found that the cat owners were, on average, 42 years old and, in the three surveys, respectively, 83%, 90% and 92% were women. Many had children: 9% had children aged 0–5 and 26% had children aged 5–15. About 23% of the cat owners were single, while the rest were married or cohabiting. The cats themselves were, on average, 5.5 years old, most of them 2–5 years, but some were up to 20 years old. These statistics are comparable with those for other western countries, as in the UK, where a survey conducted in 2021 revealed that 34% of UK cat owners were aged between 45 and 54. This is slightly higher than Westbye's average of 42. This may reflect the general ageing of the population over the intervening 20 years.

Studies show that people say they acquire cats because they want the cat's company, love and affection. Another important reason is that cats are considered independent, requiring little work to provide them with a good quality of life. We are also more likely to get a cat if we have previously owned one, especially when we were children. Westbye found the behavioural traits of the cat that were most important to the owner were (in order of priority) emotional affection and confidentiality, the cat is cuddlesome, seeks out the owner, shows its personality and intelligence, responds to the owner's signals, is independent, makes sounds, is adaptable, active and playful.

Are cat owners different from dog owners? There is certainly a commonly held belief that this is the case. Indeed, even people who do not own either species, and have no desire to, will describe themselves as a cat or dog person. But what does the science say? Since 1980, there have been several studies and the findings have been rather mixed. Some studies have found no differences between dog and cat people whilst others have. Where differences have been shown, the picture is confusing, partly reflecting differences in how the information was gathered and what aspects of personality were measured, as well as who the respondents were; they were usually current owners. To get a representative sample of dog and cat owners you need large numbers of people from as wide a range of backgrounds as possible. Older studies had relatively small numbers of participants as these had to be recruited directly or by post. Nowadays, the internet makes it possible for surveys to reach many people from many different socioeconomic backgrounds and many different countries, thereby giving more reliable and robust information.

In 2010, Samuel Gosling and colleagues ran an online survey which was designed to address these recruitment and methodological issues. They suggested that to really understand if any differences exist, we need to look beyond current owners and include those who identify as cat or dog people. They received answers from 4565 people. Participants were from various countries including the USA, Canada, UK, India, Australia and the Philippines. Though 64% identified as white/caucasian, a range of ethnicities were represented. They used a robustly tested scale that measured the 'Big Five' human personality traits (see Box 12.1), and asked people whether they saw themselves as a cat person, a dog person, both or neither. Interestingly, 45.8% (2088 respondents) considered themselves a dog person, 11.5% (527 people) a cat person, 27.7% (1264 people) identified as both, and 15% (686 people) answered that they were neither a dog nor a cat person. We may not be surprised that 27.7% identified as both, given that people will often live with a dog and a cat. In her survey of Norwegian cat owners, Eriksen found that 25% also had a dog.

Gosling and colleagues received answers from far fewer self-identified cat people than dog people, 527 versus 2088. This may reflect personality traits that influence whether people are more likely to take part in surveys and share information about themselves. Differences were certainly found between dog and cat people, and these were not influenced by gender. Overall, compared to dog people, cat people scored significantly lower on extraversion, agreeableness and conscientiousness, but significantly higher on neuroticism and openness. This means that cat owners tend to be more anxious, more reserved and more socially independent characters who are not so keen to take part in other people's lives and problems – and thus may not be so willing to do surveys. Cat people seem to be somewhat more open to engage in new activities and less likely to avoid changes to their routine compared to dog people.

In an earlier small but pioneering study, Aline and Robert Kidd found that dog owners, on average, were fonder of children and young people than were cat owners. Their data also suggested that dog owners tend to be more dependent on other people, perhaps showing a more elaborate social intelligence and more inclined to stand by their ideas and

---

Box 12.1. Human personality traits – the Big Five.

Each of the Big Five personality traits describes an aspect of human personality, across a spectrum from low to high. Individuals can be placed at a different position on each spectrum, with traits remaining stable over a lifetime (Rantanen et al., 2007). The traits are commonly known as agreeableness, conscientiousness, extraversion, neuroticism and openness to experience. In brief, these are:

Agreeableness – an individual's level of concern for social relationships and co-operation. Those higher in agreeableness are often trusting, co-operative and value others' interests. Low agreeableness is associated with lack of concern for others, often leading to the person being viewed as selfish or argumentative.

Conscientiousness – an individual's ability to control their impulses. High conscientiousness may be represented as organized but inflexible behaviour, with the person being focused. Low conscientiousness is often represented by spontaneous, disorganized behaviour, and these people may struggle to complete tasks.

Extraversion – an individual's tendency to engage with or seek out social interaction. High extraversion exhibits as outgoing, sociable, assertive, energetic and sensation-seeking, whereas an individual low in extraversion tends to be reserved and socially independent.

Neuroticism – also called emotional instability, this is the tendency of an individual towards experiencing unpleasant emotions. Highly neurotic individuals may frequently experience feelings of anxiety and hostility. They are generally more reactive and likely to interpret situations as dangerous. Low neurotic individuals display calmness and stability within their own behaviours.

Openness to Experience – an individual's willingness to engage and interact with new events or activities. Those high on this trait are often unpredictable and more likely to partake in risky behaviours. Less open individuals are likely to avoid changes to their routine, preferring what they are used to.

fight for their cause when challenged. In contrast, when cat owners face hostility or aggression, they tend to retreat and show passive resistance. On average, the cat owners were more likely to be independent, freedom-loving individuals who rely on themselves and are more emotionally concerned with their cat keeping than dog owners.

David Greene made an informal survey of art images and figures of animals in the homes of animal owners. He found that the cat owners were three times more likely to have cat decorations in their living room than dog owners were to have dog decorations. In shops, you will find far more posters and pictures of cats than of dogs. They obviously know their market (Fig. 12.1).

If we think about the needs of dogs and cats, perhaps we can see why personality influences someone's identification as a 'cat' or 'dog' person. Dogs are more sociable than cats and are dependent on their owner for regular walks and setting daily routines. Cats set their own routines and are not particularly sociable, though they can form an attachment to their owner. Their independent nature means they may well suit people who also wish greater freedom from routine. As Rudyard Kipling expressed in his book *Just So Stories*: 'The wildest of all the wild animals was the Cat. He walked by himself, and all places were alike to him.' If you do not recognize yourself in this picture of owner personality, do not worry. Remember, we all have each of the five personality traits to a greater or lesser degree, and the research results say something about the average cat or dog person, not something about you personally. Certainly, many cat owners are very sociable – as are many cats.

Personality, Attachment and Cat Ownership

Over the years there have been surveys to ascertain how many cats people keep, of what type and how they are kept. There are many different factors that influence these decisions, including our personality. A recent study of 3331 UK cat owners has looked at the relationships between owner personality and the lifestyle, behaviour and well-being of their cats (Finka *et al*., 2019). They found that owners scoring higher on neuroticism were more likely to own a non-pedigree breed and were less likely to give the cat free roaming access to the outside. These owners also seemed less satisfied with the cat, reporting more problem behaviours including anxiety, aggression and stress-related sickness behaviours, and their cat(s) being overweight. Conversely, owners scoring higher on agreeableness were more satisfied with their cats, and higher owner conscientiousness was associated with more relaxed and sociable cats. We know that our personality influences our behaviour which, in turn, influences the emotional state and behaviour of others with

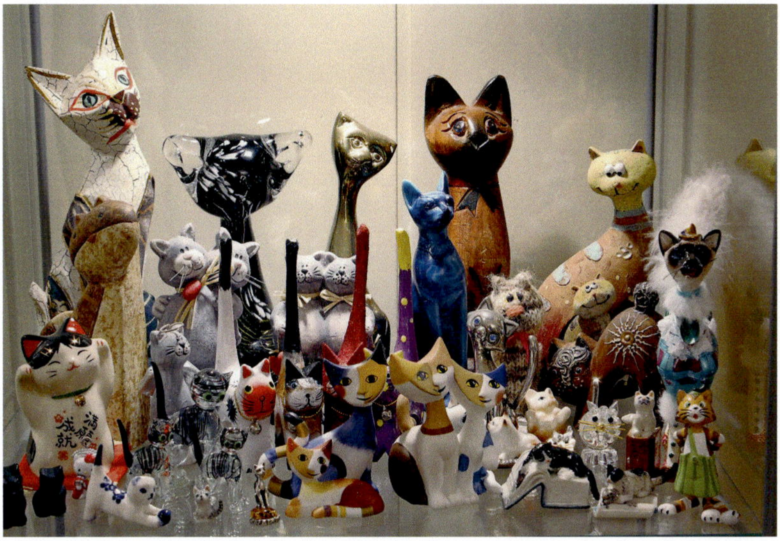

Fig. 12.1. A small selection of the numerous cat figures that cat owners often collect. (Photo: Audun Braastad, 2019)

whom we interact, and this study suggests this also applies to our cats.

The emotional relationship we have with our cats, our bond with them, is in part determined by our personality and by our attachment style. However, the bulk of research into the human–pet bond has considered attachment only in terms of how strongly attached people were to their pet. Psychologists who study human–human relationships consider this to be a blunt tool. Extensive research into how we bond and interact with our children, friends, family and romantic partners has shown that our attachment style is the thing to consider. As with personality, our adult attachment style is not an absolute, but each of us will be somewhere along the spectrum of having a secure or insecure style (Box 12.2).

Recently, and increasingly, scientists are investigating how our attachment style relates to our emotional relationship with our pets, how we care for and interact with them, the relationship our pet has with us, and the development of problem behaviours. Further, there is some evidence to suggest that it is both our personality and our attachment style that influences our pet preference, our identification as a cat or dog person (Link, 2021).

To date, most research on attachment style has focused on dog owners, for example that of Konok et al. (2015), whose findings suggest a link between those owners who score more highly on an insecure avoidant attachment style and the development of separation-related problems in their dog. This attachment style means owners are likely to be less responsive to the dog's needs, which may result in the dog developing an insecure attachment style. This is comparable to what is seen in parent–child relationships. Studies on the attachment style of cat owners or indeed the attachment style of adult cats are rare. Potter and Mills (2015) studied the attachment style of cats using a modification of a test known as the 'strange situation test'. They found, perhaps not surprisingly, that adult cats do not seem to form social bonds in the same way as dogs, and, unlike dogs, are 'not necessarily dependent on others to provide a sense of safety and security'. So links

---

Box 12.2. Human attachment styles

Our adult attachment style strongly reflects how we attached to others, especially our caregivers, when we were children. Our adult attachment style influences how we parent our children and thus influences their attachment style. In this way, attachment patterns are passed down from one generation to the next. As with children, our pets are dependent upon us to be aware of and respond appropriately to their needs, and how we do this is influenced by our attachment style and will have consequences for the animal in our care.

There are four adult attachment styles which differ in three important ways: closeness, avoidance, and anxiety. Closeness refers to how comfortable one feels being emotionally close and intimate with another. Avoidance relates to how comfortable we feel about depending on others or indeed having others depend on us. Anxiety relates to the extent to which we worry that our companion/partner will abandon and reject us.

Below are descriptions of each style in terms of how they differ in closeness, avoidance and anxiety.

Secure – low on avoidance, low on anxiety. Comfortable with intimacy; not worried about rejection or preoccupied with relationships. 'It is easy for me to get close to others, and I am comfortable depending on them and having them depend on me. I don't worry about being abandoned or about someone getting too close to me.'

Avoidant – high on avoidance, low on anxiety. Uncomfortable with closeness and primarily values independence and freedom. Not worried about partner's availability. 'I am uncomfortable being close to others. I find it difficult to trust and depend on others and prefer that others do not depend on me. It is very important that I feel independent and self-sufficient. My partner wants me to be more intimate than I am comfortable being.'

Anxious – low on avoidance, high on anxiety. Crave closeness and intimacy. Very insecure about relationships. 'I want to be extremely emotionally close (merge) with others, but others are reluctant to get as close as I would like. I often worry that my partner doesn't love or value me and will abandon me. My inordinate need for closeness scares people away.'

Anxious and avoidant – high on avoidance, high on anxiety. Uncomfortable with intimacy and worried about partner's commitment and love. 'I am uncomfortable getting close to others, and find it difficult to trust and depend on them. I worry I will be hurt if I get close to my partner.'

Adapted from Levy, T. (2017) Four styles of adult attachment (https://www.evergreenpsychotherapycenter.com/styles-adult-attachment/)

between owner attachment style and the type of problem behaviours seen in cats may be quite different to that seen in dogs.

The Changing Landscape of Cat Keeping

As we have seen, over the last 30 years, researchers have conducted surveys in various countries to understand more about who gets cats and how they are kept, as illustrated by a Norwegian survey undertaken by Bjarne and his student Silja Eriksen (see Box 12.3 and Table 12.1).

It is difficult to draw simple conclusions about the practices of cat owners as countries differ in both their culture and communities. Additionally, over time, communities change, for example due to an ageing population, and most countries have seen a dramatic rise in urbanization in recent years. More of us are now living in towns and cities, in apartments rather than in homes with gardens and easy access to green spaces. There are also cultural differences. For example, research shows that keeping a cat solely as an indoor pet is both more acceptable and more recommended in Canada and the USA than in other countries such as Norway and the UK. Likewise, there are differences in attitudes to the declawing of indoor cats. Whilst banned in New York in 2019, this is still practised in some other parts of the USA. It is illegal in the UK, Norway, Australia and many other countries where alternative methods are promoted to protect furniture and people from cats' claws, including training and generous provision of scratching posts (see Chapters 10 and 11). Reflecting the concerns about free-roaming cats being more likely to get lost, injured or stolen, 99% of respondents to a 2021 UK government consultation agreed that cats should be microchipped as a legal requirement of ownership, as it is in other places including Hawaii and Australia.

In some parts of the world, such as areas of Australia, one cannot keep a cat, or it must be taken out only on a leash or confined to the owner's property. It may be kept completely indoors, or only have access to a cat enclosure (catio) or garden from which it cannot escape. These laws aim to protect the cat, local wildlife and the local community.

As summarized in Table 11.2, a cat that is allowed to roam free is exposed to a range of risks,

---

Box 12.3. The cat's home environment in Norway

In 2014, Bjarne's student Silja Eriksen gathered data from a postal survey about the environment of 1212 cats in Norway. Where and how cats lived varied between breed groups and is shown in Table 12.1.

This survey found that, on average, there were 3.6 cats in a pedigree cat home and 2.2 in a domestic cat home. It is possible that the real figures are a bit lower since those who answered may have been more enthusiastic than the average cat owner. One in four cat households had a dog, usually only one. Other animals were also found in 23% of the cat households. Half of these had aquarium fish, and less often they had rabbits, small rodents or caged birds. Most cats had a litter tray, but one in five non-pedigree house cats did not. Please note that we have used the term non-pedigree here but they can also be called 'house cats' or 'domestic short-haired' cats.

The data about forest cats (Norwegian forest cat, Maine coon and Siberian) were separated as these were more likely to be given free access to the outdoors than other pedigree breeds and many aspects of their living environment generally seemed to be something between that of non-pedigree cats and the other breeds. The forest cats may be preferred by owners that want a more robust, longer-coated cat that can cope with the Norwegian winter weather. On farms, non-pedigree cats were the most frequently kept and they were generally more popular in rural districts than in the city, while it was the opposite for most pedigree cats. Cat owners typically lived in a house with a garden, but many owners of pedigree cats, apart from the forest cats, lived in apartment blocks. While 81% of the non-pedigree cats roamed outdoors, this applied to 42% of the forest cats and only 17% of the other breeds. Among these other breeds, Burmese and Sacred Birman were the ones most frequently allowed to roam outdoors. Rex, Persian, Oriental and Siamese cats rarely roamed outdoors. The pedigree cats, including the forest cats, were more likely to have access to an outside catio or only go out on a leash with the owner than was the case with the non-pedigree cats.

In the summer, non-pedigree cats were outdoors on average 11 hours per day, twice the time of the pedigree cats. In the winter, the non-pedigree cats were outdoors for only about three hours a day, but still five times more than the pedigree cats, which probably preferred the underfloor heating to the snowy winter terrain of Norway.

Table 12.1. Living conditions and environmental factors among non-pedigree cats, forest cat breeds (Norwegian forest cat, Maine coon and Siberian) and other pedigree breeds (N = 1212 cats). The figures are percentages within the breed groups. (Recalculated from the dataset of Eriksen, 2014.)

	Non-pedigree cats	Forest breeds	Other pedigree breeds
	N=701	N=173	N=338
Living in a city	26%	32%	49%
Living in a village	37%	41%	31%
Living in an apartment block	13%	13%	31%
Living in a free-standing house	38%	53%	36%
Living in a terraced house	18%	19%	12%
Living in rural areas	37%	27%	20%
Living on a farm	13%	7%	7%
Only indoors	7%	5%	15%
Allowed free-roaming outdoors	81%	42%	17%
In a large outdoor enclosure (>10 m^2)	0.4%	24%	12%
In a small outdoor area (≤10 m^2)	6%	17%	22%
Outdoors with the owner only	2%	3%	18%
Outdoors on leash with the owner	3%	9%	15%
Dogs in the household	25%	27%	22%
Indoor cat toilet	80%	93%	96%

be that injury in a cat fight, ingesting toxins, contracting disease, getting lost, being eaten by a larger predator, being run over by a car, or purposely injured, shot or poisoned by a person.

For wildlife, cats are a significant threat and have contributed to the decline of critically endangered species all over the world. It is estimated that cats are partly responsible for 8% of global mammal, bird and reptile extinctions that have already occurred (Trouwborst *et al.*, 2020). We may like to think this is restricted to feral, unowned cats and that our cat makes little difference. However, as we saw in Chapter 6, pet cats in both urban and suburban environments affect wildlife, and not just the unfortunate individual that is hunted and killed. The presence, even the scent of cats in the neighbourhood, can cause significant chronic stress to prey species which, in turn, reduces their health, welfare and ability to rear their young successfully. This can lead to the extinction of the local population of one or more species. In urban and suburban areas this 'local' effect will extend across the whole town or city, wherever there are free-ranging cats. This can have dramatic consequences for prey species, contributing to their decline and potentially their total extinction. Hence, there are legal requirements for cats to remain on the owner's property in parts of Australia where species vulnerable to cat predation are already endangered; that is, they are in a precarious position of survival. This is likely to become more common in other countries as the number of cats we keep increases. Such management is one way (Cecchetti *et al.*, 2022) that conservation efforts for maintaining global biodiversity can be helped, whilst still providing an excellent quality of life for the individual cat and its owner.

For the local community, a cat can be a serious neighbourhood nuisance if it bullies someone else's cat or is liable to be aggressive to people. Even friendly cats can soon make enemies by scratching people's cars and, most commonly, because of their habit of defecating in people's gardens, vegetable patches or children's sandpits. Exposure to cat faeces, or soil contaminated by it, can mean exposure to toxoplasmosis. This is a serious health risk for many pregnant women (or, rather, for the foetus they are carrying) as well as for children and those with weakened immune systems. Additionally, it is simply distressing and frustrating for someone to find their garden is repeatedly being used as the neighbour's cat's toilet. Whilst a child's sandpit can be covered every night and when it is not in use, it is also important that owners take responsible steps to manage their cats differently. When they decide not to do so, the situation can escalate into a serious neighbour dispute. It can mean that unpleasant methods are taken to deter and control the cats such as the installation of an electric cat fence, or worse.

A further issue with the keeping of cats concerns the serious problem of climate change. As calls intensify to reduce meat consumption, this could have an impact on attitudes to the keeping of carnivorous cats and dogs. Changes in meat production practices may also have an impact on cat-food formulation. As we saw in Chapter 6, cats, as obligate carnivores, are not well-adapted to the consumption of carbohydrates and increasing the dietary content of carbohydrates has been associated with increased predation of wildlife. It is therefore important to fully assess the impact of changes in food composition on cat behaviour and welfare.

Pets and Housing

As we will see in the next chapter, caring for a pet can mean a lot to people of all ages and be a positive contribution to their physical and mental health. However, there are various barriers to pet ownership in general that may mean a person cannot have a pet or at least not a cat or dog. These include time constraints, financial costs of food and upkeep, distance to veterinary care, and allergies. Additionally, not all of us live in accommodation where we are able to have a pet. Many housing providers have policies that simply say no pets or restrict the type and number of pets that can be owned. This is true for housing owned by private landlords, state or local authorities, housing associations and warden-assisted accommodation for older adults (care homes). Such restrictions cause great distress to individuals who have to choose between their pet or eviction. There are many cases of individuals having to give up their pets to keep the roof over their family. Rather than be parted from their animal companion, others choose to give up their home instead, even deciding to live on the street if they cannot find other affordable housing. Another group of concern are those wishing to escape domestic violence but remaining because they are unable to find safe shelter for themself and their pets. There are also older people who would benefit from living in sheltered accommodation or a nursing home but are unable to take their pet with them. So they may suffer alone as they struggle to look after themselves and their pet. A similar situation arises during wars and natural disasters, when people have refused to leave if that meant being separated from their pets.

It is understood that many landlords have had experience or are concerned about issues arising from pets, such as damage to property, or nuisance arising from noise or smells disturbing to other residents. On the other hand, current and potential owners consider that they have a right to own a pet and reap the benefits of a companion animal. In various countries, steps have been, and continue to be, taken to work alongside all stakeholders – housing providers, pet owners and communities – to find ways forward to facilitate the responsible keeping of pets (Fig. 12.2). The desired outcome is to encourage a Positive Pets attitude in housing providers and, ideally, Positive Pets in Housing legislation, as seen in countries including France, India and Norway, where Bjarne's expertise contributed to this pivotal change.

Pets and housing – Norway

The Norwegian Association of Cat Owners, formed by Bjarne in 1982, has had 40 years' experience of cat owners having problems with landlords. They handle many individual cases where they give advice to owners, contact the housing association or, if the case does not resolve, participate as a witness in court cases. Behind every case there are unhappy people who risk having to move, euthanize their cat or rehome it – and many have done so.

Few had the courage or funding to go to court until the owners of the Persian cat Emmeline decided to do so. Emmeline was an indoor cat who lived with her two owners in an apartment block in Oslo. The housing association had a total ban on animals. The couple knew about the ban when they moved in with Emmeline. All three had lived there for two years and no one had complained about the cat. Nevertheless, the board decided that the couple either had to move or get rid of Emmeline. The couple contacted the Norwegian Association of Cat Owners, which engaged a lawyer. The case came before the district court in Oslo, which confirmed that Emmeline should be allowed to stay since she was not a nuisance to anybody. However, the housing association did not agree with the court's decision and took it to the next highest authority – the Court of Appeal. Here it was decided that Emmeline had to be removed or the owners had to move out.

The couple did not agree. They appealed to the Norwegian Supreme Court. The renowned Supreme Court attorney, the late Tore Sverdrup Engelschiøn, was engaged on the cat owners' side and Bjarne was engaged as an expert witness. Judgement in the Supreme Court was issued in 1993, the famous

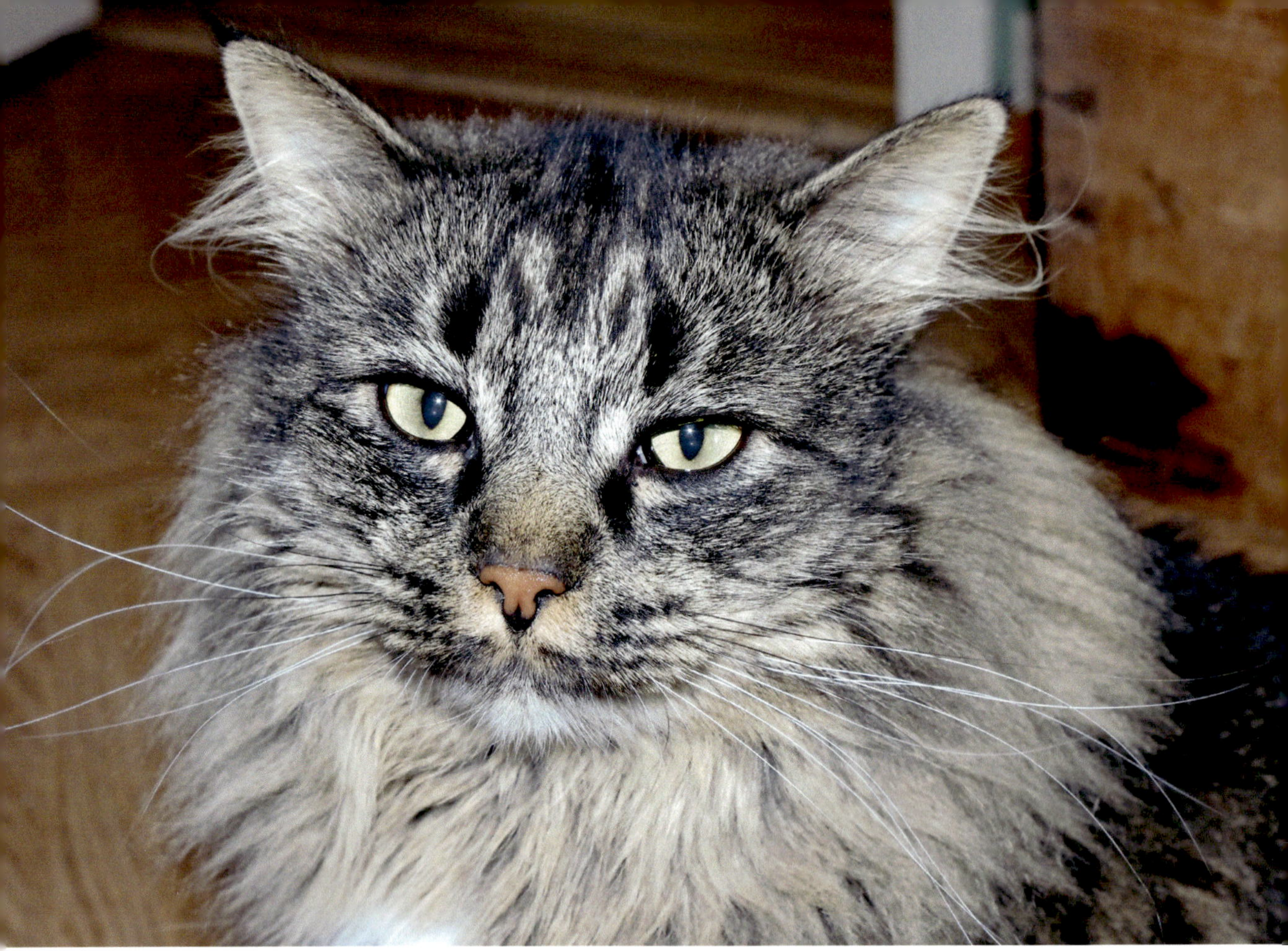

Fig. 12.2. Everyone should be allowed to keep a friendly cat like Snille if they can provide him with good care and responsible ownership. (Photo: Nina Dahl, 2019)

Emmeline judgment, in which the court ruled that Emmeline could stay. The Supreme Court stated that the housing co-operative did not have the authority to ban the keeping of an indoor cat unless there was documented evidence of the cat being a serious nuisance or causing some other disadvantage. It is worth noting that one of the neighbours, who shared the same entrance to the apartment block, was allergic to cats. However, because Emmeline was an indoor cat, this was not a problem for him, and thus not considered a disadvantage.

This was the prelude to the liberalization of the keeping of cats in Norwegian housing co-operatives. The Law on Housing Co-operatives, the Rent Act and the Ownership Section Act have been amended so that these now read: 'Even if the landlord (or the condominium) has established a ban on animal keeping, the tenant (or user of the section) can keep animals if good reasons speak for it, provided that the animal keeping is not to the detriment of the landlord or the other residents.' The Rent Act applies to all rented property and the Ownership Section Act applies to condominiums or jointly owned property. Despite the changes in the law, many landlords and housing co-operatives still have a ban and ask cat owners to apply for keeping a cat, even though such an application is not a legal requirement. This contrasts with the views of other countries, including the UK. The Norwegian law states that a person has the right to have animals in the apartment if they have good reason for keeping a pet. Nevertheless, it is unclear what is considered a good reason. If a person wants to have a cat to improve their quality of life, this should be a perfectly acceptable reason. Perhaps the legal text would have been better worded simply as 'The tenant can keep animals if the animal keeping is not to the detriment of the landlord or the other residents', to avoid the need for arguments over whether the reasons for having a pet are good enough. The Supreme Court did not allow Emmeline to stay because she was an indoor cat or because she was in single-cat household; rather, it discussed whether cat keeping was a nuisance to other residents. However, Emmeline was an indoor cat and the court judgement applied to an indoor cat. This has led to landlords, including housing co-operatives, tightening up the rules, and, where it was previously permitted to keep cats outdoors, some now only allow indoor cats or have rules to reduce the nuisance of having cats outdoors. These include the cat only being allowed out on a leash or in a catio. The Norwegian Association of Cat Owners has written a set of recommendations for owners (Box 12.4).

Pets and housing – UK

Likewise, in the UK, primarily led by the Society of Companion Animal Studies (SCAS), the last 40 years

---

Box 12.4. Norwegian Association of Cat Owners' recommendations for owners living in housing co-operatives.

The Norwegian Association of Cat Owners wrote these recommendations based on Norway's legislation, experience with the housing co-operatives and current legal practice in Norway:

1. A *general ban* on cats or dogs is not binding because the law allows animal keeping. It may be different if animal keeping is a nuisance to somebody, cf. below.

2. An order to *apply for keeping animals* does not need to be respected, since correct interpretation of the law means owners can keep an animal without any requirement for an application. However, one should inform the housing cooperative board that one keeps or intends to keep animals.

3. The law speaks of *animals without any limitations*, e.g. indoor cat, hunting dog or ferret. If the statutes of the housing cooperative try to limit the concept of animals in relation to the law, this is invalid. The housing cooperative cannot have a general ban on outdoor cats, or only allow cats that are on a leash outdoors. If this is stated as a house rule, this rule can be set aside because it is contrary to superior laws, namely the Law on Housing Cooperatives, the Rent Act, and the Ownership Section Act.

4. If animal keeping is to be limited, the *only valid requirement* is that the keeping of animals must not cause a nuisance to the landlord or residents. How should this be practised?

Firstly, *some animals are excluded* simply because keeping them always will be detrimental to others in an apartment (for example, a cow or a horse!).

Secondly, *not all types of disadvantages can be claimed*. For example, as was seen in the Emmeline judgment, allergy is not enough alone; there must be 'strong allergy reactions' due to the keeping of an animal. Disadvantages are stronger arguments than a mere nuisance. For example, should the keeper of an animal not keep the accommodation clean or not dispose of the waste properly, that can be disadvantageous for others through bad odours. Likewise, noise from frequent barking and continuous night-time courtship miaowing may represent a sufficient disadvantage. This must be discussed specifically in each case.

Thirdly, the disadvantage or nuisance must be *documented*. For ordinary cat and dog keeping, this cannot happen until the animal has lived in the apartment for a while. Only then can it be ascertained whether there is a specific disadvantage for someone due to the keeping of this individual cat or dog. Consequently, cat or dog keeping cannot normally be denied in advance of moving into the apartment and before any disadvantage is documented.

5. The law's condition that there must be *good reasons for keeping an animal* can be ignored because there will always be good reasons for having or acquiring a cat or dog. The law speaks of '*social considerations*' as sufficient. The law does not legitimate any requirement for submitting a medical certificate as the good reason to have an animal. The animal owner has the right to define his/her good reasons for having the animal.

6. No one can have their tenancy legally terminated or be thrown out of their apartment simply because one keeps animals there. *The animal must be a proven disadvantage* and not just a nuisance. The tenant can safely await the summons from the housing cooperative to go to court if the disadvantage is not established and proven.

have seen various conferences and groups of veterinary, behaviour and other experts working with stakeholders and government to improve the situation for pet owners. Anne has also had an interest in this area since the late 1980s. She co-founded, with Colette Kase – who had experienced being a homeless pet owner – a practical programme to help homeless owners with pets (HOPE). Following their involvement in a case of threatened tenant evictions, HOPE came to the attention of a national animal charity, Dogs Trust, who took up the programme in 1995, expanding it to become the Hope and Freedom Projects. These address the needs of homeless owners and those fleeing domestic abuse, respectively (see Further Reading). Anne and Colette then helped to convene a group of animal rescue charities and a major housing provider under the name Pathway. Pathway wanted to understand the current state of pet policies and, in 2003/4, sent out 1193 questionnaires to local authorities and housing associations across the UK, with 374 being returned. The results showed that there was little consistency in the types of policy. Thus, in 2007, Pathway, along with the Pets Advisory Committee, produced a comprehensive, freely available document to assist housing providers in developing positive guidelines on keeping pets in rented accommodation. This is currently being updated by SCAS. The 2007 document contained information about why pets are important to us and our health, case studies, information about key legislation, useful contacts, the needs of pets – so landlords could consider what would be appropriate in their accommodation (see Box 12.5) – and, importantly, guidelines for exemplar policy and model tenancy agreements to enable landlords to feel assured that tenants would be responsible for the pet's care and behaviour.

In January 2021, the UK government published guidance for landlords and a Model Tenancy Agreement. This actively encourages landlords to allow pets (Box 12.5) but is not a legal requirement. As in other countries, there is a growing demand for rented accommodation in the UK. This, alongside the recent dramatic COVID-19-related increase in pet ownership, has exacerbated the shortage of pet-friendly accommodation. This has now become a major reason for UK owners to relinquish their pets to a rescue centre or even abandon them.

Cats, COVID-19 and the Future

During the main COVID-19 pandemic, between the start of 2020 and the end of 2021, the numbers of pet cats have increased dramatically across the world. In the UK, pet cat numbers rose from 10.8 to 12 million and in China from 48.6 to 58 million. In Norway, the annual number of registered pedigree cats increased by 12% from 2019 to 2021. In the UK, the number of households that owned a pet had remained around 45% between 2011 and 2019, only to reach an unprecedented figure of 59% in 2020. This was a time when many countries had extended periods of lockdown, when people were restricted to their homes and only allowed to take short walks in their immediate neighbourhood; or, in some cases, not able to leave their home at all (Fig. 12.3). There have been many studies to see how this affected people, all showing that lockdown measures resulted in a general decline in the mental health of many of us. With increased feelings of loneliness, anxiety and depression, we craved companionship. Clearly, many millions of people considered that acquiring a cat, or other pet, to help them through this difficult time was a good idea. Of course, regardless of where a person lives, or the circumstances, they will only accrue the benefits of pet ownership if they choose the right sort of pet for their home and lifestyle, so that they can provide it with a good quality of life for the whole of its life.

Regrettably, that was not done in many cases, and people acquired a pet on impulse without considering how they would look after it once they returned to work or resumed their normal lifestyle post-lockdown. The outcome has been 'buyer's remorse' and a surge in pet homelessness – that is, animals that have been relinquished to rescue centres or simply abandoned. Many, if not most, abandoned pets die of parasite infections, illness, injury or starvation. They also pose a health risk to other pets and humans through disease transmission and are detrimental to wildlife. A recent survey conducted by Mars has investigated how dogs and cats have been affected. They gathered data from over 200 global and local sources, including rescue centres, and did other research on attitudes across nine countries: China, Germany, Greece, India, Mexico, Russia, South Africa, UK and USA. The researchers developed an index to measure the scale of cat and dog homelessness and identify the top factors regarding why these animals become or

Box 12.5. The UK housing guidelines.

In 2021, the UK government published guidelines that seek to deter landlords from having an outright blanket ban on allowing pets in their properties. The three main points advise that:

1. Whilst landlords are prohibited from charging a fee for keeping pets, they can require that the tenant pays a higher deposit, which can be returned when the tenant leaves, assuming the animal has not caused any damage.
   (As an aside, in a 2021 survey by the Society of Companion Animal Studies (SCAS), 40% of owners approved of pet deposits and 20% approved of landlords requiring owners to have insurance to cover any damage caused by the pet.)
2. Current or potential tenants must seek written consent from their landlord to keep an animal.
3. A landlord cannot unreasonably withhold or delay consent and should agree to such a request where they are satisfied that the tenant is a responsible pet owner *and* the property is suitable for the type (and number) of animals.

The Pathway (2007) document emphasized the need of landlords to consider the suitability for each property separately, as any particular property can responsibly accommodate a given number and size of animals. The number of animals matters because animals interact, and this needs space. Their size is relevant because every animal needs sufficient space to be able to lie comfortably in its own bed area. The document gave some guidelines for dogs and cats in respect of the size and type of accommodation. For this calculation, the floor area is calculated based on the living room(s), kitchen and utility room. Bedrooms, hallways and bathrooms are excluded.

The document goes on to say: 'The situation of a property is also relevant. In general, a property with an enclosed garden is capable of providing a more suitable environment for dogs or cats than a property with no garden. Equally, a flat in a high-rise block is less suitable for large dogs, who will find it difficult to access the property, particularly via the stairs.'

The guidance suggested is:

- If the property has a garden, add 10 m^2.
- If the property is above the fifth floor and dogs are to be allowed, deduct 10 m^2.
- The total number of animals allowed is 1 kg per square metre of living space as defined above, or one animal per 15 m^2, whichever is less.

Example calculation:
Living room	4.5 m x 4.8 m = 21.6 m^2
Kitchen	3.0 m x 3.6 m = 10.8 m^2
Utility room	3.0 m x 1.8 m = 5.4 m^2
Garden add	10 m^2
Total	47.8 m^2

The property would therefore be able to support 47.8/15 = 3 animals or 47.8 kg of animal. This would equate to two medium-sized dogs or three cats. A similar low-rise flat without a garden would support one larger dog or two cats and a high-rise flat, two cats or one smaller dog.

---

remain homeless. At the time of publication, in December 2021, the estimates were of 20 million cats and dogs in shelters, 91 million street or stray dogs and 113 million street or stray cats (www.endpethomelessness.com). These numbers only relate to the nine countries surveyed. Mars is interested to hear from other countries to expand the data collected. Clearly, pet homelessness is a massive global One Welfare issue that affects individual animals, humans and biodiversity.

We can all do our part to help improve this situation. Loving cats and being a responsible owner is clearly part of this. If we, or people we know, are considering getting a cat, we may look to rescue centres and give a young or older cat a home, rather than buying a 'purpose-bred' kitten from a breeder or pet shop. We can also use the information from this book to help inform others about what a cat needs and where to get one – perhaps you may feel able to give a talk to a local school or community group or provide information about sources of advice, such as major cat charities. You may also find posters that are free to download, such as Lili Chin's 'What a Cat Needs'.

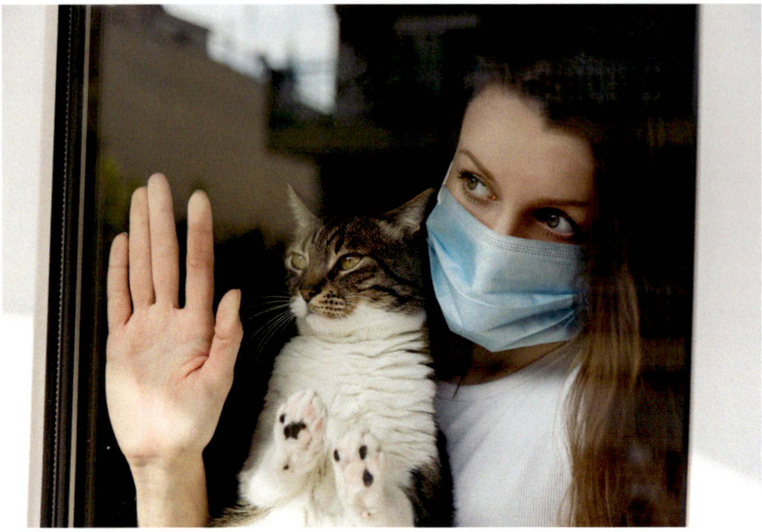

Fig. 12.3. Owner and cat in COVID-19 lockdown. (Photo: Depositphotos_326675054_XL)

Further Reading

Cecchetti, M., Crowley, S.L., Wilson-Aggarwal, J., Nelli, L. and McDonald, R.A. (2022) Spatial behavior of domestic cats and the effects of outdoor access restrictions and interventions to reduce predation of wildlife. *Conservation Science and Practice* 4(2), e597. DOI: 10.1111/csp2.597.

Chin, L. (2022) Cats need.... Available at: https://www.doggiedrawings.net/freeposters (accessed 17 July 2022).

Dogs Trust Hope and Freedom Projects. Available at: https://www.dogstrust.org.uk/help-advice/hope-project-freedom-project (accessed 22 May 2022).

Eriksen, S.C.B. (2014) Atferdsegenskaper hos rasekatter i Norge. MSc thesis, Norwegian University of Life Sciences, Ås, Norway. Available at: http://hdl.handle.net/11250/277460 (accessed 30 April 2022). [In Norwegian]

Finka, L.R., Ward, J., Farnworth, M.J. and Mills, D.S. (2019) Owner personality and the wellbeing of their cats share parallels with the parent–child relationship. *PLOS ONE* 14(2), e0211862. DOI: 10.1371/journal.pone.0211862.

Konok, V., Kosztolányi, A., Rainer, W., Mutschler, B., Halsband, U. and Miklósi, Á. (2015) Influence of owners' attachment style and personality on their dogs' (*Canis familiaris*) separation-related disorder. *PLOS ONE* 10(2), e0118375.

Link, J. (2021) People-pleasing animals: mediating factors in attachment style difference between dog people and cat people. MSc thesis, State University of New York.

Mars (2021) How data can help us end pet homelessness. Available at: https://www.mars.com/news-and-stories/articles/ending-pet-homelessness (accessed 22 May 2022).

Potter, A. and Mills, D.S. (2015) Domestic cats (*Felis silvestris catus*) do not show signs of secure attachment to their owners. *PLOS ONE* 10(9), e0135109.

Rantanen, J., Metsäpelto, R.L., Feldt, T., Pulkkinen, L.E.A. and Kokko, K. (2007) Long-term stability in the Big Five personality traits in adulthood. *Scandinavian Journal of Psychology* 48(6), 511–518.

Trouwborst, A., McCormack, P.C. and Martínez Camacho, E. (2020) Domestic cats and their impacts on biodiversity: a blind spot in the application of nature conservation law. *People and Nature* 2, 235–250.

Supplementary materials entitled 'Relationship with humans' and 'Keeping cats in housing co-operatives' can be accessed at: www.cabi.org/the-cat-behaviour-and-welfare/

13 The Cat's Contribution to Human Health

The famous English nurse Florence Nightingale (1820–1910) wrote, in 1859: 'The small pet is often an excellent companion for the sick, for long chronic cases especially'. She observed how the patients lit up when a cat walked past and maybe jumped up on their bed. In 1944, the sociologist James Bossard published an article in the journal *Mental Hygiene* where he discussed the important role that pet animals can play in the mental health of families and for child development. He suggested that an animal can give unconditional love and '…be somebody you can show your love for – it is a relationship that is unconditional, forgiving and far less complex than those we have with people'. Twenty years later, in the same journal, the psychologist Boris Levinson summed this up:

> A pet is an island of sanity in what appears to be an insane world. Friendship retains its traditional values and securities in one's relationship with one's pet. Whether a dog, cat, bird, fish, turtle, or what have you, one can rely upon the fact that one's pet will always remain a faithful, intimate, non-competitive friend – regardless of the good or ill fortune life brings us.

Levinson's work is regarded as the trigger that inspired scientists to research the significance of contact with companion animals for our physical and mental health. This knowledge helps us understand how best to facilitate good health for all – those who are 'cat people' or 'cat-and-dog people' and maybe also those who identify as neither. People may be cat owners or be unable to own a cat but still wish to benefit from interacting with them, for example by visiting a cat-café. Others can also benefit where a friendly, well socialized cat is used as part of a therapy programme or as an environmental enrichment for those who are temporarily or permanently living in institutions, such as hospitals, care homes or prisons.

Research on the Health Effects of Pets

Since the 1970s, there have been thousands of papers published about animals' effects on our health, based on research and the practical experience of therapists, teachers and others. In this chapter we consider some of the more important points and their implications. Good health is not just the absence of diseases. According to the World Health Organization (WHO), health includes physical, emotional, social and spiritual aspects of life. Regardless of our health status, interactions with companion animals can enhance our quality of life. This can be particularly so for those who suffer from a chronic illness or disorder, whether they live in their own home or in an institution.

Physically, mentally and socially, pets can help us to function better in our day-to-day lives. This seems to be the case regardless of species, but most research has looked at dogs, cats and horses. Mammals have the advantage that they are good to stroke and cuddle. Some of the information gleaned about how cats can contribute to health was described in 1984 by David Greene in his book *Incredible Cats*. If you are really interested in this area, the most important recent book on this topic is that edited by Aubrey H. Fine (2019).

It should be said that the research evidence is not always clear and can appear contradictory. This may reflect methodological issues as well as real differences in the effects on people – what may be good for one person may not be helpful or even detrimental for another. Likewise, medicines do not always work for all people. One of the challenges for further research is to clarify when and how animals benefit our health, and when and why they do not.

Given what we know already from this book, we can suggest some factors that would be influential. The cat would need to be friendly and predictable and meet the person's expectations. This is especially true if the person is the owner, as cats showing problematic behaviour are likely to increase the owner's stress. Other factors will include the person's attitudes, personality, attachment style, and external factors such as socioeconomic status.

In 1998, Glyn Collis and June McNicholas presented a model with three possible mechanisms to explain the reported link between interactions with animals and our health (Fig. 13.1). The first is that the interaction has a direct effect on our health, and the second that interacting with animals has an indirect effect on our health by facilitating our person-to-person interactions and relationships. These two effects can apply to both pet owners and non-owners who may interact with animals belonging to friends, or in animal-assisted activities or therapy. The third explanation relates only to owners and suggests that other factors influence both pet ownership and health, but that pet ownership itself is not a cause of better health. That is, it may be that people who are generally healthier are those who acquire pets. Their better health may be due to their lifestyle, better nutrition, socioeconomic status, education, or their social community networks – their social support. This model is helpful when considering explanations for research findings.

As we shall see in this chapter, our physical and psychological health is closely linked to social factors. Known as the biopsychosocial model of health, the three interconnected factors are our biology (our individual genetic make-up and any physical trauma or infection one may have suffered), psychological factors (e.g. our personality) and social influences such as our socioeconomic status, and our social support network of friends and family, including good relationships with our pets.

Cats and Our Physical Health

Cats certainly can be good for our physical health, as we shall see. However, this is not so if one is allergic to them or catches a disease from them. Diseases transmitted from animals to humans are called *zoonoses*.

Cats, allergies and zoonoses

It is well known that interacting with dogs and cats can cause allergic reactions. The number of children that develop asthma and allergies has been increasing worldwide over the last few decades. This is, in part, related to an individual's genetic predisposition, as in being allergic to some foods such as shellfish, peanuts or wheat, and to an increase in environmental allergens such as air pollution.

It was thought that cats and dogs were responsible for a lot of allergic reactions, and it is true that some people are allergic to dander in their fur, or bites from their fleas. However, research in several countries shows that children who grow up close to animals

Direct effects

Interaction with animals – may be physical or simply observational → Health benefits for **Owners and Non-Owners**, e.g. oxytocin release; increased activity – through stroking, playing with or walking animal; smiling and laughter decrease stress hormones, aids muscle relaxation and circulation

Indirect effects

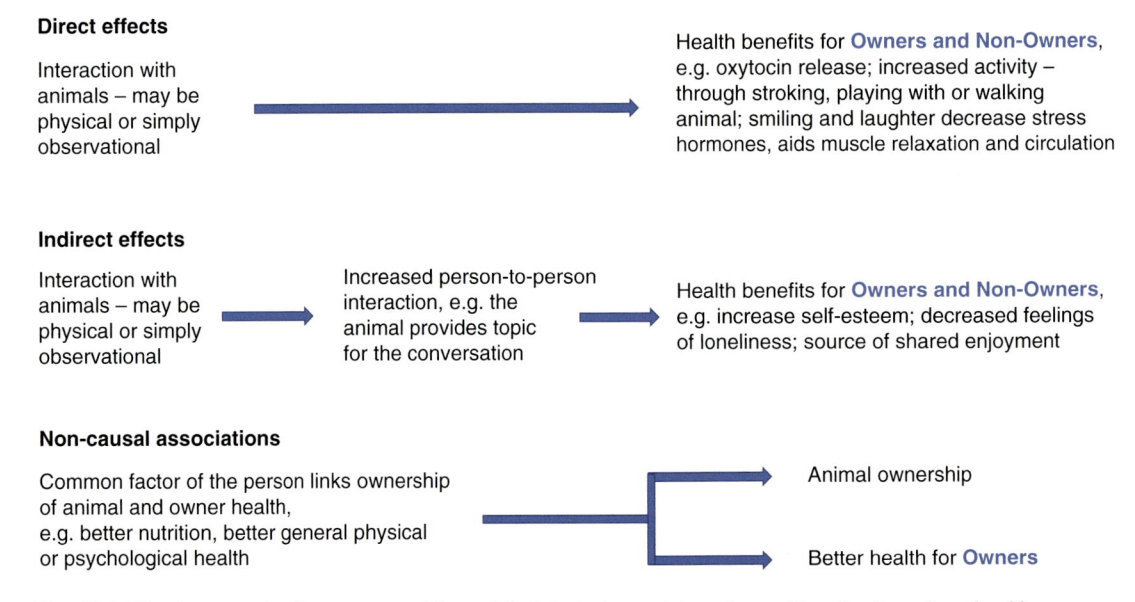

Interaction with animals – may be physical or simply observational → Increased person-to-person interaction, e.g. the animal provides topic for the conversation → Health benefits for **Owners and Non-Owners**, e.g. increase self-esteem; decreased feelings of loneliness; source of shared enjoyment

Non-causal associations

Common factor of the person links ownership of animal and owner health, e.g. better nutrition, better general physical or psychological health → Animal ownership / Better health for **Owners**

Fig. 13.1. The three mechanisms proposed to explain links between interactions with animals and our health. (Adapted from McNicholas *et al.*, 2005)

have a lower incidence of asthma and allergies – they have a stronger immune system. Moreover, this effect is enhanced the more contact children have with animals and animals of different species. This is the same reason why encouraging children to be outside playing in gardens, being out and about in woodland, meadows or parks, can also be beneficial to their immune and respiratory systems. The immune system becomes stronger when we are exposed to a multitude of bacteria and other microbiological challenges when young. If we keep our homes chemically clean, many children will not be able to develop resistance and will suffer intolerances and allergic reactions for the rest of their lives.

In respect of zoonoses, cats can carry diseases that affect people. These include rabies and toxoplasmosis. If you live in a country where there is rabies, then there is a serious risk that a cat with free-roaming outdoor access will come across wildlife that carry the virus. Likewise, free-roaming cats can catch and transmit plague to people if they are hunting rodents that are infected or carry fleas that are. Ensuring your cat has regular preventive worm and flea medication and is up-to-date with its vaccinations is essential for the health of the cat, you and other cats and people.

It has also been shown that we can transmit COVID-19 to our cats. If we are infected with COVID-19, we should be washing our hands before and after stroking our cats (or dogs) so we do not accidentally leave the virus on our hands or on their fur.

Cats and positive effects on physical health

Erika Friedmann is one of the founders of research on the positive effects of animals on human physical health. She and her colleague, Sue Thomas, showed, in 1980, that the chances of surviving a heart attack or severe angina pectoris are better if you have a cat or dog to pet. While 28% of patients without pets died within one year, only 5.7% of those who had animals died in the same period. This could be a direct consequence of the interaction with the pet or because those who had pets might have a healthier lifestyle in general or were of a calmer personality type. So, in 1995 a further, larger study was conducted, in which several physiological measures were made, and the lifestyle carefully analysed. It showed that two factors independently increased the chance of surviving myocardial infarction with subsequent irregular heartbeat: (i) pet keeping; and (ii) social support from other people. Therefore, those who lack a good social network are probably the ones who benefit most from their cat to stay healthy. But this does not seem to be the whole explanation.

Further studies have shown that blood pressure and the heart rate both decrease when a person cuddles a friendly animal, to a level otherwise only reached after several weeks of relaxation exercises. Dogs and cats are experts in both giving and receiving touches – by touching and licking us, gently sighing and purring. In many parts of the world there is far too little physical contact between people; for many men this is mostly limited to sexual situations or when their team scores a goal in football. Pets help many to meet this important biological need for touch.

In Australia, Anderson and colleagues surveyed 5700 healthy people and showed that men with pets had lower levels of cholesterol and triglycerides (fat) in their blood than men without pets. Both men and women had lower blood pressure if they had pets, but for women this was statistically significant only when they had passed 40 years of age. These differences could not be explained by smoking, exercise habits, bodyweight or socioeconomic status. There was no difference between dog owners and cat owners in this study, although the dog owners exercised more. A separate study of older people also showed that pet owners had lower fat levels in their blood. These results indicate that keeping a companion animal reduces these risk factors for cardiovascular disease. Overall, the research suggests that pet owners have a greater chance of avoiding heart attacks, and a greater chance of survival should they suffer one.

Recent studies have uncovered a likely mechanism for these results. There is a release of the hormone oxytocin when we stroke a friendly animal (Fig. 13.2). Oxytocin has long been associated with mammalian maternal behaviour, but both males and females have this hormone. It is involved in the reduction of blood pressure and cortisol and thus is an essential part of the body's system that protects us from the devastating physical and psychological consequences of stress, particularly chronic stress. Oxytocin is released by various stimuli, warmth, touch, eating, and probably when other senses are stimulated, as when we hear pleasant sounds such as birdsong or calming music, or we are in a room with 'relaxing' coloured walls and lighting. Indeed,

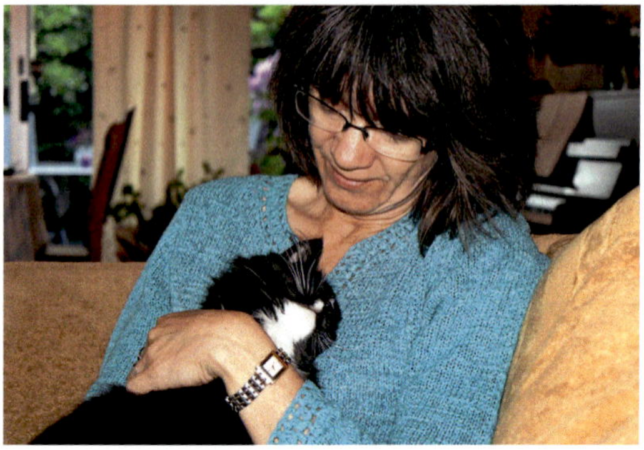

Fig. 13.2. Cuddling with a cat is good for your heart. (Photo: Bjarne O. Braastad, 2012)

oxytocin may be released when we look at something aesthetically pleasing, such as our cat playing or sleeping. Even purely psychological stimuli, as in a smile or kind word from a friend or stranger, may cause the release of oxytocin.

Studies, such as those of Curry and colleagues in 2015, suggest that our previous experience of cat ownership influences the release of oxytocin, whether we are interacting with our own or an unfamiliar cat. It appears that we benefit regardless, but we may benefit more when we have established a relationship, an attachment with the cat, whether we own it or not. In 2021, Johnson and colleagues conducted an experiment with 30 female cat owners and their cats, in the cat's own home. The findings suggest that how the owner interacts with the cat and how the cat interacts with its owners influences the release of oxytocin. For example, they found that oxytocin release was associated with cat-initiated contact, that is when the cat chose to interact, but not when the human initiated the contact. Oxytocin was also associated with specific behaviours including stroking, hugging and kissing, but not with the owners talking to the cat in a gentle or 'baby' voice, or with the cat's purring. So it seems that the benefits we can accrue from oxytocin release are affected by the quality of the relationship between the animal and the human.

James Serpell, of the University of Pennsylvania, received a research award for his work on the effects that companion animals have on minor human health problems. He examined the health of pet owners in England before they acquired the animal, and one, six and ten months afterwards, and compared them to a group of non-owners. Within a month of getting the pet, both cat and dog owners showed a significant reduction in minor ailments, including headaches, colds, insomnia, nervousness, fatigue and digestive problems. For dog owners, this effect was still highly significant after six months and still present at ten months when the study ended. The effect was not so long-lasting for cat owners. The improved health recorded at the first month did persist over the six months but had reduced to the pre-cat levels by ten months. One possible explanation is that dog owners may exercise more, as the dog needs walking, and walking the dog can also improve social connections and thus perceived social support. These benefits may not have occurred for the cat owners, who may take even less exercise, preferring to spend the time at home with their cat. Of course, there are other factors that can impact the effect pets have on our health.

Overall, the research in this area shows that owning a pet or interacting with a friendly animal is not the same for everyone. Different types of pets can affect different types of people in different ways. What is good for many people may well be irrelevant or even harmful to others.

Cats and Our Mental Health

Humans are a highly social species, and our social networks are important for our mental health, especially those of friends and family – those who provide us with friendship and love. These are the ones who care for us simply because of who we are, and thereby enhance our self-esteem and ability to withstand the inevitable stresses of being human. Loneliness is a major risk factor for poor mental health and poor physical health, and thus earlier mortality. The positive effects of pets can help combat loneliness and depression. They can promote conversation and the making of friendships, thereby increasing the owner's motivation for activities where the animal can be involved. This, then, helps the person feel more able to take decisions and initiatives for their well-being.

Studies as far back as that of Messent, in 1983, have shown that people walking a dog receive more eye contact, smiles and casual conversation than when they walk without the dog. Since 2004, there has been an increased use of social media as a way of gaining and maintaining new contacts with other people, and this has been particularly so in the last ten years as the generation that has grown up with this media reaches adulthood. It may be that this means that cat owners are able to benefit more from increased social connections based around their cat, and general interest in cats, than was suggested by earlier research. Regardless of our human support network, our pets provide physical companionship in our daily lives. For many, this is the most important aspect of pet keeping. To acknowledge this important role that they play for us, 'companion animal' is the increasingly favoured term, as opposed to pet or pet animal.

Various researchers have shown that pets provide a source of social support, but this is not a replacement for human companions. For example, the work of Reinhard Bergler of the University of Bonn with cat owners and the study of Parminder Raina and co-workers on senior community living in Canada both show that having a companion animal is particularly beneficial in stressful life situations. These are situations such as when romantic partners argue, when someone close dies, or when one is ill, work-stressed or otherwise depressed. They provide us with emotional support – after all, they do not berate us about what we ought to do or should have done. Having said that, talking to one's pet can help a person work out what to do, just as when we verbalize our problem to a close friend or counsellor.

Often, it is the many daily small problems that, over time, give rise to chronic stress and psychosomatic diseases, that is diseases that develop for psychological reasons. Here, too, the pet owners come out best. Dog owners are better at coping with stress than people without animals. Careful studies have shown that dogs can be considered as 'medication' both to prevent and alleviate everyday stress situations. The same goes for cats.

This suggests that pets may be particularly important for people whose social support system may have diminished or is not close by, such as the homeless who report how their pet has helped them avoid suicide and reduce drug and alcohol abuse (Scanlon et al., 2021). Another major, and growing, population of concern is the elderly. The elderly are particularly vulnerable to loneliness and reduced social support, namely having fewer people to turn to. They may live on their own and be unable to get out and about as easily as they once did. Their friends and partners may have died, and their children and grandchildren may live far away or have busy lives. Several studies in different countries have pointed out the importance of companion animals for the elderly.

As one gets older, the relationship with the cat often becomes ever stronger. These owners are generally more satisfied with their life situation and have better general health than elderly people without animals. Elders with pets also seem to cope more easily with psychological stress, show fewer depressive symptoms and have fewer doctor visits, even when stressed. However, such effects are not found in all studies. For example, Garrity and colleagues interviewed 1232 elderly people over 65. They found that among those who were stressed or had other serious disorders, there was a connection between stronger attachment to their animal and lower levels of depression. For healthy elderly people there was no such connection. Further research is needed to clarify under which conditions keeping of companion animals has positive health and mental effects for the elderly.

Making the link back to the physical health section above, we can revisit Friedmann and Thomas' larger (1995) study. This considered whether it is pet keeping itself that improves the health of pet-owning cardiac patients, or whether it is that people with greater resistance to diseases have a greater tendency to acquire pets. Hence, they considered psychosocial factors that buffer us against illness, including social support. They found that the higher the psychosocial status of the pet owners, the stronger their attachment to the pet. The greater the fondness for the pet, the more social support the owners experienced from family members and other people. In line with other research, it appears the companion animal was more of an extra social support than a substitute for social relationships with humans. The authors suggested that pet owners may more easily perceive the social support they receive from people than those who do not have pets. The study also revealed that the more time the owners spent with the pet, the less anxiety they had. Owners who spent more time with the animal demonstrated a less hurried pace and were less competitive than those who spent less time with the animal. All these findings likely reflect individual differences, possibly in personality and attachment style. There is much more to learn. However, spending time with your cat and relaxing from the hustle and bustle of everyday life is good advice (Fig. 13.3).

It is not just adults who benefit from interaction with cats; children, too, can benefit from having a pet cat in the family.

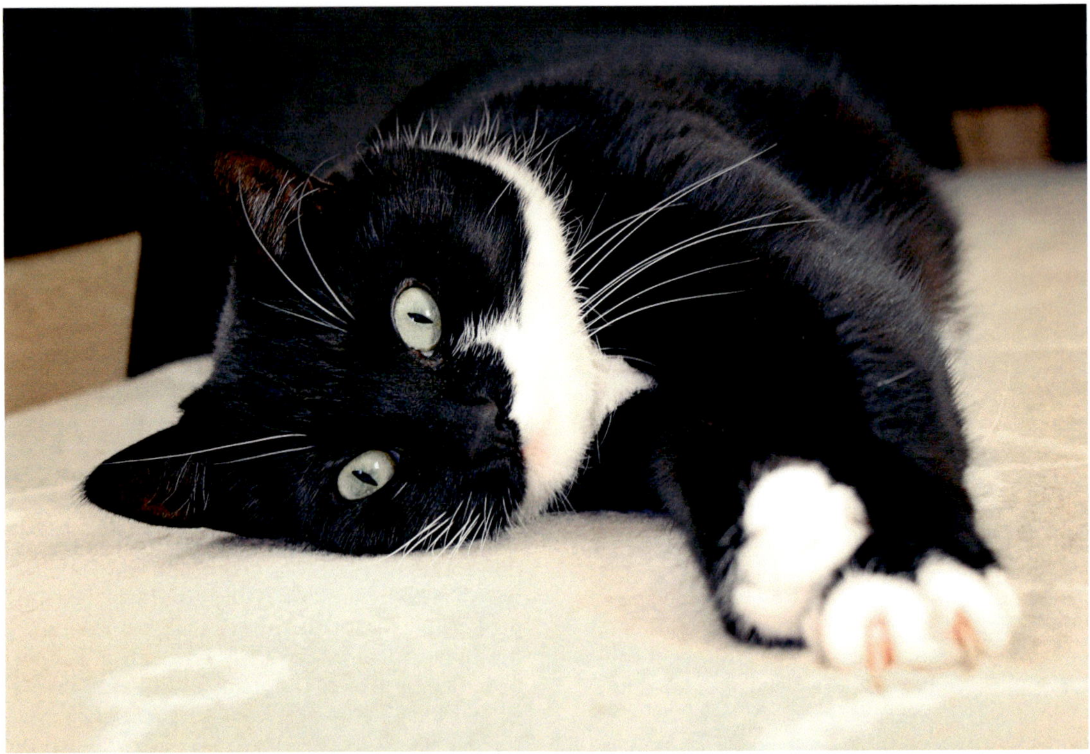

Fig. 13.3. A relaxed cat that thrives with you is beneficial to your mental health. (Photo: Christin Klös, 2019)

Pet Cats May Positively Affect Children's Development

Extensive studies in child psychology suggest that pets can act as good companions for children and can help their development. Children are attracted to animals and by the age of six months will smile, hold, 'chat' with and follow their pets with their eyes, and bodies as soon as they start to crawl. Only 45–50% of children aged 3–5 believe that animals can communicate, but they miss the pet if it dies. At age 6–9, children can have developed a strong emotional bond with the animal, and 10–13-year-old children understand more of their pet's mental abilities and have good general knowledge about its management, likes and dislikes. Adolescence begins around 13 years of age, and adolescents are mentally of an age to develop an ethical awareness of animal welfare and expand their knowledge about the ecological needs of animals.

There is evidence that suggests that children with pets are more popular with schoolmates and are more socially adept and empathic than those without pets at home. Interaction with pets may help the child develop a better ability to interpret non-verbal communication signals and emotions in humans, i.e. body language and facial expressions. These skills are enhanced by learning about the animal's communication – if the child misinterprets the cat slashing its tail, then he can get a lesson he will remember for a long time. Lessons from the animal, as in walking away when it does not want to play, or reprimanding the child for being too persistent, can help the child learn tolerance and self-control. Parents also need to guide the child so they do not get frustrated but are taught how to interact appropriately with the pet. So the cat does not ever need to get to the point of lashing out.

Animals can give children the experience of caring. Again, this does not happen without parental guidance, for example giving the child simple animal-care tasks that they can master according to their age, and overseeing that these are done. For a young child, this may be helping prepare the cat's meal and filling the water bowl. For older children it may involve grooming the cat and being responsible for ensuring the litter tray is clean. All of the above, plus the cat's companionship, can enhance a child's self-image (Fig.13.4).

Of course, there are individual differences, and simply having a cat or other pet in the home does not automatically mean the child will be interested in it or benefit from it. Likewise, not having a pet does not mean that the child is deprived. In 2017, Miles and colleagues surveyed 5191 Californian households with children. 2236 had a cat or dog that was allowed in the house and 2995 had neither. This study set out to investigate the true 'pet effect' by taking into consideration potential confounding factors. These included, but were not limited to, measures of socioeconomic status, how many hours the parents worked and if the child was limited in ability to do age-appropriate tasks. Analysing the data before accounting for these factors showed that children with pets were significantly different in terms of better general health, being more active, and their parents being less concerned about the child's mood, behaviour and learning ability. However, once the possible confounding variables were considered in the analysis, the differences between the two groups of children were much smaller and no longer significant. Pets are not magic, they can add to our children's lives, but they are not a substitute for parental guidance, good nutrition, education, friends or exercise.

However, the relationship a child has with a pet can be an indicator of the child's well-being. For example, a child may show an unusually intense relationship with a pet to the extent that they constantly want to play with the cat rather than with their friends. This may indicate the child is being bullied or is otherwise worried about something.

Sadly, another reason for this type of behaviour may be that the child is worried for the pet's safety. It is not uncommon in situations of family abuse that the pet is targeted as a way of controlling the partner and children (see Freedom Project, Chapter 12). Indeed, it is well recognized that there is a strong likelihood that where a pet is being abused, so are the children in the family, and *vice versa*. In the UK, there is an organization called the Links Group (thelinksgroup.org.uk) whose mission is to raise awareness of the link between people and animal abuse through support, training and interagency working – between veterinary professionals, animal rescue, and human social and health services.

Should a child have to leave the family home for any reason to go into care, a foster home or long-term medical care, they are likely also leaving their pet. The pet may have been a very close companion, their friend. This loss, the associated grief, and concern for the pet can be very distressing. It is important that this is recognized and that the child is supported. Of course, this also applies to adults who have had to leave pets behind, be that because of ill-health, abuse, going to prison, escaping from a fire, flood or other disaster, or fleeing a situation of war.

For people suffering trauma or other aspect of poor mental health, therapeutic options may include animals.

Animal-assisted Therapy

Animals can be used as an assistance in many forms of therapy. We distinguish between the animal triggering a positive emotional response in humans (recreation, entertainment), and the animal providing a therapeutic effect. Therapy can be defined as a process involving a particular relationship between a person seeking help to solve a physical or mental problem and a person who is trained to provide such assistance. Therefore, a distinction is made between *animal-assisted therapy* (AAT) and *animal-assisted activities* (AAA).

AAT involves a systematic use of the animal to help the patient reach a particular goal in their therapy or treatment. So it is designed to have a relatively predictable and measurable effect. It is a targeted intervention where an animal that meets certain criteria is an integral part of a treatment programme, and the process is documented and evaluated. Such treatment is chiefly provided to people with physical, neuromotor, and mental conditions. In some cases, the animal will be part of the triad comprising patient, therapist and animal. In other situations, there may be an additional person who has responsibility for the animal, enabling the therapist to focus fully on the patient. AAT is used by a range of health professionals including psychologists, psychiatrists, nurses, occupational therapists and physiotherapists.

In contrast, AAA is much more flexible and has no specific goals other than helping people relax and get that rush of oxytocin. It is used with both those in good health and those currently suffering ill-health. AAA is used in many different contexts, including schools, hospitals, care and nursing homes, and prisons. The animal handler may be a specially trained professional or a volunteer layperson.

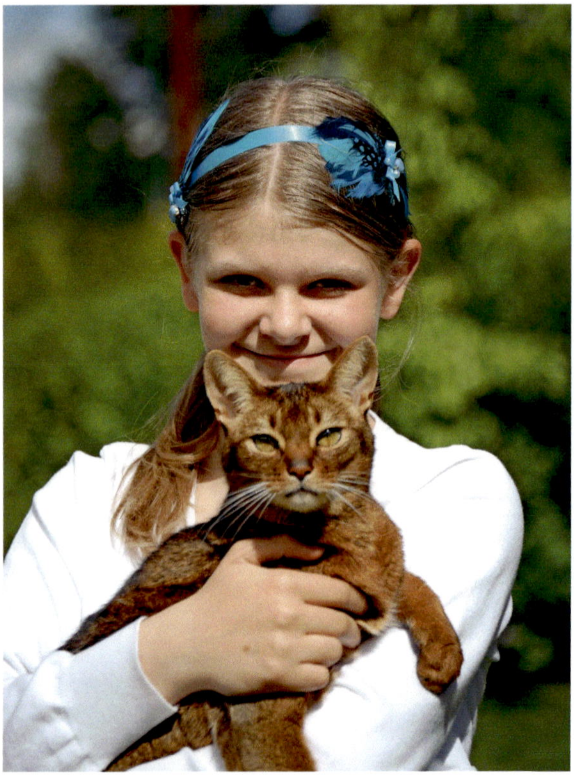

Fig. 13.4. A girl proudly shows her cat. (Photo: Gry Løberg, 2019)

These activities can have positive health effects, as well as generally improving the recipient's quality of life.

In many countries, AAA schemes have been introduced where volunteers can bring a dog to visit in a hospital or nursing home. Likewise, some schools will keep animals or bring a dog into class to give children a more relaxed atmosphere in which to read aloud. More recently, some universities are setting up opportunities for students to interact with animals when they are stressed, such as when first leaving home to attend university, and during exam periods. Several studies show that people appreciate such activities. Their mood is temporarily lifted; they have a pleasant experience that can help promote conversation with others and feel more relaxed when they remember it later. Box 13.1 describes the benefits and concerns relating to animals in nursing (care) homes for the elderly.

There can be overlap between AAA and AAT, and therefore it is now more common to use the collective term *Animal-assisted Interventions* (AAI).

Animal-assisted Interventions – responsible implementation

One group of working animals, usually dogs, that provide both AAA and AAT to the person are known as *assistance animals*. They assist a person who has deafness or blindness, or uses a wheelchair, with aspects of daily life. More recently, dogs are being partnered with people who have psychological needs such as autism or post-traumatic stress disorder. In assistance animal roles, the animal must be selected carefully for temperament and undergo substantial training, ideally by professional trainers using reward-based methods. This is to ensure not only that they perform in a manner that is safe for the person, but also that they are fully prepared to be able to cope with the role and do not suffer in so doing. Likewise, the recipients of these dogs must be educated in all aspects of the animal's care and handling.

As Fine *et al.* (2019) clarify in their excellent handbook, whether animals are to be used for AAI

> **Box 13.1.** Cats as therapists in nursing homes.
>
> Elderly people who move from their home to an institution easily develop what is called the translocation syndrome. This consists of depression, loneliness and low morale. If a caged bird is given to an elderly person who just moved into a nursing home, they show less depression. Earlier, it was most common for the home to keep aquarium fish and caged birds; nowadays, many have a resident cat or dog.
>
> Several studies report on the benefits and disadvantages of introducing companion animals into nursing homes. One study was that of Ida Myren (2010) who examined attitudes to and experience of having animals at nursing homes in Norway, by sending questionnaires to the senior staff. Among the 282 nursing homes, 80 of them had animals. This accounted for 28% of the nursing homes in which 44% (35) had a cat and 23% (18) had a resident dog. Many others had visiting dogs. Fourteen of them used a cat actively as a therapeutic animal, not just as an environmental enrichment. The cat was usually owned by the home and was present on the ward or in the common living-room area.
>
> Among those in charge of the nursing home, more than two-thirds believed that the animals contributed to a better social environment, better mood and quality of life, and better health among the residents. This is important for the challenges in nursing homes, as a large proportion of the residents have depressive disorders, cognitive problems or dementia, where language functions may be reduced and there are issues with distress, and verbal and physical aggression may be exhibited by some residents. The survey also showed that animals in nursing homes may improve the well-being of the employees. The work environment becomes more homely, and when the residents thrive better, the job becomes easier for the staff.
>
> Problems with allergies are often used as an argument for banning animals in nursing homes. In the Myren survey, 45% of the nursing homes that did not have animals stated risk of allergies as a major concern. Among those who had animals, only about 24% had experienced allergy problems. This suggests that many non-animal nursing homes over-estimate this risk. One way to accommodate this is to have animals in some wards and place allergic residents and staff in wards without animals. More than half of the nursing homes that did not have animals reported that they would like to have animals and had great faith in the health benefits of animals to the elderly.
>
> Many care homes now allow the residents to bring their own pet with them when they move to the institution. The main social benefits reported are that the person has a familiar companion they can talk to, which provides a homely and friendly atmosphere, and means that the person more readily accepts medication. Other beneficial effects noted in studies are that residents seemed more relaxed, were more active, were distracted from thinking about their aches and pains and showed fewer and less-intense symptoms, including less pain. The disadvantages are that some other people, including staff, do not like or are afraid of the person's animal, or that animals belonging to different people do not like each other and may fight. There are also practical problems regarding the pet when the owner of the animal dies. Problems with cleanliness and hygiene, in general, have been found to be negligible, but some studies mentioned fleas, loose animal hairs and that some animals ate the residents' food. Other disadvantages were that some animals were not friendly, could be noisy or cause allergic reactions. But all these situations can be managed with planning and agreed conditions regarding how the animal is provided for.

or AAT, both professional or volunteer practitioners have the same level of ethical responsibility to ensure the welfare of both the human recipient *and* the animal. In terms of the recipient's welfare, it is important that volunteers are accompanied by a professional and have been given relevant information to enable them, as well as the animal, to make a good connection with the recipient. It is also important that potential recipients have agreed to an animal interaction. Whilst dogs are the most popular species used, not all patients or nursing home residents like dogs. People who offer therapy or are hospital volunteers with a pet can have a strong preference for an animal. It is a common mistake to forget that the patient may have completely different preferences.

If AAI is to be carried out in a responsible manner, owners should first pass a course in this topic and the animal be assessed for its suitability. This may be organized by a relevant charity such as Pet Partners in the USA or Pets as Therapy in the UK, or through an education provider such as the International Centre of Anthrozoology, a Norwegian-initiated foundation (icofa-community.com). The International Society for Animal Assisted Therapy (ISAAT) has a growing list of such providers available in various countries (isaat.org). Even those health professionals working with a handler and animal should understand the animal's behaviour, needs and capabilities and be guided by the handler if the animal needs a rest break, for example.

A range of species are used in AAI, in particular horses, donkeys, dogs, rabbits and cats. Indeed, from the animal welfare perspective, wild species, and even other domesticated species, such as cows, goats and sheep, unless they are well socialized to humans, are likely to find the experience of interacting with lots of different people stressful and it is not advised that they are used. The ISAAT provides a comprehensive list of the pros and cons of using different species (isaat.org). Regardless of species, the individual animal's welfare must always be central to any intervention. Only then can the well-being of all involved be protected.

All animals are individuals, and there is not one type that is suitable for all patients or users. When planning an intervention, it is important to think hard about what is required of the animal and then consider what species and breed is appropriate, before looking for the right individual. Planning also must ensure that it is clear who will be caring for the animal throughout its life even when it is retired from the role. Useful guidelines are provided by the UK Society for Companion Animal Studies AAI Code of Practice (scas.org.uk).

Let us use the context of a nursing home for elderly people as an example. Though dogs may often be the first thought, studies show that what people prefer is often closely related to what kind of animals one's parents and grandparents had. Since so many have had cats earlier in life, cats should be considered. A brief set of planning considerations is given in Box 13.2.

One must consider questions such as:

- Should it be a visiting animal or a resident 'pet' for the home? A well socialized and trained cat can certainly be a visiting animal.
- Should the animal motivate the residents to be more active? If so, a cat that enjoys playing would be appropriate.
- Should the animal be able to provide safety and security to an anxious resident? If so, the cat needs to be able to be calm and enjoy being stroked, and a more mature adult cat may be perfect.

Box 13.2. Some advice notes on cats in nursing homes.

While it is good for the elderly to be in contact with animals, it is important that the administration at nursing homes has considered in advance the purpose of, and the organization of, the cat-keeping.

- It is important to inform residents, employees and any relatives in advance, so that they agree to the keeping of a cat at the nursing home.
- Consider having a resident cat only on certain wards if there is resistance among some residents or employees.
- To achieve the best possible effects, it is important to consider the type of animal-assisted intervention, whether the cat should work as an environmental enrichment for everyone, cuddling for some residents, or be actively used in therapy situations.
- It is important to choose the right individual cat that is fit for the purpose. The cat should be assessed by a person with professional competence in such assessments, for example a clinical animal behaviourist or other cat specialist (see Chapter 11). The cat must be adult, social and mentally robust. It must be controllable, reliable and have predictable behaviour. It must have the ability to create confidence and the feeling of security among the residents.
- A cat is easier to keep as an environmental enrichment than a dog and often arouses less fear among the residents.
- Good routines must be established to give the animal optimal health and well-being, and proper nutrition. Do not let the residents feed the cat uncontrollably as it can become overweight. The cat should be seen regularly by a vet, be vaccinated and be de-wormed if it is allowed outdoors.
- For positive health effects to occur between animals and humans, it is a prerequisite that the relationship is without serious problems. A cat with poor welfare will not benefit the residents. Any concerns regarding changes in the cat's behaviour should be addressed without delay, initially with a health check by a vet.
- Risk management, prevention and treatment of accidents should be central parts of the action plan, in respect of bites, scratches, allergies and zoonoses.

- Is it desired that the cat stimulates social contacts and communication between residents and with staff? This requires a cat who actively initiates contact, and the staff can encourage conversations with and between residents about its activities. Basically, the cat must be sociable towards other people, not show fear, not bite or scratch, and be happy to be picked up and carried.

Cats have the advantage that they require less from those responsible for their care, are less expensive to keep, beautiful to watch, and are relaxing, soothing and entertaining companions. A cat is especially suitable for persons who are not very mobile and when more constant contact is not required. The cat will bring benefit to the residents, their visitors and the staff.

In summary, having interactions with cats can be good for our health and well-being. In turn, we must ensure that we provide them with all they need to ensure their health and well-being is the best it can be.

Further Reading

Anderson, W.P., Reid, C.M. and Jennings, G.L. (1992) Pet ownership and risk factors for cardiovascular disease. *The Medical Journal of Australia* 157, 298–301.

Bossard, J.H. (1944) The mental hygiene of owning a dog. *Mental Hygiene* 28, 408–413.

Collis, G.M. and McNicholas, J. (1998) A theoretical basis for health benefits of pet ownership: attachment versus social support. In: Wilson, C.C. and Turner, D.C. (eds) *Companion Animals in Human Health*. Sage, Thousand Oaks, California, pp. 105–122.

Curry, B.A., Donaldson, B., Vercoe, M., Filippo, M. and Zak, P.J. (2015) Oxytocin responses after dog and cat interactions depend on pet ownership and may affect interpersonal trust. *Human–Animal Interaction Bulletin* 3(2), 56–71.

Fine, A.H. (ed.) (2019) *Handbook on Animal-Assisted Therapy: Foundations and Guidelines for Animal-Assisted Interventions*, 5th edn. Academic Press, San Diego, California.

Friedmann, E. and Thomas, S.A. (1995) Pet ownership, social support, and one-year survival after acute myocardial infarction in the Cardiac Arrhythmia Suppression Trial (CAST). *American Journal of Cardiology* 76, 1213–1217.

Garrity, T.F., Stallones, L.F., Marx, M.B. and Johnson, T.P. (1989) Pet ownership and attachment as supportive factors in the health of the elderly. *Anthrozoös* 3, 35–44.

Johnson, E.A., Portillo, A., Bennett, N.E. and Gray, P.B. (2021) Exploring women's oxytocin responses to interactions with their pet cats. *PeerJ* 9: e12393. DOI: 10.7717/peerj.12393.

Levinson, B.M. (1962) The dog as a co-therapist. *Mental Hygiene* 46, 59–65.

McNicholas, J., Gilbey, A., Rennie, A., Ahmedzai, S., Dono, J.A. et al. (2005) Pet ownership and human health: a brief review of evidence and issues. *British Medical Journal* 331(7527), 1252–1254.

Messent, P.R. (1983) Social facilitation of contact with other people by pet dogs. In: Katcher, A.H. and Beck, A.M. (eds) *New Perspectives on Our Lives with Companion Animals*. University of Pennsylvania Press, Philadelphia, Pennsylvania, pp. 351–359.

Miles, J.N., Parast, L., Babey, S.H., Griffin, B.A. and Saunders, J.M. (2017) A propensity-score-weighted population-based study of the health benefits of dogs and cats for children. *Anthrozoös* 30, 429–440.

Raina, P., Waltner-Toews, D., Bonnett, B., Woodward, C. and Abernathy, T. (1999) Influence of companion animals on the physical and psychological health of older people: an analysis of a one-year longitudinal study. *Journal of the American Geriatrics Society* 47, 323–329.

Scanlon, L., Hobson-West, P., Cobb, K., McBride, A. and Stavisky, J. (2021) Homeless people and their dogs: exploring the nature and impact of the human–companion animal bond. *Anthrozoös* 34, 77–92.

Serpell, J.A. (1991) Beneficial effects of pet ownership on some aspects of human health and behaviour. *Journal of the Royal Society of Medicine* 84, 717–720.

Supplementary material entitled 'How can the cat benefit human health' can be accessed at: www.cabi.org/the-cat-behaviour-and-welfare/

14 Conclusions: How to Develop a Harmonious, Well-functioning Adult Cat

Like all other characteristics of animals, the individual's behaviour and mental and physical health are developed as a function of genes and environmental experience. The goal must be that the breeding and experience kittens obtain during kittenhood and adolescence results in the development of a well-functioning adult cat. Particularly when breeding for pedigree cats, the choice of breeding animals is entirely down to the breeder, not the cat. It is essential that healthy, confident parents are chosen to increase the chance that the kitten has a genotype that favours good health and normal behaviour. The type of early experience that the kitten gets before it is sold or given away will further develop the behaviour and the kitten's ability to cope with life and have a good quality of life. Both factors are the responsibility of the cat breeders. Owners of free-roaming cats, be they pedigree or non-pedigree, cannot influence the breeding. However, if their female cat is not neutered or given contraceptive pills, owners can at least contribute to a good kittenhood.

Breeding

Selecting breeding animals traditionally involves conscientious breeders avoiding individuals with anatomical or health disorders, or individuals with genetically-related susceptibility for certain diseases. But the behaviour of the parents must not be forgotten when selecting breeding animals.

Activity level, playfulness, sociability and behaviour related to nervousness and anxiety are the behavioural traits showing the highest heritabilities. In her Master's thesis, Ingrid Westbye of the Norwegian University of Life Sciences investigated the heritability of behavioural traits in Persians and Siamese, two quite different breeds. This was based on half-siblings from the same father (paternal half-sibs) to avoid any confounding influence of the maternal environment between conception and weaning. The highest heritability was found for the degree to which the cat was active and playful. High heritabilities were also found for the cat's tendency to approach unfamiliar children or adults, and anxiety or fear of strong sounds and unfamiliar people.

Cat breeders can use this knowledge to select against undesired behavioural traits and select for desired traits. In particular, they can promote features that contribute to improved animal welfare. In the longer term, this will contribute to better-balanced cats and more satisfied cat owners. If behaviour traits that are desirable for the owner and beneficial to the cat are included in the breeding work, this will have wide consequences. Behavioural problems will decrease, and by knowing more about breed-typical behaviour, cat buyers will be able to better assess which breed to acquire. The expectations of the owner will be more consistent with the actual behaviour of the kitten. In the next generation, kittens that show desirable behavioural traits will be preferred in the further breeding.

Based on the heritability estimates presented above, it is feasible to include activity, playfulness, the absence of extreme anxiety/fear towards people and the environment, and a reasonable level of friendliness rather than aggressiveness towards unfamiliar people in the breeding goals of pedigree cats. Also, keep in mind that moderation in selection goals is preferable to breeding for extremes in either direction. So while we don't want an extremely active cat that destroys the house through its rampages in three dimensions, neither do we want one so placid that it becomes obese and at risk of cardiac and skeletal disorders. While we don't want a terrified cat that spends most of its time hiding, neither do we want one that is so trusting that it fails to avoid traffic and predators when outdoors. Furthermore, multiple behavioural and health traits should be included in the breeding index rather than the current preoccupation with a handful of traits affecting appearance. This maintains balance and avoids the risk of inadvertently selecting for unwanted traits that come along with the desired ones.

From Kittenhood to Adulthood

The development of the kittens starts before birth, at the embryonic stage. Experiments in many animal species show that if a pregnant female is exposed to severe stress, this may cause the offspring to develop hypersensitive stress mechanisms – meaning they are more nervous and reactive. This is due to the stress hormone cortisol being secreted by the mother and entering the bloodstream of the foetus. This *prenatal stress* causes a permanent change in how the offspring's brain responds to stress. This is an example of an *epigenetic effect*, i.e. that environmental factors affect how the genes are expressed. As a result of prenatal stress, the offspring may have impaired learning abilities, poor social coping ability, and an increased risk of mental disturbances. In female offspring, this can detrimentally affect their maternal behaviour towards their own young – so what happens to the mother can also affect her grandchildren. Epigenetic effects can also occur after birth and throughout life but especially when young, in both males and females. So we should not only consider the maternal line but the paternal line, too, as sperm can carry epigenetic marks to the offspring. As such effects are widely described in mammals (and in domestic fowl and salmonid fish), and also reported in humans, they can be expected in cats as well.

The best things one can do to contribute to favourable behavioural development in kittens are to ensure that breeding tomcats and pregnant and nursing queens are well fed, in good health, live in an enriched environment and are allowed privacy when they want it. The latter means providing queens with a safe, secluded nest, and both toms and queens with continuously accessible, safe, quiet resting places.

Kittens do not thrive alone. Experiments show that kittens taken from the mother two weeks after

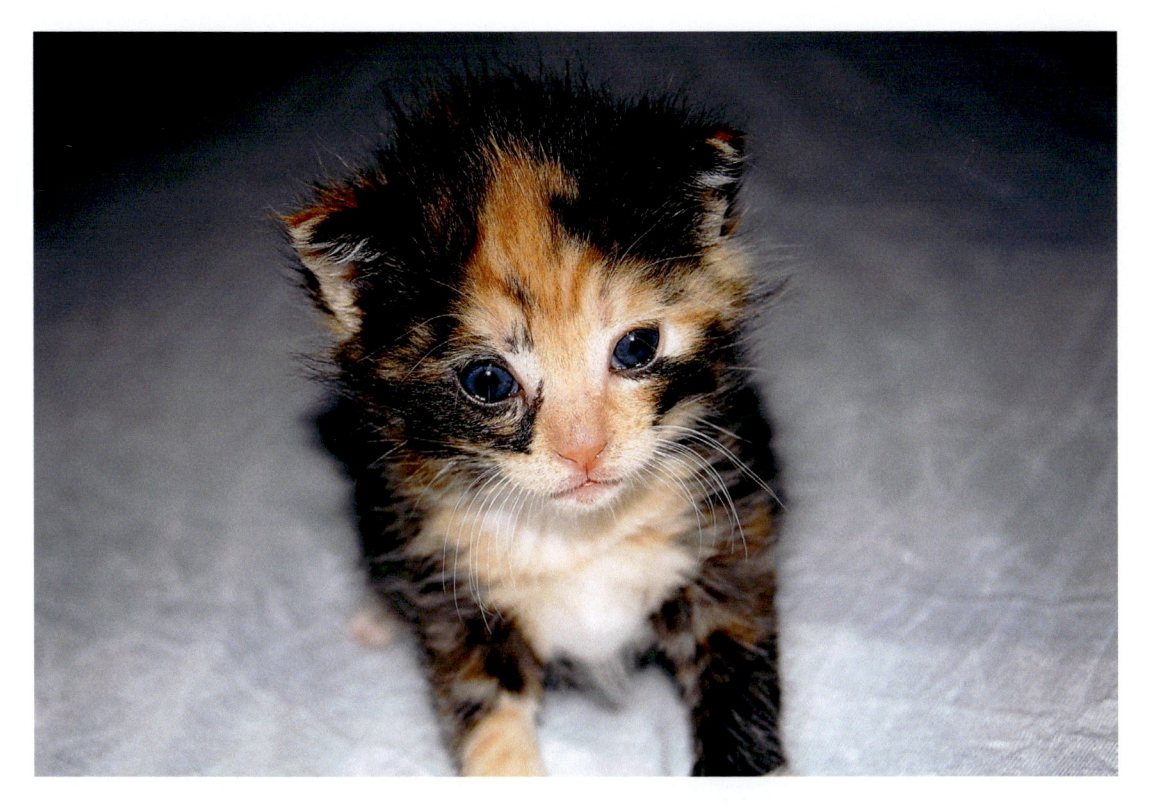

Fig. 14.1. The breeder is responsible for giving the kitten a good start in life. (Photo: Linda Iren Jensen, 2019)

birth and kept without the opportunity to interact with their mother and littermates developed emotional disturbances. They were more fearful in new situations, less trusting, more aggressive and more inflexible. Such kittens become very timid in social relations.

The kitten's social behaviour begins to develop at three weeks of age. At this age, the senses are well developed, and they begin to crawl around more. This is also when they start playing with their mother and siblings. Through this *social play*, they learn details of cat social behaviour and how to use language signals in the right way and in the right context. They send a signal, a sound or an ear signal, and record how the others respond to this. Now the kittens are learning the characteristics of the individuals with whom they have social contact. Just like the dog, the cat also has a *socialization period* when this initial learning must take place. Although lifelong social experience is valuable, its success depends on what happens during this period when the building blocks are established. The most sensitive part of this period is 3–7 weeks of age, after which the kittens' openness to learning the basics about 'cat language' and about the social environment gradually decreases – with the socialization period ending at approximately three months of age. Continuing the social contact with the mother and siblings until the kittens are at least 14 weeks of age helps to prevent later behavioural problems.

Furthermore, if the cat does not have positive experiences with humans during this period from 3–12 weeks of age, it will remain shy towards humans and very difficult to tame later. The breeder has a great responsibility here. It is an advantage for the kitten to get to know different people during this socialization period, both women and men, children and adults. It will then acquire a more generalized image of what humans are. Many cats who have only lived with a woman are scared of men, especially when they hear the deeper voice of a man.

To ensure that the kitten learns what it needs to know about social behaviour, it should not be taken from its mother and littermates until it is at least 12–14 weeks old, depending on the behavioural development of the individual kitten. Especially if the cat breeder is a single person, it will be a great advantage if the new owners can visit and have contact with the kitten a few times before it is old enough to move to its new family.

Both before and after separation from its mother and littermates, the cat must face challenges it can learn to master. Experience with mild stress-eliciting stimuli (stressors) stimulates the cat and contributes to learning and good stress-coping ability. This means giving it novel experiences such as different toys, objects, puzzle feeders, surfaces, scents and noises. Brief reward-based training sessions add to this experience. Every time the cat succeeds with something, self-confidence will increase and make it more robust when it meets challenges later in life. This must be done at the cat's own pace, as overstimulation, like under-stimulation, will defeat this objective.

The cat breeder and the new owner need basic competence, knowledge and understanding of the cat's normal behaviour, motivation, physical and behavioural needs, and learning mechanisms. Only then can they design a proper home environment, respond adequately to the cat's behaviour and signals, and know how to handle behavioural problems if they arise.

Box 14.1. Breeding for good qualities.

- Behaviour, and mental and physical health, are functions of genes and the environment, including the cat's experiences.
- In pedigree cats, the choice of breeding animals is essential:
    - You should avoid breeding individuals that are very fearful of people and the environment.
    - In addition, highly aggressive behavioural traits towards people and other cats should be avoided.
    - Remember that the temperament of both parents affects the offspring.
- Early experience that the kitten acquires before it is sold or given away will further develop desirable, harmonious behaviour.

Box 14.2. Care and handling of kittens and adult cats.

- The kitten's development starts during the embryonic stage. Prenatal stress may cause the offspring to develop hypersensitive stress mechanisms.
- To ensure that the kitten learns what it needs about social behaviour, it should not be taken from its mother and littermates until it is at least 12–14 weeks old.
- Both before and after weaning, the kitten needs opportunities to face gentle challenges it can learn to cope with. This builds confidence and emotional resilience. Whenever the cat succeeds in doing something, self-confidence will increase and make it more robust in facing later challenges.
- The cat owner must acquire basic competence in understanding cat behaviour, motivation, needs and learning mechanisms. This is essential to provide cats with a proper environment, prevent behavioural problems and solve them if and when they arise.

Supplementary material entitled 'How can you develop kittens into well-functioning adult cats' can be accessed at: www.cabi.org/the-cat-behaviour-and-welfare/

Literature

This is a list of important sources as well as recommended literature for those who wish to learn more about the cat's behaviour, welfare and relationship with people.

Books, articles and reports

Ahola, M.K., Vapalahti, K. and Lohi, H. (2017) Early weaning increases aggression and stereotypic behaviour in cats. *Scientific Reports* 7: 10412. DOI: 10.1038/s41598-017-11173-5.

Amat, A., Ruiz de la Torre, J.L., Fatjó, J., Mariotti, V.M., van Wijk S. *et al.* (2009) Potential risk factors associated with feline behaviour problems. *Applied Animal Behaviour Science* 121, 134–139.

Anderson, W.P., Reid, C.M. and Jennings, G.L. (1992) Pet ownership and risk factors for cardiovascular disease. *The Medical Journal of Australia* 157, 298–301.

Atkinson, T. (2018) *Practical Feline Behaviour: Understanding Cat Behaviour and Improving Welfare*. CAB International, Wallingford, UK.

Australian Government, Department of the Environment (2015) Background document for the threat abatement plan for predation by feral cats. Available at: www.environment.gov.au/system/files/resources/78f3dea5-c278-4273-8923-fa0de27aacfb/files/tap-predation-feral-cats-2015-background.pdf (accessed 9 April 2022).

Baker, R.R. (1980) Goal orientation by blindfolded humans after long-distance displacement: possible involvement of a magnetic sense. *Science* 210, 555–557.

Baker, R.R., Mather, J.G. and Kennaugh, J.H. (1983) Magnetic bones in human sinuses. *Nature* 301 (5895), 79–80.

Baugh, S. and McBride, E.A. (2022) Animal welfare in context: historical, scientific, ethical, moral and One Welfare perspectives. In: Vitale, A. and Pollo, S. (eds) *Human/Animal Relationships in Transformation – Scientific, Moral and Legal Perspectives*. Palgrave Macmillan, London.

Bekoff, M. (2010) *The Emotional Lives of Animals: A Leading Scientist Explores Animal Joy, Sorrow, and Empathy – and Why They Matter*. New World Library, Novato, California.

Berget, B., Krøger, E. and Thorød, A.B. (eds) (2018) *Antrozoologi – Samspill mellom dyr og menneske*. Universitetsforlaget, Oslo. [In Norwegian]

Bergler, R. (1991) *Man and Cat: The Benefits of Cat Ownership*. Blackwell, Oxford, UK.

Bessant, C. (2002) *Boarding Cattery Manual*. Feline Advisory Bureau, Tisbury, UK.

Bessant, C. (2006) *Feral Cat Manual*. Feline Advisory Bureau, Tisbury, UK.

Bischof, R., Hansen, N.R., Nyheim, Ø.S., Kisen, A., Prestmoen, L. *et al.* (2022) Mapping the 'catscape' formed by a population of pet cats with outdoor access. *Scientific Reports* 12, 5964. DOI: 10.1038/ s41598- 022- 09694-9.

Bossard, J.H. (1944) The mental hygiene of owning a dog. *Mental Hygiene* 28, 408–413.

Braastad, B.O. (1980) Kattens orienteringsevne og atferd i ukjent terreng. MSc thesis, the University of Trondheim, Norway. [In Norwegian]

Braastad, B.O. (2011) Katten som predator – en fare for norsk fauna? *Fauna* 64(1), 2–8. [In Norwegian]

Braastad, B.O. and Heggelund, P. (1984) Eye-opening in kittens: effects of light and some biological factors. *Developmental Psychobiology* 17, 675–681.

Bradshaw, J. and Ellis, S. (2016) *The Trainable Cat: How to Make Life Happier for You and Your Cat*. Basic Books, New York.

Broom, D.M. (2014) *Sentience and Animal Welfare*. CAB International, Wallingford, UK.

Bru, A. (2019) *I love Happy Cats - Guide for a Happy Cat*. Schiffer Publishing, Atglen, Pennsylvania.

Cabanac, M. (2002) What is emotion? *Behavioural Processes* 60, 69–83.

Casey, R.A. and Bradshaw, J.W.S. (2008) The effects of additional socialization for kittens in a rescue centre on their behaviour and suitability as a pet. *Applied Animal Behaviour Science* 114, 196–205.

Cecchetti, M., Crowley, S.L., Goodwin, C.E.D. and McDonald, R.A. (2021) Provision of high meat content food and object play reduce predation of wild animals by domestic cats *Felis catus*. *Current Biology* 31, 1107–1111.e5. DOI: 10.1016/j.cub.2020.12.044.

Cecchetti, M., Crowley, S.L., Wilson-Aggarwal, J., Nelli, L. and McDonald, R.A. (2022) Spatial behavior of domestic cats and the effects of outdoor access restrictions and interventions to reduce predation of wildlife. *Conservation Science and Practice* 4(2), e597. DOI: 10.1111/csp2.597.

Collis, G.M. and McNicholas, J. (1998) A theoretical basis for health benefits of pet ownership: attachment versus social support. In: Wilson, C.C. and Turner, D.C. (eds) *Companion Animals in Human Health*. Sage, Thousand Oaks, California, pp. 105–122.

Council of Europe (1987) European Convention for the Protection of Pet Animals. Council of Europe, Strasbourg, 13 November 1987. Available at: https://rm.coe.int/09000016800ca43a (accessed 30 April 2022).

Curry, B.A., Donaldson, B., Vercoe, M., Filippo, M. and Zak, P.J. (2015) Oxytocin responses after dog and cat interactions depend on pet ownership and may affect interpersonal trust. *Human–Animal Interaction Bulletin* 3(2), 56–71.

Davies, Z.G., Fuller, R.A., Loram, A., Irvine, K.N., Sims, V. *et al.* (2009) A national scale inventory of resource provision for biodiversity within domestic gardens. *Biological Conservation* 142(4), 761–771.

Dogs Trust Hope and Freedom Projects. Available at: https://www.dogstrust.org.uk/help-advice/hope-project-freedom-project (accessed 17 July 2022).

Driscoll C.A., Menotti-Raymond, M., Roca, A.L., Hupe, K., Johnson, W.E. *et al.* (2007) The Near Eastern origin of cat domestication. *Science* 317, 519–523.

Driscoll, C.A., Clutton-Brock, J., Kitchener, A.C. and O'Brien, S.J. (2009) The taming of the cat: genetic and archaeological findings hint that wildcats became housecats earlier – and in a different place – than previously thought. *Scientific American* 300(6), 68–75.

Duffy, D.L., Diniz de Moura, R.T. and Serpell, J.A. (2017) Development and evaluation of the Fe-BARQ: A new survey instrument for measuring behavior in domestic cats (Felis s. catus). *Behavioural Processes* 141, 329–341. DOI: 10.1016/j.beproc.2017.02.010.

Ellis, S. (2009) Environmental enrichment: practical strategies for improving feline welfare. *Journal of Feline Medicine and Surgery* 11, 901–912.

Ellis, S. and Sparkes, A.H. (eds) (2016) *ISFM Guide to Feline Stress and Health: Managing Negative Emotions to Improve Feline Health and Wellbeing*. International Cat Care, UK. For purchase at: https://icatcare.org/shop/isfm-guide-to-feline-stress-and-health-pdf/ (accessed 17 July 2022).

Emmelinedommen (1993) Høyesterettsdom 29.10.1993. *Rettstidende* 1260, 466–493. [In Norwegian]

Endenburg, N. and Baarda, B. (1995) The role of pets in enhancing human well-being: effects on child development. In: Robinson, I. (ed.) *The Waltham Book of Human–Animal Interaction: Benefits and Responsibilities of Pet Ownership*. Elsevier, Kidlington, UK, pp. 7–17.

Eriksen, S.C.B. (2014) Atferdsegenskaper hos rasekatter i Norge. MSc thesis, Norwegian University of Life Sciences, Ås, Norway. Available at: http://hdl.handle.net/11250/277460 (accessed 30 April 2022). [In Norwegian]

FEDIAF (2021) Facts & figures 2021. European overview. Available at: https://europeanpetfood.org/about/statistics/ (accessed 23 September 2022).

Feuerstein, N. and Terkel, J. (2008) Interrelationships of dogs (*Canis familiaris*) and cats (*Felis catus* L.) living under the same roof. *Applied Animal Behaviour Science* 113, 150–165.

Fine, A.H. (ed.) (2019) *Handbook on Animal-Assisted Therapy: Foundations and Guidelines for Animal-Assisted Interventions*, 5th edn. Academic Press, San Diego, California.

Finka, L.R., Ward, J., Farnworth, M.J. and Mills, D.S. (2019) Owner personality and the well-being of their cats share parallels with the parent–child relationship. *PLOS ONE* 14(2), e0211862. DOI: 10.1371/journal.pone.0211862.

Fitzgerald, B.M. and Turner, D.C. (2000) Hunting behaviour of domestic cats and their impact on prey populations. In: Turner, D.C. and Bateson,

P. (eds) *The Domestic Cat: The Biology of Its Behaviour*, 2nd edn. Cambridge University Press, Cambridge, pp. 151–175.

Friedmann, E. (1995) The role of pets in enhancing human well-being: physiological effects. In: Robinson, I. (ed.) *The Waltham Book of Human–Animal Interaction: Benefits and Responsibilities of Pet Ownership*. Elsevier, Kidlington, UK, Chapter 4.

Friedmann, E. and Thomas, S.A. (1995) Pet ownership, social support, and one-year survival after acute myocardial infarction in the Cardiac Arrhythmia Suppression Trial (CAST). *American Journal of Cardiology* 76, 1213–1217.

Friedmann, E., Katcher, A.H., Lynch, J.J. and Thomas, S.A. (1980) Animal companions and one-year survival of patients after discharge from a coronary care unit. *Public Health Reports* 95, 307–312.

Fugazza, C., Sommese, A., Pogány, Á. and Miklósi, Á. (2021) Did we find a copycat? Do as I do in a domestic cat (*Felis catus*). *Animal Cognition* 24, 121–131. DOI: 10.1007/s10071-020-01428-6.

Garrity, T.F. and Stallones, L. (1998) Effects of pet contact on human well-being: review of recent research. In: Wilson, C.C. and Turner, D.C. (eds) *Companion Animals in Human Health*. Sage Publications, Thousand Oaks, California, pp. 3–22.

Garrity, T.F., Stallones, L.F., Marx, M.B. and Johnson, T.P. (1989) Pet ownership and attachment as supportive factors in the health of the elderly. *Anthrozoös* 3, 35–44.

Geiger, M., Kistler, C., Mattmann, P., Jenni, L., Hegglin, D. *et al.* (2022) Colorful collar-covers and bells reduce wildlife predation by domestic cats in a continental European setting. *Frontiers in Ecology and Evolution* 10: 850442. DOI: 10.3389/fevo.2022.850442.

Gosling, S.D., Sandy, C.J. and Potter, J. (2010) Personalities of self-identified 'dog people' and 'cat people'. *Anthrozoös* 23(3), 213–222.

Gray, J.A. (1987) *The Psychology of Fear and Stress*, 2nd edn. Cambridge University Press, Cambridge.

Greene, D. and Braastad, B.O. (1986) *Utrolige katter. Om katters fantastiske evner og psykologi*. Aventura, Oslo. [In Norwegian; extended version of Greene, D. (1984) *Incredible Cats: The Secret Powers of Your Pet*. Methuen, London]

Hart, B.L. and Hart, L.A. (2013) *Your Ideal Cat: Insights into Breed and Gender Differences in Cat Behavior*. Purdue University Press, West Lafayette, Indiana.

Heath, S. (1993) *Why Does My Cat…?* Souvenir Press, London.

Herrick, F.H. (1922) Homing powers of the cat. *The Scientific Monthly* 14, 525–539.

Horwitz, D.F. (ed.) (2018) *Blackwell's Five-Minute Veterinary Consult Clinical Companion: Canine and Feline Behavior*, 2nd edn. Wiley, Ames, Iowa.

Horwitz, D.F. and Mills, D.S. (eds) (2009) *BSAVA Manual of Canine and Feline Behavioural Medicine*, 2nd edn. British Small Animal Veterinary Association, Quedgeley, UK.

Houston, K. (2014) *21 Days to the Perfect Cat*. Hamlyn, London.

Johnson, E.A., Portillo, A., Bennett, N.E. and Gray, P.B. (2021) Exploring women's oxytocin responses to interactions with their pet cats. *PeerJ* 9: e12393. DOI: 10.7717/peerj.12393.

Kessler, M.R. and Turner, D.C. (1997) Stress and adaptation of cats (*Felis silvestris catus*) housed singly, in pairs and in groups in boarding catteries. *Animal Welfare* 6, 243–254.

Kessler, M.R. and Turner, D.C. (1999) Socialization and stress in cats (*Felis silvestris catus*) housed singly and in groups in animal shelters. *Animal Welfare* 8, 15–26.

Kidd, A.H. and Kidd, R.M. (1980) Personality characteristics and preferences in pet ownership. *Psychological Reports* 46, 939–949.

Konok, V., Kosztolányi, A., Rainer, W., Mutschler, B., Halsband, U. and Miklósi, Á. (2015) Influence of owners' attachment style and personality on their dogs' (*Canis familiaris*) separation-related disorder. *PLOS ONE* 10(2), e0118375.

Kotrschal, K., Day, J., McCune, S. and Wedl, M. (2014) Human and cat personalities: building the bond from both sides. In: Turner, D.C. and Bateson, P. (eds) *The Domestic Cat: The Biology of Its Behaviour*, 3rd edn. Cambridge University Press, Cambridge, pp. 113–127.

Kristiansen, K.B. and Landfald, O. (2013) Atferd hos katter (*Felis silvestris catus*) på omplasseringssentre og etter adopsjon. MSc thesis, Norwegian University of Life Sciences, Ås, Norway. Available at: http://hdl.handle.net/11250/186185 (accessed 30 April 2022). [In Norwegian]

Landsberg, G.M. and Denenberg, S. (2009) Behaviour problems in the senior pet. In: Horwitz, D.F. and Mills, D.S. (eds) *BSAVA Manual of Canine and Feline Behavioural Medicine*, 2nd edn. British Small Animal

Veterinary Association, Quedgeley, UK, pp. 127–135.
Lawrence, C.E. (1981) Individual differences in the mother–kitten relationship in the domestic cat, *Felis catus*. PhD thesis, University of Edinburgh, UK.
Levine, E., Perry, P., Scarlett, J. and Houpt, K.A. (2005) Intercat aggression in households following the introduction of a new cat. *Applied Animal Behaviour Science* 90, 325–336.
Levinson, B.M. (1962) The dog as a co-therapist. *Mental Hygiene* 46, 59–65.
Levy, T. (2017) Four styles of adult attachment. Available at: https://www.evergreenpsychotherapycenter.com/styles-adult-attachment (accessed 31 May 2022).
Leyhausen, P. (1979) *Cat Behavior: The Predatory and Social Behavior of Domestic and Wild Cats*. Garland STPM Press, New York.
Link, J. (2021) People-pleasing animals: mediating factors in attachment style difference between dog people and cat people. MSc thesis, State University of New York.
Litchfield, C.A. *et al.* (2017) The 'Feline Five': An exploration of personality in pet cats (Felis catus). *PLOS ONE* 12(8): e0183455. DOI: 10.1371/journal.pone.0183455
Little, S.E. (2012) Female reproduction. *The Cat*, 1195–1227. DOI: 10.1016/B978-1-4377-0660-4.00040-5.
Macdonald, D.W, Yamaguchi, N. and Kerby, G. (2000) Group-living in the domestic cat: its sociobiology and epidemiology. In: Turner, D.C. and Bateson, P. (eds) *The Domestic Cat: The Biology of Its Behaviour*, 2nd edn. Cambridge University Press, Cambridge, pp. 95–118.
Marchei, P., Diverio, S., Falocci, N., Fatjó, J., Ruiz de la Torre, J.L. *et al.* (2009) Breed differences in behavioural development in kittens. *Physiology and Behaviour* 96, 522–531.
Mars (2021) How data can help us end pet homelessness. Available at: https://www.mars.com/news-and-stories/articles/ending-pet-homelessness (accessed 22 May 2022).
McComb, K., Taylor, A.M., Wilson C. and Charlton, B.D. (2009) The cry embedded within the purr. *Current Biology* 13, R507–R508. DOI: 10.1016/j.cub.2009.05.033
McCoy, D.E., Schiestl, M., Neilands, P., Hassall, R., Gray, R.D. and Taylor, A.H. (2019) New Caledonian crows behave optimistically after using tools. *Current Biology* 29, 2737–2742.

McCune, S. (1992) Temperament and the welfare of caged cats. PhD thesis, University of Cambridge, Cambridge.
McCune, S. (1995) The impact of paternity and early socialisation on the development of cats' behaviour to people and novel objects. *Applied Animal Behaviour Science* 45, 109–124.
McMillan, F.D. (2020) Mental health and well-being benefits of personal control in animals. In: McMillan, F.D. (ed.) *Mental Health and Well-Being in Animals*, 2nd edn. CAB International, Wallingford, UK, Chapter 6.
McNicholas, J., Gilbey, A., Rennie, A., Ahmedzai, S., Dono, J.A. *et al.* (2005) Pet ownership and human health: a brief review of evidence and issues. *British Medical Journal* 331(7527), 1252–1254.
Mendl, M. and Harcourt, R. (2000) Individuality in the domestic cat: origins, development and stability. In: Turner, D.C. and Bateson, P. (eds) *The Domestic Cat: The Biology of Its Behaviour*, 2nd edn. Cambridge University Press, Cambridge, pp. 47–64.
Menotti-Raymond, M., David, V.A., Pflueger, S.M., Lindblad-Toh, K., Wade, C.M. *et al.* (2008) Patterns of molecular genetic variation among cat breeds. *Genomics* 91, 1–11.
Messent, P.R. (1983) Social facilitation of contact with other people by pet dogs. In: Katcher, A.H. and Beck, A.M. (eds.) *New Perspectives on Our Lives with Companion Animals*. University of Pennsylvania Press, Philadelphia, Pennsylvania, pp. 351–359.
Miles, J.N., Parast, L., Babey, S.H., Griffin, B.A. and Saunders, J.M. (2017) A propensity-score-weighted population-based study of the health benefits of dogs and cats for children. *Anthrozoös*, 30, 429–440.
Moelk, M. (1944) Vocalizing in the house-cat: a phonetic and functional study. *American Journal of Psychology* 57, 184–205.
Moser, E.I., Moser, M.-B. and McNaughton, B.L. (2017) Spatial representation in the hippocampal formation: a history. *Nature Neuroscience* 20(11), 1448–1464. DOI: 10.1038/nn.4653.
Myren, I.K. (2010) Terapi- og selskapsdyr i norske sykehjem – en kartleggingsstudie. MSc thesis. Norwegian University of Life Sciences, Ås, Norway. [In Norwegian]
Myren, I.K., Kvaal, K. and Braastad, B.O. (2011) Hund og katt i sykehjem – et bidrag i miljøbehandling? *Demens & Alderspsykiatri* 15(2), 24–26. [In Norwegian]

Natoli, E. and De Vito, E. (1991) Agonistic behaviour, dominance rank and copulatory success in a large multi-male feral cat, *Felis catus* L., colony in central Rome. *Animal Behaviour* 42, 227–241.

Nightingale, F. (1859) *Notes on Nursing*. Harrison & Sons, London.

Norwegian Scientific Committee for Food and Environment (2022) Assessment of the risk of negative impact on biodiversity and animal welfare from keeping domestic cat (*Felis catus*) in Norway. Scientific Opinion of the Panel on Alien Organisms and Trade in Endangered Species of the Norwegian Scientific Committee for Food and Environment. VKM Report 2022. Available at: https://vkm.no/english (accessed 1 October 2022).

O'Neill, D.G., Romans, C., Brodbelt, D.C., Church, D.B., Černá, P. *et al.* (2019) Persian cats under first opinion veterinary care in the UK: demography, mortality and disorders. *Scientific Reports* 9, 12952. DOI: 10.1038/s41598-019-49317-4.

Ottoni, C., Van Neer, W., De Cupere, B., Daligault, J., Guimaraes, S. *et al.* (2017) The palaeogenetics of cat dispersal in the ancient world. *Nature Ecology & Evolution* 1, 0139. DOI: 10.1038/s41559-017-0139.

Panksepp, J. (2004) *Affective Neuroscience: The Foundations of Human and Animal Emotions*. Oxford University Press, Oxford.

Petersen, M.L. and Farrington, D.P. (2007) Cruelty to animals and violence to people. *Victims & Offenders* 2(1), 21–43.

Potter, A. and Mills, D.S. (2015) Domestic cats (*Felis silvestris catus*) do not show signs of secure attachment to their owners. *PLOS ONE* 10(9), e0135109.

Precht, H. and Lindenlaub, E. (1954) Über das Heimfindevermögen von Säugetieren. I: Versuche an Katzen. *Zeitschrift für Tierpsychologie* 11, 485–494. [In German]

Pryor, K. (2003) *Getting Started: Clicker Training for Cats*. Sunshine Books, Waltham, Massachusetts.

Raina, P., Waltner-Toews, D., Bonnett, B., Woodward, C. and Abernathy, T. (1999) Influence of companion animals on the physical and psychological health of older people: an analysis of a one-year longitudinal study. *Journal of the American Geriatrics Society* 47, 323–329.

Rantanen, J., Metsäpelto, R.L., Feldt, T., Pulkkinen, L.E.A. and Kokko, K. (2007) Long-term stability in the Big Five personality traits in adulthood. *Scandinavian Journal of Psychology* 48(6), 511–518.

Robertson, S.A. (2008) A review of feral cat control. *Journal of Feline Medicine and Surgery* 10, 366–375.

Rochlitz, I. (ed.) (2007) *The Welfare of Cats*. Springer, Dordrecht, The Netherlands.

Rodan, I. and Heath, S. (eds) (2016) *Feline Behavioural Health and Welfare*. Elsevier, St. Louis, Missouri.

Royal Society for the Protection of Birds (n.d.) Birds of conservation concern 5. Available at: https://www.rspb.org.uk/globalassets/downloads/bocc5/bocc5-report.pdf (accessed 19 May 2022). A full report is available at: https://britishbirds.co.uk/sites/default/files/BB_Dec21-BoCC5-IUCN2.pdf (accessed 19 May 2022).

Sandem, A.I. (1998) Det sosiale båndet mellom katt og menneske. MSc thesis, Norwegian University of Life Sciences, Ås, Norway. Available at: http://hdl.handle.net/11250/2378892 (accessed 30 April 2022). [In Norwegian]

Scanlon, L., Hobson-West, P., Cobb, K., McBride, A. and Stavisky, J. (2021) Homeless people and their dogs: exploring the nature and impact of the human–companion animal bond. *Anthrozoös* 34, 77–92.

Seitz, P.F.D. (1959) Infantile experience and adult behaviour in animal subjects. II. Age of separation from the mother and adult behaviour in the cat. *Psychosomatic Medicine* 21, 353–378.

Serpell, J.A. (1991) Beneficial effects of pet ownership on some aspects of human health and behaviour. *Journal of the Royal Society of Medicine* 84, 717–720.

Serpell, J.A. (2014) Domestication and history of the cat. In: Turner, D.C. and Bateson, P. (eds) *The Domestic Cat: The Biology of Its Behaviour*, 3rd edn. Cambridge University Press, Cambridge, pp. 83–100.

Slater, M.R. (2007) The welfare of feral cats. In: Rochlitz, I. (ed.) *The Welfare of Cats*. Springer, Dordrecht, The Netherlands, pp. 141–175.

Steiger, A. (2007) Breeding and welfare. In: Rochlitz, I. (ed.) *The Welfare of Cats*. Springer, Dordrecht, The Netherlands, pp. 259–276.

Stenevik, I.H. and Mejdell, C.M. (2011) *Dyrevelferdsloven. Kommentarutgave*. Universitetsforlaget, Oslo. [In Norwegian]

Trouwborst, A., McCormack, P.C. and Martínez Camacho, E. (2020) Domestic cats and their impacts on biodiversity: a blind spot in the application of nature conservation law. *People and Nature* 2, 235–250.

Turner, D.C. and Bateson, P. (eds) (2000) *The Domestic Cat: The Biology of Its Behaviour*, 2nd edn. Cambridge University Press, Cambridge.

Turner, D.C. and Bateson, P. (eds.) (2014) *The Domestic Cat: The Biology of Its Behaviour*, 3rd edn. Cambridge University Press, Cambridge.

Turner, D.C., Feaver, J., Mendl, M. and Bateson, P.P.G. (1986) Variation in domestic cat behaviour towards humans – a paternal effect. *Animal Behaviour* 34, 1890–1901.

Uenoyama, R., Miyazaki, T., Hurst, J.L., Beynon, R.J., Adachi, M. *et al.* (2021) The characteristic response of domestic cats to plant iridoids allows them to gain chemical defense against mosquitoes. *Science Advances* 7(4), eabd9135. DOI: 10.1126/sciadv.abd9135.

Vigne, J.-D., Guilaine, J., Debue, K., Haye, L. and Gérard, P. (2004) Early taming of the cat in Cypros. *Science* 304, 259.

Walker, B. (2009) *The Cats' House*. National Cat Protection Society, Newport Beach, California.

Westbye, I. (1998) Forskjeller i atferd mellom tre katteraser. Arvbarhet av noen atferdsegenskaper, og eierens forhold til sin katt. MSc thesis, Norwegian University of Life Sciences, Ås, Norway. Available at: http://hdl.handle.net/11250/2378902 (accessed 30 April 2022). [In Norwegian]

Videos

Fugazza, C., Sommese, A., Pogány, Á. and Miklosi, A. Did we find a copycat? Imitation in a domestic cat [the video of Eibsu]. Available at: www.youtube.com/watch?v=-BU4tmyidpg (accessed 21 April 2022).

Linda Ryan, a UK cat behaviourist, has some helpful videos on how to train your cat:

Cat carrier training
https://www.facebook.com/watch/?v=297576148513494&_rdr (published 11 May 2021; accessed 13 May 2022).

Handling training
https://www.facebook.com/watch/?v=244803293382860 (published 26 April 2020; accessed 13 May 2022).

Oral handling basics (mouth checks)
https://www.facebook.com/watch/?v=729445687996613 (published 28 November 2020; accessed 13 May 2022).

Poster

Chin, L. (2022) Cats need... Available at: https://www.doggiedrawings.net/freeposters (accessed 22 May 2022).

Index

Note: Page numbers in bold type refer to figures
Page numbers in italic type refer to tables
Page numbers followed by 'B' refer to Box

abandoned cats 90–92, 160
absolute hierarchy 55
abuse
    domestic 160
    pet 169
Abyssinian cat
    aggression 30, 32
    amyloidosis 97
acoustic communication 36–41
acoustic map 73
activity, breed differences 29–30, **32**
activity feeders 148
ad libitum feeding 146
adoption, rescue cats 113
adrenaline 79, 123
adult cats, care and handling of 176B
affective states, emotions 81–87
African wildcat (*Felis lybica*) 1, 2, 3, 35, 59
age, behaviour differences 26–27
aggregation, of single cats 56
aggression 25, 137, 142–147
    Abyssinian cat 30, 32
    between males 58
    and coat colour 28, **28**
    defensive 41, 84, **85**, 142
        towards people 142–143
    extinction-induced 114
    intra-/inter-specific 142
    in multi-cat household 60
        case 128–129
    non-pedigree house cats 29
    offensive 146
    redirected 144–146
    social, between neighbouring cats **135**
    towards people, case study 145
aggressive behaviour 137, 146–147
aggressive signals 35, 57
agonistic signals, aggressive/defensive 35
agreeableness, owner 152B, 153
Aktivait® 149
alert, duty to 91B
allergies 164–165, 171B
alliances, co-operative 58
allo-grooming 142

American Bengal cats 30
American breeds 7
Americas 5
amyloidosis 97
anatomical disorders 98
ancient times 2–4
animal hoarding 96
animal-assisted activities (AAA) 169–170
    schemes 170
animal-assisted interventions (AAI) 170
    responsible implementation 170–173
    species used 172
animal-assisted therapy (AAT) 169–173
    treatment programme 169
anti-predator behaviour 66
anticipation 86, 90
anxiety 84–86, 117, 125
    association 145
    generalized 131
        explanation/solution 131
    and pica 140–141
    specific 131–135
        explanation 133
        solutions 133–135
anxious adult attachment style 154B
anxious and avoidant adult attachment
    style 154B
Anxitane™ 149
appeasement 84
arousal 108, **109**
Asian breeds 7
assaults 106
assistance animals, dogs 170
association
    fear 110, 111–112, 117
    learning by 109–115
    rules 111
asthma 164–165
attachment style, human 154–155, 154B
attachment-related problems 140
    solutions 140
attack 54, 133
attention-seeking 129, 137, 147
aunting behaviour 57

Australia 5, 155
    CatBib® 67–68
    endangered species 156
    exotic/invasive species 66
    feral cats 66
    hunting by imported carnivores 66
    physical health benefits 165
avoidant adult attachment style 154B

Balinese cat 7
Bastet 4, **4**
    cult 4
BBC2, *Horizon*, *The Secret Life of the Cat* 133B
begging
    for food 39
    vocalization 37, 40
behaviour
    choice 81
    drivers 130
    first three weeks 16
    patterns 27, 123
        consequence 80–81
    problem, categorizing 124
    traits 25, **26**, 123, 151
        and age 26–27
        heritability 174
        inheritance 27
        undesired/desired 174–175
    types 123
        response to cat outside the window 123, *124*, **124**
behavioural phenotype 79
behaviouralists 126–127
Belgium 6
bell 67, 124, 148
belly exposing 45–46
Bengal cat 2, **3**, 30, 98
    separation problems 30, *32*
bib 67
biodiversity 156
biological environment 89
biological function 88, **89**
biopsychosocial model of health 164
birds
    catching 63
    endangered species 65
    vulnerable passerine 66
Birdsbesafe® 67, **68**, 124, 148
birth control (pills) 11, 95, 100
birthing den 13
biting 16, 18
black cats 6, 28
black redstart (*Phoenicurus ochruros*) 66
blink signal 51
blood pressure 165
boarding cattery 104, **105**
    requirements 104–106, **105**

body
    contact 127
    language 41–46
    postures 43–46, **44**, 57
        offensive/defensive signals 43–44, **43**
    wraps 149
bodyweight
    gain, kittens 14–15
    loss 14
boldness 28
bond
    human–cat 119, **119**
    human–pet 154
boredom 128–129, 130, 135
boundaries, territorial 50
brachycephalia 97
brain 82
    cells, grid/nerve/place 74
    GPS 74
    hippocampus 31, 74
breeders
    pedigree cats 30
    seasonal 11–12
breeding 92B, 174–175
    behavioural traits consideration 27
    effects 96–97
    goal-oriented for colour/shape 97
    for good qualities 176B
    pedigree, side-effects 93
    random 6
    season 11
    selective, fancy breeds 7
breeding cats, care guidelines 102B
breeds
    behavioural differences 29–30
    emergence 6–10
    fancy 7
    groups 7
    international standards 29
    most popular 7, *8*
    natural 7–8
    relationships between 7–10
    standards 97
British shorthair cat *8*
bully cats 143, 144
Burmese cat 30, *32*
buyer's remorse 160

call signal 24, 51
calling, vocalizations/miaows 40
Canada, effects on fauna 65
cannibalization, by queen 14
care 88
    good, guidelines (NRR) 99, 101–102B
    of kittens and adult cats 176B
    professional, of animals belonging to others 92B

care homes 171B
carrying basket 22–23, 112–113
castrated males 59, 94
castration 11, 94
cat flap 24, 84, 86, 111, 115, 128, 144
cat people 151–152
CatBib® 67–68, 124, 148
catching
    prey 19
    runaway cat 76
catio 100, 124, **130**, 145, 148
catnip (*Nepeta cataria*) 99, **100**
catscape, Norwegian village 133B
ceasefire, body posture 44, **45**
chatters 41
Chausie 98
cheek
    rubbing 46, 48, 50, **50**
    stroking 50, **50**
children 19, 21
    and allergies 164–165
    development, and pet cats 168–169
    immune system 165
    self-image 169, **170**
China 5
    cat numbers 160
Chinese mountain cat (*Felis bieti*) 1, 2
chirps 41
choice, of kitten 21
cholesterol 165
classic tabby 6, 7
classical conditioning (learning) 86, 108–110, 111, **112**, **119**, 143
    extinction in 111–114
classification 1
clawing 137
cleanliness 102B
clicker training 118–119, 121
climate change 156–157
co-operative alliances 58
coat
    colour, and aggression 28–29, **28**
    patterns, tabby 6–7, **6**, **7**
cognitive dysfunction 121, 139–140, 150
cognitive impairment 27
collaboration, kitten care 57
collar
    bell 67, 124, 148
    cover 67, **68**, 124, 148
    quick-release 77, 94
colony of cats 56, 57, 58
colostrum 13
communal nursing 57
communication 35
    acoustic 36–41
    humans with cats 49–50
    olfactory 46–48

    signals 18, 35–36
    tactile 49
    visual 41–46
community, ethical responsibility for homeless cats 93
companion animal 63, 93, 160, 163, 167
    effects on minor health problems 166
    in nursing homes 171B
    right to own 157, **158**
competence 91B
competing motivation 80, 83
competition, sexual 146
conditioned stimulus (CS) 110
conditioned (learnt) response (CR) 110
conditioning 110
    see also classical conditioning (learning); operant conditioning (learning)
confidence 28, 52
conflict
    between males 58
    body posture 43, **45**
conscientiousness, owner 152B
consequence
    of behaviour pattern 79–80
        desirable 80
        thwarting of desired 81
        undesirable 81
continuous reinforcement schedule 120
contraceptive pills 11, 95, 100
coping, with stress 83
coprophagy 14
copulation 12
copycat 122
core group 56, 57
cortisol 33, 79, 90, 123, 175
Council of Europe 98
counsellors 127
counter-conditioning 108, 112, 113, 135, 140, 145
courtship 12
COVID-19 160–161, **161**, 165
crossbreeding 92
crossed eyes 97
cruelty 106
cuddling 165, **166**
cues 115
cultural difference, and cat keeping 155
Cyprus 2–3
Cystophan® 149

de-clawing 155
deafness 96
decorations, cat 153, **153**
defence, local resource 52, 53
defensive aggression 41, 84, **85**, 142
    territory 52
    towards other cats 143–144
    towards people 142–143
        solutions 143

defensive signals 35
    body postures 43–44, **43**
    facial expression 41–42, **41**
delivery 12–14
dementia
    older cats 27
        prevention 27
dental problems 125
depression 83, 118, 167
desensitization 108, 112, 113, 140, 145
    for fear of men 133–135
Devon rex cat 8
diet 68–69, 147–148
directional summation 74
disappearance 75
discrimination learning 115
disease 93
    hereditary 96–97
    symptoms 96
    zoonotic 6
    see also zoonoses
displacement activity 81, 83
distress 131
divine cat 3–4
DNA testing 98
dog people 151–152
dogs
    assistance animals 170
    and cats together 61–62, **61**
    kitten socialization to 18
    as 'medication' for stress 167
    owners 152–153
    owning effects, on minor health problems 166
    tracking 76
    walking 166
domestic abuse 160
domestic cats *see* non-pedigree cats
domestication 1, 3
    early stages 6
    multiple events 1–2
dominance 55
    males 57–58, 75, **75**
dopamine 16, 86
drugs 149–150
    anxiety-reducing 131
        and behaviour modification 150
    nutraceuticals 140, 142, 149
duty, to help/alert 91B

ear, tattooing 94, **94**
ears-back signal 41–42
East African breeds 10
eating, reduced 125
Egyptian mau cat 8–9, 30, *32*
Egyptians 3–4
elderly 167

embalming 4
Emmeline judgment (Norwegian Supreme Court) 157–158
emotional relationship, with pets 154
emotional states 131–137
emotional support 167
emotions 81–87
    appetitive 86
    aversive 82–85
    and behaviour problems 130, *136*
    conflicting 81
    relationship between 82, **82**
empathy 88
endorphins 37, 142
England, effects on fauna 65
enjoyment **93**
enrichment 121
    environmental 33, 98, 163
    training as 121
environment 89, 123, 126
    early 125
    enrichment 98, 163
        for pre-natal stress remedy 32
    home 126, 155B
    impact on behaviour 30–32
    living 91B, 155–156, *156*
environmental conditions **103**
    of mother's pregnancy 27–28
environmental factors, living conditions 155–156, *156*
environmental needs 98–103
epigenetic effect 33, 175
ethical obligation, for ensuring welfare 90, 91–92B
ethical responsibility, for homeless cats, community 93
Europe
    effects on fauna 65
    western, prey predation 66
European breeds 7, 8
European Pet Food Industry (FEDIAF) 6
European wildcat (*Felis silvestris*) 1, **2**
euthanasia 91–92B
Exotic shorthair cat 8
expectation, positive 89
experience 27
    early 131, 174
    frightening 125, **125**, 131–133
    subjective 88, **89**
exploration, prevention from 99
exploratory behaviour 79, 90
export 4
expulsion, by dominant males 75, **75**
extinction 111–114, 147
    in classical learning 111–113
    in operant learning 113–114
extinction burst 113–114, **114**, 116, 119
extinction-induced aggression 114
extraversion, owner 152B
extrovert owners 25

eye opening 15–16
eyelids position 51
eyes
    crossed 96
    half-closed 51, **51**
    newborn closed 15–16, **17**

facial expressions 41–43, **42**
faeces 14, 65
    scent marking 47
fancy breeds 7
father 58–59
    friendliness of 28
fauna
    effects on 65–69
    threat to 63
fear 84, 110, 125, 131, 131–135
    association 111–112, 118
    aversion 111
    response, freeze/flee/fight 84, **85**
    solutions 133–135
fear–relief–anxiety training method **116**, 117
Fédération Internationale Féline (FIFe) 19, 96, 97, 98
feeders
    activity 148
    puzzle 99, 121, 122, 147–148
feeding regime 147–148
feelings 82
    see also emotions
feet, as toys 146–147
Feline Grimace Scale© 89–90
felinin 47
Felis
    bieti 1, 2
    catus 1
    lybica 1, 2, 3, 59
    silvestris 1, **2**
        catus 1
Feliscratch® 138, 149
Feliway® Classic 137–138, 149
Feliway® Friends (Felifriends) 149
Feliway® Optimum 149
females
    central 56
    social behaviour 56–57
fencing, cat-proof 144
feral cats 68, 92, 93
    Australia 66
    control 94
    predation by 66
feralization 5
fertility 11
fights, between males 57, 58
figures, cat 153, **153**
Finland, transfer to new owner survey 21
flap *see* cat flap

flehmen response 47
flight 35
fold-ears (osteochondrodysplasia) 96
food 22, 110
    availability 56
    begging for 39
    composition changes 157
    fit for carnivores 68–69
    queuing system 58
    solid 15
    see also feeders
forest cats *see* Maine coon cat, Norwegian forest cat, and Siberian cat
France 6
free-roaming cats 52, 56, 155, 165, 174
    insect catching 63–65
    Norway 65
    prey-catching variation 65
    risks to 155–156
Freya 5, **5**
friendliness, and father with same trait 28
frightening experience 125, **125**, 131–133
frustration 82–83, **83**, 100, 103, 113–114, 116
    external neighbourhood cat 145
    problem behaviour causing 128–129, 135–137
        explanation 135
        solution 135–137
frustration burst 114, 147
furniture 98

gangliosidosis 96
gender
    and behavioural development 21
    behavioural differences 29
generalization learning 114–115
genes, and behaviour 27–29
genetic basis, of behaviours 79
genetic defects 7
genetic disorders, reduction 97
genetics 123
geriatric cats 26–27
gestation, period 12–13
gods, cat 4, **4**
GPS (global positioning system)
    of brain 74
    tracker 63–65, 78
grass 69, **69**
greeting cats, by humans 49–50, **49**
grid cells 74
grief, of losing pet 169
grooming 125
    of kittens 14
group-living cats 54
    females 56–57
    indoors 55
growling 40–41

habituation learning 107–108
hair colour, and behaviour 28
handling 125
    and defensive aggression 142–143
    kind, anxiety-reducing 131
    of kittens and adult cats 176B
hands, as toys 146–147, **146**
harmony
    human–cat 123
    living in 10, 60, 129–130, 149
    'messages' 129
health
    check 96
    effects of pets, research 163–164
    minor problems, effects of companion animals 166
    problems, pedigree cats 96
hearing 15, 73
heart attacks, reduction and survival 165
heart rate 165
heat (oestrus) 11–12, **12**, 56
    silent 12
    synchronized 12, 57
help, duty to 91B
helper system 57
hereditary disease 96–97
heritability, of behavioural traits 174
Herodotus 4
hiding 22, 85, **85**
hierarchy, absolute/relative 55
Himalayan cat 8
hippocampus 33, 74
hissing 41
hoarding, animal 96
holidays 77–78, 103
home
    bringing to new 22–23
    environment 126
        Norway 155B
    good start in new 21–24
    see also environment
home range 52–53, 103
    core area 53, 57, 129
    female 53, 56, 57
    intact males 57
homeless
    cats 90–96, **93**, 160–161
    dogs 160–161
    owners 160, 167
homing 70
    ability 73
    pigeons 73
hope 86
hormones 79, 123
    reproductive 79
hospitals, AAA 170
house cats *see* non-pedigree cats
housing
    complexes, indoor cats 98
    and pets 157–160
        no-pet policy 157
housing co-operatives
    Norway 157–159
        liberalization of cat keeping 158
humans, social experience with 18–19
hunting 63, 75
    area 63
    body posture 43, **43**
    outdoors 54
    skills 33
    training, and object play 19
husbandry training 119
hybrid cats 98

iCatCare (International Cat Care) 94
ID
    marking 22, 76–77, 94
        microchip 22, 77, **77**, 94, 155
    tagging 94, 100
idiopathic cystitis 125
illness 36, 125
imitation learning 121–122
immune system, human 165
inappropriate play 129, 146–147, **146**
    solutions 147, **147**
inbreeding, avoidance 12
Incredible Cats (Greene) 163
independence 6, 21, 30, 63, 101, 103, 140, 151
    owners 152, 153, 154
indoor cats 12, 27, 130
    care guidelines 101B
    group-living 55
    and housing complexes 99
    toileting 138
indoor pen 140, 143
indoors
    keeping in 100
    at night 67
infanticide
    by males 4, 14, 58
    by queen 14
inheritance, of behavioural traits 29
injury 36
inquisitive nature 107
insects, nocturnal, catching 63–65
insight, learning by 122
intact males 40, 47, 52, 59, 95
    home range 57
    scent marking 36, 47, 48
intention movement 45
inter-individual distance 54
interactions 127–128
    with animals, health link mechanisms 164, **164**
interdigital glands 48, **48**
international breed standards 29

International Centre of Anthrozoology (ICofA) 171
International Society for Animal Assisted Therapy
        (ISAAT) 171–172
International Union for Conservation of Nature (IUCN) 1
internet 121
interval reinforcement schedule 120
iridoids 99
islands, species eradication 66
Italy, mating and coat colour survey 28

Japan 5
    mythology 6
joy 86, 87, 93, **93**
Just So Stories (Kipling) 153

keeping
    changing landscape 155–157
    guidelines (NRR) 101–102B
Kellas cats 1
killing 93
    campaigns 93–94
    skills 121
kin selection 57
kitten-time 22
kittens
    born in shelters 104
    care
        collaboration 57
        and handling 176B
        by males 58–59
    choice 21
    development, to adulthood 175–176
    emotional disturbance 176
    good start in life **175**
    growth 14–15
    mother
        effects of her stress 32–33, 175
        licking 49
    newborn 14, 15–16, **17**
    separation from mother/litter 21, **22**
    social behaviour 176
    socialization 16–19
    toleration by males 57
knowledge
    new owner 21
    for problem behaviour prevention 147
Korat cat 96

lactase 15
landlords 157
    problems with 157–158
    UK 160
language
    body 41–46
    cat 176
    odour 46–48

touch 49
    see also signals; marking
latent (hidden) learning 121
learning
    ability, and pre-natal stress 33
    discrimination 114–115
    generalization 114–115
    imitation 121–122
    by insight 122
    latent 121
    non-associative 107–108
    see also classical conditioning (learning); operant
        conditioning (learning)
learnt helplessness 118
leash 23, 100, 129, **131**
'leave' training 120, **120**, 144–145
licking
    of kittens 49
    lip 43
    social 49
lifestyles 129–130
    likelihood of problem behaviour by
        130, *134*, 137
    outdoor cats 133B
    welfare benefits 130, *132*
lifting 127–128, 143
lions 58
litter tray 138, 139, **139**
littermates 60
litters 11
    size 11, 57
living environment/conditions 89, 155–156, *156*
local resource defence 52, 53
locomotory play 16
loneliness 166, 167
lordosis 12
lost cat
    advertising 76
    finding 74–77

mackerel tabby 6, **6**
Madagascar 5
magnetic sense 73–74
Maine coon cat 7, **8**
mainland leopard cat (*Prionailurus bengalensis*)
        1, 2, 30
males
    care of kittens 58–59
    castrated 59
    conflict between 58
    dominance 57–58
    infanticide by 4, 14
    intact, home range 57
    quarrel 57–58
    social behaviour 57–58
    toleration of kittens 57
    tom 12
    see also intact males

marking 137–138
    of behaviour 118–119
    scent 36, 47–48, 52, 52, 103, 137–138
    urine 46–47
Mars 160, 161
maternal behaviour 13–15
mating 12, 58
    and coat colour 28
medical problems 130
Mediterranean basin group 8–9
men, fear-provoking stimuli 133–135
mental health 97
    and cats 166–167
        benefit 167, **168**
mental states 88–89
mental stimulation 148
miaowing 35–36, 37–40, 113–114
    calling 40
    types 37–40, **38**
microchip *see* ID, marking
Middle Ages, persecution 6
Middle East 3
milk
    finding 15
    from pipette 14, **14**
    nursing 11, 14–15, 57
    production 11
    specially-made mix 14, **14**
mink farms 56
monoamine oxidase inhibitors (MAOI) 150
mother cats 53
    social contact with 176
    stress in, effect on kittens 32–33
mother–kitten bond 37
motivation 79–81, 108, **109**
    competing 80, 83
multi-cat household 54, 60–61, 129–130
    harmony 60, **60**
    introducing newcomer 60–61
    litter trays 138
    resources 128, 130
        case study 128–129
myocardial infarction survival 165
mythology
    Egyptian 4
    Japanese 6
    Norse 5

natural breeds 7–8
natural life 88, **89**
natural selection 5
    for tameness and sociability 3
navigation 21
    to home 72
    in unfamiliar terrain 72–73
navigational ability 72

needs
    behavioural 79–81
        definition 79–80
    environmental 98–103
negative punishment, and positive reinforcement
        116–117, **116**, 118
negative reinforcement, and positive
        punishment **116**, 117
neighbourhood, nuisance 156
neighbouring cats 12, 19, 54, 58, 89, 123, *124*, **124**
    social aggression between 28, **135**, 143, 145B, 156
    stress causing 145–146, 156
neighbours
    difficulty with 6
    good 76, 96, 103
neoteny 35–36
nerve cells 74
nest 57
neurotic owners 25–26
neuroticism, owner 152B, 153
neutering 11, 22, 59, 93, 94, 99
    early 94
new home 20–24
new owners
    for kittens 21
        knowledge and information needed 21–22
New Zealand 5
newborn kittens 14
    closed eyes 15–16, **17**
newcomer, to multi-cat household, introduction 60–61
night vision 16
noise **125**, 133
non-associative learning 107–108
non-pedigree cats 1, 3
    behaviour 30
    home environment, Norway 155B
    personality axes 25
    signals 35–36
Norse mythology 5, **5**
Norway
    behaviour survey (2014) 25, **26**
    bird predation 67
    cat numbers 160
    home environment 155B
    Law on Housing Co-operatives 158
    most common breeds, behaviour
        differences 30, *32*
    Ownership Section Act 158
    pets and housing 157–158
    Rent Act 158
    Trondheim, males caring for kittens 58–59
    village, catscape 133B
    wading bird catching 65
Norwegian Animal Welfare Act (2009) 90, 91–92B
Norwegian Association of Cat Owners 157, 159
    recommendations for owners living in housing
        co-operatives 159B

Norwegian forest cat **6**, 7
    behaviour 30, 32
        development 8, 30, **31**
    home environment 155B
novelty 110
nuisance, neighbourhood 156
numbers
    of breeds 7
    owned 6, 160
    per household, limiting 96
    stray and feral 6
nursing 11
    communal 57
    period 14–15
nursing homes
    AAA 170
    cats in
        advice notes 172–173, 172B
        as therapists – benefits and concerns 171B
nutraceuticals 142, 149
    for cognitive dysfunction 140

object (predatory) play 16, 19–20, **20**, 26, 68, 146–147
    for dementia prevention 27
    and hunting training 19
odour language 46–48
oestrus (heat) 11–12, **12**, 56, 57
offensive aggression 146
    solutions 146
offensive signals 57
    body postures 43–44, **43**
    facial expression 42–43, **42**
older cats 26–27
    dementia 27
    toileting 138
older owners, physical health benefits 165
olfactory communication 46–48
olfactory orientation 73
openness
    of owners 25–26
    to experience 152B
operant conditioning (learning) 108–110, 111, 115–121, **119**, 133
    extinction in 113–114
opioids 99
orange coat colour 7, 28
oriental breeds, behavioural development 30
Oriental shorthair cat 7
orientation 24
    ability 73
    research 71–72
    olfactory 73
    skills 73
osteochondrodysplasia 96
outdoor cats **103**
    care guidelines 101–102B
    home range 53
    lifestyle 133B
    social organization 56
outdoors 22, **23**, 155B
    access 130, 148
    and prey taking 65
    hunting 54
over-attachment 140
over-grooming 83, **84**, 140, 141–142
    solutions 142
over-population 11
ovulation 12
owned cats 53
    prey predation 66
owners 153
    acquisition reasons 151
    characteristics 151–153
    dog 152–153
    extrovert 23
    homeless 160
    new, kittens to 21
    openness 25–26
    personality affecting cats 25–26
    sociability to 25
ownership barriers 157
owner–cat bond 127
oxytocin 76, 165–166, 169

parturition 13–14
paternal instinct 59
paternity, and response to strangers 29, 33
paw lifting 45
pedigree cats 65, 95
    breeders 30
    breeding, side-effects 96
    health problems 96
    home environment, Norway 155B
pellets, food 15
penis 12, **13**
performance **109**
peripheral cats 56
persecution, Middle Ages 6
Persian cat 7, 8
    behaviour 29, **29**, 30, 32
    brachycephalia 7
    heritability of behavioural traits 29
personal space 54
personality 79
    axes, domestic cats 25
    differences 25–26
    of owner
        affecting cat 25–26, 153–155
        traits 152, 152B
    traits and characteristics 123
    types 25, 123, *124*
    and unwanted behaviour 125–126

'pet effect' 169
pets 3
    health effects of 163–164
    and housing 157–160
        Norway 157–158
        UK 159–160
pheromones 12, 46–47, **48**, 129, 146
    as anxiety solution 131
    for cognitive dysfunction 140
    messages 149
    as scratching solution 137–138
    social system role 46–47
phobias 85
physical environment 89
physical health, of owner, and cats 164–166
physical states 89
physical stimulation 148
physiological stress 90, 108
pica 140–142, **141**
    solutions 142
picking up 125, 127–128, 143, **144**
piloerection 42
place cells 74
play 86, 90, 123
    inappropriate 129, 146–147, **146**, **147**
    kitten 16–17
    locomotory 16
    owner initiation 147
    social (play-fighting) 16–17, **18**, 176
    see also object (predatory) play
play-fighting see play, social
playfulness, breed differences 30, **32**
pleasure 86, 116, **119**, 130
pleasure–frustration training method 116–117, **116**
polycystic kidney disease (PKD) 97
popularity 151
Positive Pets 157
positive punishment 127
    and negative reinforcement **116**, 117
    should it be used? 117–118
positive reinforcement, and negative
        punishment 116–117, **116**, 118
poster pets 98
prey-catching behaviour 63
prenatal stress 32–33, 175
    remedy 33
predators, super 67
predatory behaviour 63–65, 146
    reduction measures 67–68
predatory play see object (predatory) play
predictors, of events, scary 112
preferences 80
pregnant cat 12–13
'presents' 124
prey
    brought home 65, 67, 69, 138
    catching 19

species
    caught 65
    eradication by cats 66–67, 156
    substitute 141
problem behaviour
    categories 123
    likelihood, by lifestyle 130, *134*
progressive retinal atrophy (PRA) 97
propagation control 95
protest signals 40
psychosomatic diseases 167
punishers 115
punishment 115–116, 127
    negative, and positive reinforcement 116–117, **116**, 118
    positive
        and negative reinforcement **116**, 117
        should it be used? 117–118
pupils 42
purring 36, 37
    demanding 37
puzzle feeders 99, 121, 122, 147–148

quarantine 33–34
queen 11, 12, 13
quick-release collar 77, 94

rabies 165
radio
    tracking 65
    transmitter 72, **72**
Ragdoll cat **9**
random breeding 6
rank order 55–56
rat catchers 3–4, 67
ratio reinforcement schedule 120
rearing 45
red/orange gene variant 28
redirected aggression 144–146
reflex 107
rehoming 129
reinforcement 115–116
    negative, and positive punishment **116**, 117
    positive, and negative punishment 116–117, **116**, 118
    schedules 120–121
        continuous 120
        interval 120
        ratio 120
reinforcers 114, **117**
relationship
    with cat, strengthening with age 167
    damage to 118
    reinforcement 119, **119**
relative hierarchy 55

relief 86, 117
reproductive hormones 79
rescue cats, adoption 113
resources 128–129, **130**
    choice and access 128, 130, 138, 143–144, 145
    for multi-household cats 130
    for problem behaviour prevention 147–150
response
    spontaneous recovery of 111, **112**
    to strangers 33
responsibility 91B
resting 14, 15, **83**, 90, **93**
    place 53, **55**, 58
restlessness 83
reward **116**
reward-based training 118–120, 131, 135, 176
reward/no reward pairing 116–117, **116**
roaming 70–71
    outdoors 98, **103**
rodent hunting 63, **64**
runaway cat, catching 76, **76**
rural cats 65
rut 12

Sacred Birman cat 8, **9**
satisfaction 80, 90
Savannah cat 98
Scandinavia 4–5
scarers 117
scary predictors of events 112
scary stimuli 110
scent
    map 72
    marking 47–48, 52, 54, 98–99, 137–138
        faeces 47
        intact males 36, 47, 48
    skin glands 48
schools, AAA 170
Scottish fold cat 96, 97
scouting 73
scratching 16, 18, 48, **48**, 137, **137**
scratching posts 99, 124–125, 137
seasonal breeders 11–12
secure adult attachment style 154B
selection, kin 57
selective breeding 174
    and behavioural differences 30
    of fancy breeds 7
selective serotonin reuptake inhibitors (SSRI) 150
self-confidence 29
self-mutilation 140, 141–142, **141**
sense of place 24
senses, development 15–16
sensitization 16
sensory information 4
sentience 89

separation problems, Bengal cat 30, 32
sex, behavioural differences 27
sexual competition 146
shaping 114, 119, **119**
shelters, requirements 104–106, **105**
shock 84
show-oriented ideals 97
shows, cat 93, 97
Siamese cat 7, 12, 65
    amyloidosis 97
    behaviour 29–30, **29**
    heritability of behavioural traits 29
    visual pathways error 97
Siberian cat 8, **8**
siblings, social contact with 176
sight 16
signals
    aggressive 35, 57
    agonistic 35
    of anticipated pleasure 86, **87**
    blink 51
    calling 51
    communication 16, 35–36
    defensive
        body postures 43–44, **43**
        facial expression 42–43, **42**
    language 35
    offensive 57
        body postures 43–44, **43**
        facial expression 42–43, **42**
    protest 40
    sound 36–37
    tail 46
    visual 36
silent heat (oestrus) 12
silver vine (*Actinidia polygama*) 99
single cats 56, 129
single life 54
skin glands, scents 48
skins, as commodity 5
sleeping, excessive 83
smell 15, 72, **72**
snake killers 4, 65
sniffing 48
sociability 3, 26, 27, 29
    breed differences 30, 32
    and prenatal stress 32
social behaviour, kittens 176
social contact, with mother and siblings 176
social contest, body posture 44
social environment 89
social experience 18–19
social interactions, and emotions 82
social issues 123
social learning 121–122
social licking 49
social life 54

social media 166–167
social memory 74
social play 16–17, **17**, 176
social status 35
social support 167
socialization
    kitten 16–19, 176
        prenatal stress remedy 33
        to cats 16–18
        to dogs 19
        to people 18–19
Sokoke cat 10
solicitation purrs 37
Solliquin® 149
Somali cat 8
sound map 73
sound signals 36–41
spatial mapping ability 74
spatial memory 74
spaying 11, 22, 94
Sphynx cat 7
spitting 41
spontaneous recovery, of response 111, **112**
spotted tabby 6, **7**
spraying 46–47, 137
    cleaning 138
spread of cats 4–6
standards
    breed 96
    international breed 29
startle 84
status 93
stereotypies
    behavioural 83, 140
    passive 83
stillborn kittens 14
stimulation, mental and physical 148
stimuli 108, 110
    environmental 131
    external 79, 123
    internal 79, 123
    mild stress-eliciting 176
    pleasant 110
    scary 110
    unpleasant 117
strange situation test 154–155
strangers, response to 28, 33
stray cats 90, 161
    control 94
    predation by 66
stress 79, 98, 125, **125**, **126**
    continuous (chronic) 79, 81, 118, 167
    coping 83
    dogs as 'medication' for 167
    hormones 123
    physiological 89, 108
    prenatal 32–33, 175

response, pupils 42
    short (acute) 78, 81
stress therapy 90
stroking 128, 165, **166**
    cheek 50, **50**
subjective experience 88, **89**
suburban cats 65
super predators 67
superstition 111
surprise 86
survival 115
    skills 121
sweat glands 48
Sweden, bird predation 66
Switzerland
    collar covers 67
    prey predation 66
synthetic breeds 98

tabby
    classic 6, **7**
    coat patterns 6–7, **6**, **7**
    mackerel 6, **6**
    spotted 6, **7**
tactile communication 49
tail signals, up/over the head/lashing/slight/rub 46
tameness 3
taste 15
    aversion 111
tattooing 77
    ear 94, **94**
taurine 68
teat order 53–57
terrain
    unfamiliar
        behaviour in 72–73
        navigation in 73–74
        timidity 75–76
territory 52, **53**
therapy
    animal-assisted 169–173
    definition 169
threat 84
    to fauna 63
thundershirt 149
thyroxine 123
time sense 74
timidity, in unfamiliar terrain 75–76
TNR (trap/neuter/return) method 94
TNVR (trap/neuter/vaccinate/return) method 94
toileting 124–125
    inappropriate 138–139
        in gardens/sandpits 156
    solutions 138–139
tomcat 12, 53
    home range 57

urine marking 47
    wanderings 75
torment 106
torture 106
touch 15, 165, **166**
    language 49
toxoplasmosis 156, 165
toys 98, 116, 119, 146
    for appropriate play 147, **147**
tracker dog 76
tracking 73
trading 92B
traffic, cat 54
training 107, 115
    clicker 118–119, 121
    easy 25
    fear–relief–anxiety method **116**, 117
    'leave' 120, **120**, 144–145
    reward-based 118–120, 131, 135, 176
trap 76
trapping 94
treatment of animals 91B
trees 99
trial-and-error 110–111
'tricks' 119, 135
tricyclic anti-depressants (TCA) 150
triglycerides 165
trust **119**, 127
TTVARR (trap/test/vaccinate/alter/rehome or release)
    method 94
Turkish angora cat 8
Turkish van cat 8–9
tying up 102–103
typical behaviour 25

UK
    cat numbers 160
    Dogs Trust 160
    Governing Council of the Cat Fancy (GCCF) 97
    Hope and Freedom Projects 160
    HOPE (Help Homeless Owners with Pets) 160
    Links Group 169
    Model Tenancy Agreement guidance 160, 161B
    Pathway 160
    Pets Advisory Committee 160
    pets and housing 159–160
    Pets as Therapy 171
    Society of Companion Animal Studies
        (SCAS) 159–160, 172
ultrasound devices 67
umbilical cord 13–14
umbilical hernia 97
unacceptable behaviour 51, 124
    toileting 138–139
unconditioned stimulus (US) 110
under-attachment 140
understanding, for problem behaviour prevention 147

university, AAA 170
unpleasant feelings 81
unwanted behaviour 123, 124
urban cats 65
urbanization 155
urination, methods 47
urine 12
    marking 47–48
    spraying 46–47, 137, 138
USA
    effects on fauna 65
    Pet Partners 171

vaccination 21
vector addition principle 74
veterinary involvement 126
veterinary visits 112, 133
video camera 63, 65
Vikings 5, 7
visual communication 41–46
visual pathways error 97
visual signals 36
vocalizations 36
    calling 40
vomeronasal organ 47
vulnerable species, caught by cats 65–66

wading bird catching 65
walking, dog 166
wanderings 75
    tales 70–71
water spray/gun 118
weaning 14, 15
welfare
    definition 88
    dimensions 88, **89**
    good **90**
    indicators for mental and physical states 89–90
    in nursing homes, recipient and animal 171
    scale 89–90
well-being, child 169
wet food 15
whistle 51
wild cats 92
wildcat species 92–93
wildlife, threat to 156
witchcraft 6
World Health Organization (WHO) 163

Yerkes-Dodson Law 108, **109**, 113
yowling 40, **40**, 57

Zoom Groom 125
zoonoses 6, 164–165
Zylkene® 149

CABI – who we are and what we do

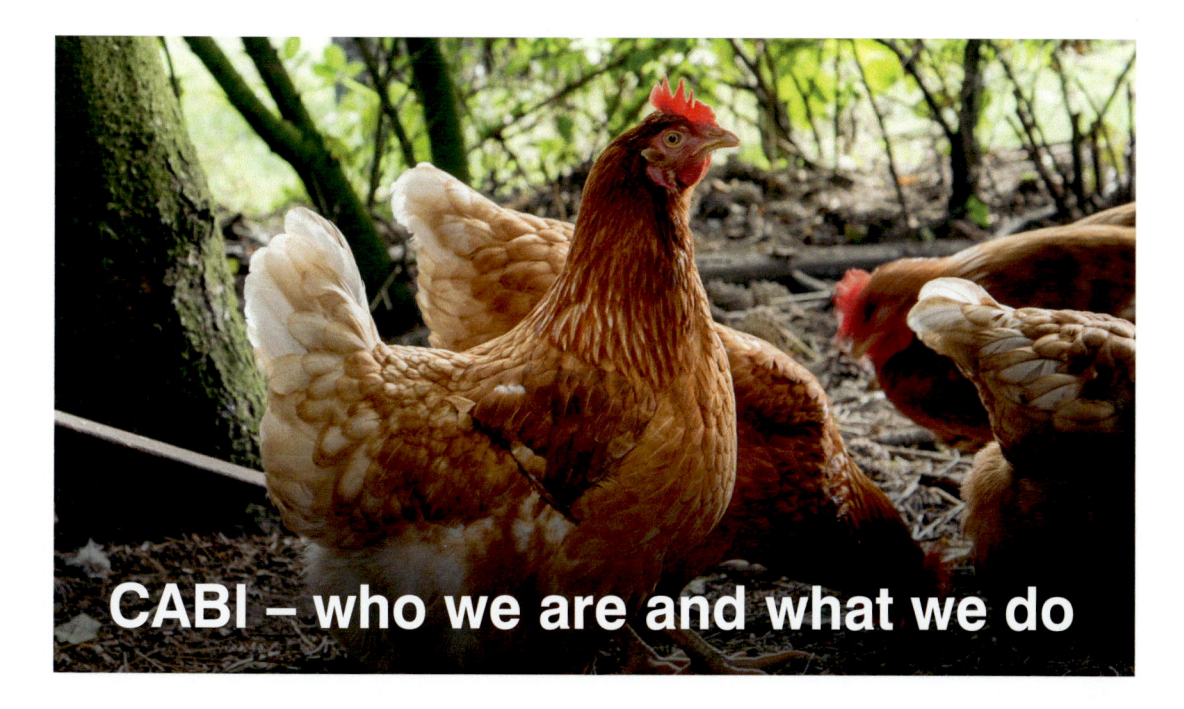

This book is published by **CABI**, an international not-for-profit organisation that improves people's lives worldwide by providing information and applying scientific expertise to solve problems in agriculture and the environment.

CABI is also a global publisher producing key scientific publications, including world renowned databases, as well as compendia, books, ebooks and full text electronic resources. We publish content in a wide range of subject areas including: agriculture and crop science / animal and veterinary sciences / ecology and conservation / environmental science / horticulture and plant sciences / human health, food science and nutrition / international development / leisure and tourism.

The profits from CABI's publishing activities enable us to work with farming communities around the world, supporting them as they battle with poor soil, invasive species and pests and diseases, to improve their livelihoods and help provide food for an ever growing population.

CABI is an international intergovernmental organisation, and we gratefully acknowledge the core financial support from our member countries (and lead agencies) including:

UKaid from the British people

Ministry of Agriculture People's Republic of China

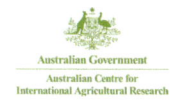

Australian Government Australian Centre for International Agricultural Research

Agriculture and Agri-Food Canada

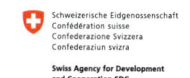

Ministry of Foreign Affairs of the Netherlands

Schweizerische Eidgenossenschaft Confédération suisse Confederazione Svizzera Confederaziun svizra
Swiss Agency for Development and Cooperation SDC

Discover more

To read more about CABI's work, please visit: **www.cabi.org**

Browse our books at: **www.cabi.org/bookshop**, or explore our online products at: **www.cabi.org/publishing-products**

Interested in writing for CABI? Find our author guidelines here: **www.cabi.org/publishing-products/information-for-authors/**